Illness and Culture
in the Postmodern Age

Illness and Culture in the Postmodern Age

DAVID B. MORRIS

UNIVERSITY OF CALIFORNIA PRESS

Berkeley   Los Angeles   London

University of California Press
Berkeley and Los Angeles, California

University of California Press, Ltd.
London, England

First Paperback Printing 2000
© 1998 by
The Regents of the University of California

Grateful acknowledgment is made for permission to quote from
"Ceremony," from *Ceremony* by Leslie Marmon Silko. Copyright © 1977
by Leslie Silko. Used by permission of Viking Penguin, a division of
Penguin Putnam Inc. In addition, Janet F. Boyd's "A Snowball" and
Marvin Bell's "A Healthy Life" are reprinted by permission of their
respective authors. Finally, for permission to reprint portions of his
previous articles in revised form, the author wishes to thank the editors
of *Daedalus, Literature and Medicine,* and *The Wilson Quarterly,* as well as
Harvard University Press, the Johns Hopkins University Press, and the
University of Michigan Press.

Library of Congress Cataloging-in-Publication Data

Morris, David B.
    Illness and culture in the postmodern age / David B. Morris.
        p.   cm.
    Includes bibliographical references and index.
    ISBN 0-520-22689-5 (pbk. : alk. paper)
        1. Diseases—Social aspects.   2. Social medicine—Philosophy.
    3. Postmodernism.   I. Title.
    RA418.M68   1998
    306.4'61—dc21   98-7092
                                                           CIP

Printed in the United States of America

08 07 06 05 04 03 02 01 00
9 8 7 6 5 4 3 2 1

For
Emily, Ruth, and Ellen

Contents

Illustrations

I came packed in oils, the residue of Eden.
Some said that grief made me.
Some said it was the death of a child.
Or a passion so dense no light escaped.
Some said it was sin.
They told me stories to account for disease.
Of heavy elements that kept me from rising.
Of the ribbed wings of angels.
Of cells that changed.
I trusted the world to be natural. The voice
Of disease was the white noise I slept by.

What happened to me happened to you.
I ate too much or little, the water was unclean.
I saw the face of illness mature in the mirror.
Everything that had been outside me
Came to be inside me.
I was equally well and unwell.
I was my own medicine.
And now the endless remedies
Became the white noise I slept by, deeply.
For such and so many are the body's afflictions,
That to live is to die.

MARVIN BELL,
"A Healthy Life" (1998)

Introduction

Man is more sick, uncertain, changeable,

indeterminate than any other animal, there is no

doubt of that—he is *the* sick animal.

FRIEDRICH NIETZSCHE,
On the Genealogy of Morals (1887)[1]

Illness somehow defines us. It tells us who we are. It informs us, in a
sense Nietzsche understood in his bones, that we are creatures
marked by a uniquely unstable relation to health. Unlike robots or
rabbits, humans possess a tendency toward repeated and often protracted illnesses that seem finally less a flaw in our design than a
mysterious signature. Walk through any suburban mall, however,
and you cannot avoid seductive displays promising miracle cures,
ageless bodies, and perpetual well-being, as if our main task in life
were to defeat mortality. The search for perfect health and vigor is an
ancient impulse. Ponce de León pursued tales of a youth-restoring
fountain all the way into the swamps of sixteenth-century Florida.
Few people today believe that fitness gurus, herbs, hormone therapies, and weekend yoga classes offer something so literal as everlast-

ing youth, yet as a distant prospect or utopian glimmer, the promise of living forever—or at least for a very long time—increasingly fires the imagination of an audience eagerly consuming news of each fresh medical triumph over disease. The dream has a notably postmodern grain. Although various religions propose an eternal afterlife, it took secular Western civilization to invent cryonics, which deep-freezes the diseased body until a cure is found. More than a scheme to exploit our fears of death, cryonics employs a futuristic technology to extend ad infinitum the curative agenda of contemporary biomedicine. The goal is consistent with wider cultural fantasies that (without the need for religion or the inconvenience of a soul) project the flesh into an indefinitely expanded future-perfect state devoid of illness. In a move that the prescientific Europe of Ponce de León would have found sacrilegious or incomprehensible, our culture has declared war on biology.

I do not mean to misrepresent the medical struggle against illness and impairment as inevitably a form of warfare, although a militaristic vocabulary of battles and counterattacks still dominates medicine. The miniature electronic hearing aid, for example, represents a huge advance beyond the clumsy ear trumpets of Victorian times. It is a gain for the human spirit; it enhances the biology of hearing rather than assails or supersedes it. Who would wish to do without antibiotics, skin grafts, or kidney dialysis? Several days ago, however, I listened to a prominent specialist in geriatrics describe his frustration over an elderly patient who had fallen and broken her hip. The woman—frail, ill, bedridden, alone—announced she was through with life. She wanted nothing done for her hip. Just give her medications to keep her comfortable, she insisted, and let her die in peace. Nothing in her manner or medical history indicated that she was unable to make a rational choice. What happened? The doctor sighed as several nurses in the audience guessed the answer. Other specialists had intervened with a hip-replacement operation. Now she was back in surgery because two screws securing the artificial hip had come loose. The episode, a sadly familiar skirmish in what seems genuine warfare against the biology of old age, suggests how all of us, not just the elderly and infirm, live in the grip of cultural forces unprecedented in the age of ear trumpets—cultural forces that now decisively shape our fates.

This book explores the changing relationship between culture and biology as they reconfigure our experience of illness. The argument can be stated briefly. Illness has changed in the last fifty years, during the transition from modern to postmodern times. We fall sick from unheard-of ailments, we pass through undreamed-of treatments, we die in unsettling new ways and places. Postmodern illness—my term for our changed and still changing experience of human affliction—is as distinctive as the films, cars, computers, and space shuttles that help define the era following World War II. It takes shape from specific historical convergences between biology and culture. We must explore these complex relations between biology and culture if we hope to understand the contemporary experience of illness and ultimately (as Nietzsche suggests) ourselves. In the process, we may come to look somewhat differently upon the quest to live forever.

The historical changes that have brought us to the present state are so immense that they defy enumeration. Consider the year 1872. Nietzsche had just written *The Birth of Tragedy*. Remington and Sons, famous for the rifles that helped to win the American West, had begun to work on a new technology: the typewriter. The Brooklyn Bridge had just opened for traffic. Alexander Graham Bell was putting the finishing touches on the telephone, and Viennese surgeon Theodor Billroth (the founder of modern abdominal surgery) was about to report his discovery of potentially infectious streptococci and staphylococci. As the contemporary world struggled into being, a nine-year-old boy named Black Elk lay seriously ill in his parents' tipi, his face and arms swollen, his legs so weak he could not walk. For twelve days he lay on his back, motionless, as if dead.

In this state of suspended life, some things were very clear to the boy as he looked at the sky through the opening at the top of the tipi. Two men were coming from the clouds, headfirst "like arrows slanting down." He had seen the men before, he knew, but this time they looked different: "Each now carried a long spear, and from the points of these a jagged lightning flashed. They came clear down to the ground this time and stood a little way off . . . and said: 'Hurry! Come! Your Grandfathers are calling you!'" Black Elk describes how he followed the two men to a place where a small cloud lifted him off the ground and sped away. "And when I looked down," he said, "I could see my mother and my father yonder, and I felt sorry to be leaving them."[2]

With the help of a Sioux medicine man named Whirlwind Chaser, Black Elk recovered from his twelve-day, near-death sickness. (As a boy, he would take a scalp at the last stand of General George Custer, and as a young man he performed before Queen Victoria with Buffalo Bill's Wild West Show, on his return surviving the infamous massacre at Wounded Knee.) What he retained, once the illness had passed, was the magnificent and frightening vision imparted during his journey into the clouds. The vision, he claimed, gave him the power to cure, but he did not dwell upon his skills as a medicine man. "If a man or woman or child dies," he said as an old man, now confined to a reservation, "it does not matter long, for the nation lives on. It was the nation that was dying, and the vision was for the nation; but I have done nothing with it."[3]

Black Elk's frank self-condemnation puts a personal face on the larger tragedy that Native Americans faced in the legalized seizure or outright theft of their lands and in the systematic assault on their cultures. It is hard to imagine how anyone could have stopped the sweep of European immigration or blocked the advance of modern industrial society. Sioux legends had foretold such a conquest, but what Black Elk could not have foreseen was the simultaneous conquest of traditional medicine by a science-based biomedical model that effectively reduces illness to the operation of mechanical processes. Illness, inside this biomedical model, is pure biology, and Black Elk's momentous visionary experience is no more than a feverish delusion. While the scientific biomedicine that accompanied the birth of the modern world would see in Black Elk's traditional ceremonies and cures simply the practice of superstition, I offer a different story—or the fragments of a story—about health and illness. In this story, although the power of the biomedical model continues almost unabated, we are feeling our way toward a new and still uncertain understanding of illness. This new understanding respects the wisdom in nonscientific traditions of healing, such as the one Black Elk inherited, and finds in our growing passion for alternative therapies an impulse to recover lost knowledge about health. Indirectly and even inadvertently, Black Elk shows us in his practice as a Sioux medicine man, even as a scientist does working on the latest vaccine, how illness is always constructed at the crossroads of biology and culture.

It is important to respect the continuing power of the biomedical model, which (in addition to being an entrenched institution) has a record of brilliant success, from the eradication of smallpox to heart-bypass surgery. It will be modified, perhaps drastically, but not soon rejected. We have learned its lessons too well. Unlike Black Elk, most people in the industrialized world have grown up in a culture dominated by the belief that illness comes from microbes, toxins, and internal malfunctions. We consult doctors who perform tests tracing our discomfort back to its source in a recognized pathology, objective and concrete. This is the perfection of twentieth-century medical science. Illness, however, is not strictly speaking an object. It is not something we can know inside and out, through an inventory of its material properties, like a moon rock. Even when caused by a toxin, by a microbe, or by the dysfunction of an organ, illness is a fluid process that changes as we change, enigmatic, insubordinate, subjective. It captures bodies, minds, and emotions, remains at its deepest level inaccessible to language, and alters under the influence of nonmedical events from divorce to climate change. What biomedicine finds hard to recognize or to accept is that different observers—patient, spouse, doctor, pastor, insurance provider, hospital administrator, epidemiologist, to name a few—examining the same illness from their separate perspectives will observe different aspects of its truth.

This book traces a historically new way of understanding illness, one that has emerged during the last fifty years of the twentieth century. It calls into question various beliefs basic to the still reigning biomedical model, reflecting an imperfect but widespread and growing recognition that illness depends not solely on biological mechanisms, no matter how crucial they are, but on convergences between biology and culture. Such convergences are ultimately irreducible to a mechanistic model. They signal the end of the machine age and perhaps the advent of systems theory as a dominant metaphor for illness. They define the specific and complex ways in which we in the postmodern era continue to reinvent ourselves as (in Nietzsche's incisive phrase) *"the* sick animal."

Every road taken implies roads not taken. Let me thus say clearly what this book is *not*. It is not meant as a contribution to theories of postmodernism. Illness, not postmodernism, is my subject. Recent theorists can show us how illness constitutes a "social text": something at least partly created by the densely interwoven network of experiences and interpretations we bring to it. Illnesses, like texts, are amenable to various traditions of reading, both medical and nonmedical, so that a Native American shaman will interpret them differently than does a Western physician. Yet, illness is unique among social texts. It touches each of us, in our flesh, as we fall under the spell of internal events. Illness too is often thrust upon us, capable of interrupting every plan. It is a text we cannot put down or put off. One day it will likely kill us. So powerful is its hold that few contemporary maladies from racism to crime have not been described as an epidemic. It is a pool in which we behold the reflection of every evil. Illness, further, is never strictly a matter for theorists but always contains deeply practical imperatives: something must be *done,* often quickly and with imperfect knowledge. Anyone who longs for sustained theoretical analysis of postmodernism has a rich harvest to choose from elsewhere, which seems reason enough to sidestep the philosophical agendas and technical dialects common among theorists.[4] My explanation for preferring a more concrete approach—I cannot write as a philosopher or theorist anyway—is very basic. Our health as individuals may depend directly on how we understand crucial, specific changes implicit in the experience of postmodern illness.

We can safely defer the question of just what the troublesome term *postmodern* means. It is notoriously vague. It took a flashy, breakneck run up the stock market of academe—peaking from, say, 1975 to 1985—and now appears to be in a modest decline, as conference organizers search for less overworked topics. Some scholars are beginning to reappraise their relation to postmodern thought, to put it at arm's length, to criticize postmodernity both as an intellectual style (associated with ideas about the meaning of texts as inherently indeterminate) and as a social force (associated with a multiculturalism that threatens to undermine all nonlocal values). The result has been a gradual erosion of prestige for a concept that once inspired an almost unstoppable flow of articles, books, and symposia. My aim is, if possible, to extract *postmodern* from a context of academic fashion. It remains a term useful in identifying the relatively coherent period in the development of Westernized industrial nations that begins, roughly, at the end of World War II. Its vagueness in fact recommends *postmodern* as applied to a period of rapid transition when values and styles are losing their familiar shape. There is no term half so serviceable to replace it. Even its critics, even televangelists or conservative commentators impassioned in their defense of traditional virtues, stand within the stream they oppose, taking calls on their cell phones, eating in franchised restaurants owned by multinational corporations, raising kids who speak computerese. We are all, like it or not, postmodern.

This book shares something of a postmodern spirit in its disregard for claims to originality. It does not seek to be first in line or to write something never before written or thought. Its main purpose could be described as rethinking and extending the disorganized minority tradition that argues for the importance of cultural influences upon health and illness. Many readers will recognize the contributions of such distinguished figures in this tradition as René Dubos, George L. Engel, Oliver Sacks, Melvin Konner, Arthur Kleinman, and (preeminently) Michel Foucault.[5] Some will know the work of equally important, if less celebrated, historians, sociologists, anthropologists, philosophers, and literary critics, who help to show how various bio-

logical states—from menopause to post-traumatic stress disorder—
are shaped by historical and cultural forces.[6] This minority tradition
has even spun off a few popular television specials and coffee table
books. The bulk of such work has appeared within the last fifty years,
in the period, if not always in the spirit, known as postmodern. A few
scholars have even begun to explore specific ways in which postmodernism as a style and postmodernity as a period affect the individual experience of illness. (The work of Zygmunt Bauman,
Nicholas J. Fox, Arthur W. Frank, and Elaine Showalter is important
here.)[7] My aim is to provide a deployment rather than an archaeology of this recent minority tradition and to emphasize the proliferating connections between biology and culture. It is the emergent literature (growing more robust daily) on the connections between
biology and culture that creates a context within which my arguments about postmodern illness stand as far more significant than
were they simply the unprecedented thoughts of a solitary writer.

Haven't people always believed or hoped they could live forever?
The answer is no. Even the pharaohs—stocking their tombs for the
afterlife—had to face up to their own mortality. For centuries, the
graveyards beside every parish church reminded the faithful that
they, too, must die. The current assault upon biology expresses not a
permanent disposition of human nature but an impulse with specific
historical roots. In fact, postmodern thinking can rank among its
most important accomplishments a rejection of Enlightenment arguments that human nature is always and everywhere the same, universal and absolute. Unfortunately, in exploding myths about universal human nature and about purportedly changeless essences such as
justice or sexuality, postmodern thinkers have emphasized cultural
differences at the cost of neglecting the equally strong evidence of biological sameness or consistency. They write as if we were beings
wholly constructed by culture, rather than social creatures endowed
by the long prehistoric processes of evolution with nervous systems,
hormones, genes, and a biological heritage that we share not only
with fellow humans but also (approaching within a whisker-thin

margin of complete overlap) with various chimps, apes, and other
higher primates. Culture plays a crucial role in human affairs; but its
power is far from total, and biology often combines with culture to
produce colorful local variations in our behavior, from courtship rituals to eating disorders. In a rare condition called gourmand syndrome, researchers recently discovered that lesions of the front right
cerebral hemisphere produce a compulsive preoccupation with gour-
met food.[8] Hunger, thirst, and sexual desire, no matter how elegantly
we stylize their satisfaction, proceed from a level beyond culture.

We are beginning to discover the evolutionary implications in the
concept that humans are social animals. This book aligns itself with
the sometimes inaudible voices within postmodern thought that emphasize the intricate relations between our animal heritage and our
social experience. One example must suffice. The much touted differences between women and men, as Deborah Blum shows, while
shaped by cultural practices rooted in time-bound and place-bound
ideologies of gender, also have biological underpinnings rooted in
human evolution. Even mice, it turns out, manage to develop de-
fenses against incest, based on a system of immune-system proteins
that govern female mating patterns. (Mice also appear to possess a
gene that facilitates social behavior.) The balance between biological
and cultural sources of our sexual behavior is not static, Blum
demonstrates, but in constant change.[9] So, too, with illness. Historical
differences in our experience cannot be fully understood apart from
the biology of nerves, neurotransmitters, microbes, and genes that
gives human affliction a degree of sameness across disparate times
and cultures. The delicate balance between biology and culture, as it
alters in a continuous flow, is what constitutes the elusive truth of illness.

Skeptics may contend that an exploration of convergences between biology and culture does not truly add to our knowledge of illness but simply rearranges it. Two brief responses are thus in order.
First, knowledge often advances by strategic rearrangements. Science
tends to prosper precisely because we set established facts in the context of sounder hypotheses or theories. Individual studies that may

have minor impact in isolation gain significant power when brought together with other studies that reinforce major changes in thinking. Second, established facts are altered—sometimes decisively—by the new context in which they are set. Lung cancer has for years remained securely enclosed within a biomedical discourse that relegates social practices to the status of "risk factors." Risk factors, in this way of thinking, do not "cause" a disease (at least not all the time) and so do not really belong to it: they are outriders on biology. Suppose, however, that we rearrange the facts slightly and move the cultural practice of smoking cigarettes toward the center of our thinking about lung cancer. The rearrangement, in turn, allows other established but neglected facts to snap into focus: facts about suppressed research into nicotine addiction, about advertising campaigns targeted at children, about government subsidies for tobacco. Suddenly the biology of lung cancer appears inseparable from the culture in which it occurs, with the result that serious improvements in public health are at last possible.

The importance of understanding such convergences between biology and culture cannot explain away every complication. This book does not offer the medical equivalent of a unified field theory, sweeping up every possible illness, past and future, into a single explanatory model. My claims are limited. Convergences between biology and culture help to clarify many illnesses, but not all. Some maladies are wholly genetic in origin, extremely rare, or so rapid and deadly in their onset that the influence of culture barely registers. Further, for millions of years disease worked its way through the animal kingdom before the arrival of humans and their cultural activities. The current status of disease in animals of course illustrates how hard it is to escape the grip of culture: pets and livestock are prey to diseases that come with domestication, while wild animals also suffer ailments related to human activities, like the endangered Florida panthers whose malformed hearts result from the inbreeding of populations severely depleted as we destroy their habitat. Still, convergences between biology and culture, no matter how extensive, do not constitute a master key to all illness. A master key would eliminate the need for further inquiry, as one answer fits every question. What this book offers instead is the exploration of an unfamiliar and still unfolding way of thought.

The way of thinking about illness explored here, in its rejection of a single theory or model that will explain every illness, shares at least one feature with much postmodern analysis. Postmodernism has generated a distrust of the comprehensive explanations that French theorist Jean-François Lyotard calls "grand narratives"—vast encompassing megabodies such as Christianity and Marxism that reduce other stories and historical details to mere satellites within their all-encompassing gravitational field. "The grand narrative," writes Lyotard in *The Postmodern Condition: A Report on Knowledge* (1979), "has lost its credibility."[10] From a postmodern perspective, the long-dominant biomedical model provides one such comprehensive and dubious grand narrative: a theory that reduces every illness to a biological mechanism of cause and effect. By contrast, my argument—that postmodern illness is defined by an awareness of the elaborate interconnections between biology and culture—does not aspire to the stature of a grand narrative. It does not seek to explain every affliction on the planet, but rather to describe a new, transitional, and unfinished understanding of illness that typifies numerous industrial societies during the second half of the twentieth century. Whatever power this understanding may possess, a postmodern model of illness will no doubt (such is the inner logic of postmodernism) need to be supplemented by other compatible and similarly limited models.[11] The main point here—setting aside the questions about the value of grand narratives—is that we can best grasp what makes postmodern illness distinctive if we examine various specific instances (in all their irreducibly rich, local details) where biology and culture converge.

No single study can fully address a topic that is as immense as postmodern culture and as sprawling as postmodern illness. This book, by virtue of its subject, cannot fail to be incomplete. Its gaps are required or at least inevitable features—although all authors have blind spots. Where completeness is impossible, moreover, an emphasis on one illness inevitably slights another. Inclusion or omission here does not signify relative importance; it is not as if illnesses competed for space to reflect which is more serious or weighty. Is AIDS more serious than breast cancer? Is Tourette syndrome less weighty than asthma? My purpose is not to rank incommensurate forms of suffering but to tell a highly selective, nonlinear story about the distinctive qualities of postmodern illness. It is, ultimately, a story about a transition from the biomedical model that has served us well for over a century to a new, incomplete, unnamed model that I am calling *biocultural*.[12]

The incompleteness implicit in this inquiry into the development of a biocultural model at least acknowledges the open-endedness of this period in which experiences of illness continue to change. The end of postmodern illness, I believe, will not arrive until the human genome project and biotechnology (both in early stages) have advanced far enough to offer a radically altered vision and a vast new array of effective treatments. The old distinction between genetic disease and nongenetic disease, for example, is breaking down as researchers show a genetic component in most diseases.[13] (We recently learned that a form of the gene known as apolipoprotein E may predispose boxers to develop chronic traumatic brain injury and that another gene, when defective, causes a hereditary form of Parkinson's disease.)[14] The world will see momentous change when genetic engineering permits us not only to transplant healthy genes into a person who is ill but also to prevent illnesses by altering the genetic makeup of human embryos. At this future point, genetic medicine will have actively redesigned—not merely influenced or redirected—the biology of illness. This post-postmodern world will face presently unknown diseases—some doubtless introduced by the widespread use of DNA technologies to create genetically modified microorganisms, like the synthetic bacteria engineered to clean up oil spills at sea. Such far-reaching manipulations will ultimately rewrite both illness and culture. Meanwhile, it will take many voices to tell the ongoing story of postmodern illness. I prefer to think of my voice as aspiring to the virtues of a prologue—or maybe an extended introductory essay—rather than providing a definitive scholarly exposition.

One major omission—from the perspective of medicine in the United States—is an account of the recent transition to a system of so-called managed care. The huge health maintenance organizations (HMOs) that have sprung up to negotiate contracts with hospitals and doctors (and often to set the terms of treatment) reflect far more than a change in medical economics. Many doctors feel their decision-making autonomy threatened as choices about proper medical treatment end up on the desks of cost-conscious bureaucrats. Many patients feel their health undermined and their trust in doctors eroded as HMOs decide—in some cases, wrongly or illegally—to withhold access to care.[15] In the United States today, an illness does not count as an illness unless an HMO will certify it. (So much for biology alone.) The danger in an account that focuses on managed care is that we will lose sight of larger interrelations between illness and culture. The United States, as Robert H. Blank points out, is the only Western industrialized nation that fails to guarantee universal health care. "The core problems of American health care," he contends, "are not solely economic or even political but instead emerge from a set of uniquely American illusions about health, health care, and the role of government."[16] Managed care represents a unique subplot that contributes to the confusion and powerlessness that frustrate many American doctors and patients today, but its significance lies within the larger and inherently international narrative of convergences between biology and culture. Managed care, as a national problem resolvable by legislation, remains less important to a knowledge of postmodern illness than the unresolved cultural illusions about health (illusions by no means unique to the United States) that stand behind it. Although the illustrations and data in this book come primarily from the United States, which is the culture I know best, a similar study of postmodern illness—adjusted for local differences—could be written in almost any industrial nation. Americans, with or without HMOs, are not alone in their fantasies of living forever.

Narratives of unfinished change are often unwelcome. Already preoccupied with crowded waiting rooms and the daily proliferating biomedical literature, as well as with threats to their income and autonomy, many doctors would prefer not to think about a new vision of illness. The biomedical model works pretty well, much of the time. Do we really need an account of illness that requires us to confront immense and perhaps irremediable problems of culture and public health? Patients as well as doctors remain deeply attached to a biomedical model that has helped to prolong life expectancy, to eradicate lethal diseases, and to develop effective plans of treatment for once debilitating illnesses. Many people take comfort in thinking about the body as a machine that requires merely an occasional trip to the repair shop: the analogy allows us to postpone troublesome questions about illness because we assume that the medical profession will know exactly what to do when an emergency arises. This is a good assumption.

The intensive care unit, the burn unit, and the emergency room save numerous lives that just a few years ago would have been inescapably destroyed. Almost all patients who need such care are awed by the medical skill and cutting-edge technology that permit their survival, and nothing in this book should be interpreted as a contribution to the popular pastime of doctor bashing. A few criminals with medical degrees are among the people responsible for billions of dollars lost annually to Medicare and Medicaid fraud in the United States, but the health care profession (although occasionally dishonored) has a remarkable record of helping us get through crises that otherwise would be insurmountable. The problem lies less with individual doctors than with the biomedical model that still controls a great deal of medical education and clinical practice. Significantly, the assumptions that underlie the biomedical model work best for patients whose lives are in jeopardy from a clear organic cause where surgical interventions or drugs provide an effective response. Medicine today, however, must also deal with illnesses that last for decades. It must treat patients with difficult chronic conditions such as alcoholism, arthritis, diabetes, hypertension, heart disease, and nonmalignant pain, to name just a few common maladies. It must address the needs of a swiftly aging population whose complicated illnesses cannot be reduced to a short-term emergency or to a curable malfunction.

Here, beyond the emergency room and intensive care unit, as doctors respond to the changing world that medicine has helped to create, the biomedical model and the mechanistic thinking behind it run up against nearly fatal limitations. Worse, in ignoring these limitations, medicine at times pursues its own research agenda and economic interests at the patient's expense. When patients do not openly opt for alternative healers or for non-Western systems of care, from Chinese acupuncture to the ancient medicine from India known as Ayurveda, they often prove the staunchest defenders of the same mechanistic biomedicine in which the pursuit of cure reinforces an illusion that our lives can be indefinitely extended by means of continuous high-tech repairs. In effect, patients and doctors collude in this fiction. "A strong presumption throughout my medical education," writes physician Ira Byock of the period extending into the 1980s, "was that all seriously ill people required vigorous life-prolonging treatment, including those who were expected to die, even patients with advanced chronic illness such as widespread cancer, end-stage congestive heart failure, and kidney or liver failure. It even extended to patients who saw death as a relief from the suffering caused by their illness."[17] Death is a scandal in postmodern times partly because it unmasks the illusion that we can live forever.

A good index to the character and limitations of biomedicine is what happens when the hope of cure is gone. When all their vigorous invasive procedures prove futile, when the patient can no longer sustain either the curative assault of medicine or the punishment of illness, the cardiologist and the nephrologist and the other specialists are suddenly and curiously absent—not even a courtesy visit is paid—or at least such was my experience during one especially difficult episode. Well-known surgeon and author Sherwin B. Nuland, who teaches the history of medicine at Yale University, sees something similar in today's high-tech biomedicine. "The diagnosis of disease and the quest for overcoming it with his intellect," he writes, "are the challenges that motivate every specialist who is any good at what he does. He is fascinated with pathology. When faced by the certainty of his own impotence to treat it, the would-be healer too often turns away. If a riddle is by its nature insoluble, it cannot long hold the interest of any but a tiny fraction of the doctors who treat specific organ systems and disease categories."[18] This is not good news for patients, who may feel disinclined to have their illness reduced to a riddle on which the male intellect (note Nuland's telltale masculine pronouns) can exorcise its fears of impotence. The one stalwart health care figure, almost invariably female, who does stay and care until the end while the highly paid professionals often turn away, not surprisingly occupies the lowest status and earns the most meager income in the entire hierarchy of medical expertise: the nurse's aide.[19]

The dying patient, if not wholly abandoned by medical experts, is often left the casualty of a mechanistic dream of cure so tattered and threadbare that it cannot allay fears of a painful, humiliating death in the grip of the same life-extending technology that is a trademark of postmodern medicine. Our anxieties about death have shifted from the fact of dying to the methods that medicine will use to keep us alive. "Don't let me die on a machine," patients now whisper to their physicians or assert in advance directives. The widespread call for physician-assisted suicide is not simply the result of documented medical failures in pain management, failures that come despite an abundance of powerful opioids that guarantee almost no patient should die in pain. It is a logical extension of the biomedical model. When the biomedical "continuous repair" job inevitably fails, many people reasonably (but incorrectly) suppose that doctors have nothing left to offer except one last drug or high-tech mechanism that will quickly and painlessly dispatch us.

The public taste for quick fixes through drugs and surgery, as deeply rooted as the taste for fast food and the fifteen-minute oil change, helps keep the biomedical model in business at a time when a number of doctors and caregivers are coming to recognize its limitations. The desire for instant cure should probably rank right after rapid weight loss and world-class sex on the list of contemporary fantasies. What proves ultimately in our best interests, however, is not the biomedical delusion of cure—as irresistible as the lottery—but a down-to-earth understanding of illness that corresponds to the chronic conditions and complicated ailments for which continuous repairs seem unavailable. Postmodern illness, as I describe it here, does not fit the pattern of mechanistic biomedical thought that was so prevalent in the first half of the twentieth century—and is still going strong. It calls for a vision more complex than modernist views that found the best model for sickness in a malfunctioning machine.

An account of postmodern illness will need to encompass the anxieties created by rapid and uncertain change, the anxieties of a period in which both patients and doctors may feel adrift, as once stable forms (the house call, the family physician, the biomedical model) fall under intense pressure, straining, dissolving, emerging in altered shapes. It will need to reflect the confusing welter of self-help programs, group therapies, alternative healers, and experimental drugs. It will need to recognize how doctors as well as patients are caught in the turmoil of shifting times.

One evening at our local university I ran into a well-regarded young neurologist. When I asked what had brought him, he replied he was taking night classes to earn an master's degree in business. Why? His malpractice premiums had lit up like a jackpot. His partners were tangled in lawsuits. If he lost his license or got squeezed out by insurance costs, he would need the new business credentials for a fallback position as hospital administrator. Here, I thought, was someone caught in a system disordered (or hyperorganized) to the point of giddiness. Many people feel a similar vertigo as HMOs and group practice reshape an earlier, more personal relation between doctors and, what shall we call them now, clients? The complaints go far beyond grousing. They betray a sense that medicine has embarked upon a dangerously uncharted course, where hyperactive schoolchildren are routinely drugged into good behavior, where physicians must plead with insurance executives in distant cities to approve a necessary treatment, where old diseases disappear and new ones arrive overnight: a quietly desperate scene of disarray, upheaval, and lost direction.

A vision appropriate to the age of postmodern illness, however, must not focus solely on disarray and upheaval. It must also convey the sense of a complex new order coming into view within the turmoil, controversy, and bewilderment, as we learn how to recognize the intricate interactions set in motion when biology and culture converge. The forces that make up culture are as complicated as the interacting forces behind the weather—jet stream, ocean currents, sun spots, land masses, wind, and volcanic eruptions, for a start—and, like the weather, they are in continuous change. An understanding of the interrelations between culture and biology will require a tolerance for ambiguities far greater than any medical school today is likely to test for and certify in its graduates. It also demands an awareness of unusual new patterns where traditional observers see mere randomness or a confusion of unconnected data. Scientists now use the postmodern tool known as chaos theory (which came to public attention in the 1980s) as a means of uncovering mathematical laws at work within forms so bizarre that they resemble swirls, moonscapes, ink blots, squiggles, and tiny jagged chains. Physicists use chaos theory to study hidden order in the motion of electrons. There is a strong, if sporadic, interest in chaos theory among the life sciences, where epidemiologists detect invisible patterns within the oscillations of epidemics such as measles, polio, and rubella. Even the metabolism of cells and the propagation of nerve impulses are illuminated by the new science of chaos, while postmodern novelists, directly or indirectly influenced by science, have begun to explore the emergence of strange, complex harmonies within apparently random experience.[20] Chaos theory, with its base in mathematics, can provide no more than a metaphor to describe the nonmathematical coherences at work within irregular, multilevel, turbulent scenes of change. It may, however, as eminent gerontologist James S. Goodwin writes, prove helpful in giving us "the concepts and vocabulary to articulate the fact that much of the practice of medicine is outside the realm of the modernist reductionist model of science."[21] It also suggests that what looks chaotic or disorderly in the twilight of the biomedical model may be an intricate and unusual new order in the making.

This new order will take some getting used to. The complications of a biocultural perspective—which are beyond the power of computerized logarithms to represent—may excuse (or even demand) an exploration as many-sided and asymmetrical as the fragmentary nonfiction narrative I offer here. Such a narrative, although less satisfying than a rounded history or a statistical demonstration, has much to tell about the difficult changes we are living through—changes that help to shape and, inescapably, to define us. It can help us recognize the outlines of our emerging future.

An understanding of illness as biocultural—the subject of this book—goes a long way toward illuminating the changes, conflicts, and confusions of postmodern medicine. It clarifies an outlook not fully developed or fully accepted either inside or outside the medical community. Knowledge of this new outlook should be standard equipment for anyone who enters a doctor's office. It will not help us live forever—nothing will—but it just might reorient our thinking about health, prevent a disastrous medical error, and keep us from wasting our lifeblood in the pursuit of a shopworn mechanistic illusion. The potential benefits in improved public health and in reduced costs that flow from a biocultural outlook are immense, if as yet unrealized: a legacy of the future. Fifty years ago, only a few mavericks or visionaries within mainstream medicine would have risked describing illness as a mental, emotional, bodily event constructed at the crossroads of biology and culture. For many people, the description remains no more than another flawed, unworkable, disruptive, crackpot, postmodern idea. Let us see where it might lead.

chapter one

The Country of the Ill

Illness is the night-side of life, a more onerous

citizenship. Everyone who is born holds dual

citizenship, in the kingdom of the well and in the

kingdom of the sick.

SUSAN SONTAG,
Illness as Metaphor (1978)

Illness is our common fate. Although we inevitably experience it with our idiosyncrasies intact, it is something almost everyone shares. Black or white, Hindu, Muslim, or Jew, we all sooner or later take our turn in the country of the ill. The sojourn is often deeply distressing. Drawing breath may require conscious struggle; fever and chills sweep through the body; your head hurts, your limbs ache, your disposition sours. It is easy to see why the adjective *cranky* shares a root with the German word for *disease*. Illness not only makes us irritable, or as we say, ill-tempered, but can also make us feel alienated from ourselves, as if we had been replaced by a pain-filled, seriously flawed, charmless replica. Unsoundness is not just a state of body. "To be sick is already to be disordered in your mind as well," writes editor and critic Anatole Broyard of his struggle with prostate cancer, which at times evoked an irrationality so deep that he calls it "a patient's madness." "Illness," he confides in his journal, "is a kind of incoherence." [1]

Like any struggle, illness may call forth a latent courage or wisdom (almost a hidden truth) in people who face adversity with exceptional resilience, but it also has a long association with falsity. The bedridden "invalid"—a term that links ill health with illogic—is not merely sick but somehow fallacious at the core. "I couldn't be the person I needed to be," says novelist Reynolds Price of the terrible ordeal that followed his diagnosis with spinal cancer. [2] It is not just that we mistrust the judgment of the sick. Illness threatens to undo our sense of who we are. Its darkest power lies in showing us a picture of ourselves—false, damaged, unreliable, and inescapably mortal—that we desperately do not want to see. A serious and protracted illness constitutes an immersion in an alien reality where almost everything changes. At its most dire, it can wreck the body, unstring the mind, and paralyze the emotions, plunging entire families into bankruptcy and chaos. Fortunately, most illnesses do not last long enough to create a permanent schism in our sense of self or to change our vision of the world. We quickly reenter our former lives and put the illness behind us, consigning people who cannot stop talking about their ailments to the first rank of bores. Still, no matter how fast we forget a recent affliction, few experiences are so disorienting as our glimpses into the counterworld that opens up whenever we cross over from health to illness. Such glimpses, dimly recalled, are what make visiting the sick something we usually find innumerable reasons to defer.

The country of the ill, no matter how widely shared its terrain, is not a universal realm located outside the influence of space and time. Our common fate, it turns out, is entry into a region that regularly, if sometimes very slowly, shifts its features, like a populous valley once covered by primal seas. Illness depends on relatively stable biological features—a cough in every culture uses the same muscles and respiratory organs—but it is also deeply historical, no less changing than the microbes that surround and interpenetrate us. Indeed, the country of the ill assumes the distinctive features of whatever nation or social group inhabits it. It is a slippery place in which our condition depends not only on biological processes but also on our gender, race, and income. Black patients in the United States, for example, get measurably worse care than white patients—including care as specific as standard procedures for heart disease and chest pain—and they die sooner.[3] (Overall, blacks in the United States are 4.5 times more likely than whites to die of medically preventable conditions.)[4] The vast social changes during the last fifty years of the twentieth century—the period usually designated postmodern—have in effect reshaped the experience of illness.

POSTMODERNISM UNDEFINED

The upstart term *postmodern* makes many people edgy. It has been so overused as to mean almost anything. Some employ it as a sign of intellectual power, as if it contained a secret erudite meaning, and the urge to dump such a troublesome term is hard to resist. As two American sociologists write, "Postmodernism is everywhere. It has become the hip, the in, the trendy catchword of the late 1980s. There is even a 'Postmodern Hour' on MTV."[5] The spell of the postmodern extends well beyond the 1980s, so the main issue is how to understand a concept that will not go away. Some analysts prefer to rush in with a definition, but it is folly to provide a firm definition for something still in flux, a flux that encompasses the definer. A more useful approach is to accept some degree of indefiniteness, with the irritation it inspires, as intrinsic to postmodernism.[6] After all, the postmodern world almost reinvented uncertainty—in quantum physics and cross-dressing, for example—and such a shifting quarry is bound to resist a perfect definition. Instead of seeking to capture it whole, we will do better to examine some of the postmodern fragments that have helped to reshape the contemporary experience of

illness, and meanwhile we can validly employ postmodern in its
most restricted sense to denote the unfinished period that com-
mences (roughly) with the second half of the twentieth century.

Of course, even employed to designate the period after World
War II, postmodern will inevitably include people and events ahead
of their times, or behind, spanning or resisting categories. Marcel
Duchamp helped invent modernist art, although his works—especially the famous "readymades," such as the porcelain urinal that he
exhibited under the title *Fountain* (1917)—exude a distinctly postmodern spirit. Samuel Beckett? Is he an early postmodern or, as he
has been called, the last modernist?[7] Borderline cases highlight another question. Does postmodernism represent a decisive break with
the past—or an extension and development of modernist programs?
In some fields (architecture, for example) differences between postmodern and modern are obvious, but elsewhere the relationship is
much harder to sort out.[8] Even cultural trends that analysts agree to
call postmodern are divided by disagreement and conflict. In short,
there is not one postmodernism, monolithic and homogeneous, but a
dialogue of postmodern voices.[9] Postmodernism is self-consciously
pluralistic and multicultural, a freewheeling consortium of heterogeneous parts, where underlying consistencies are often less visible
than the outward play of difference.

One benefit of resisting a definition—of using postmodern at the
start to indicate the relatively cohesive historical period of Western
industrial development commencing about 1950—lies in avoiding a
tedious demonstration of how all the current theoretical definitions
of postmodernism at some point founder or fall short. Postmodernism in its copious variety cannot be captured in slogans about the
failures of Enlightenment rationality, about the loss of foundations,
or about a linguistic turn in philosophy. It is equally hard to pin
down as it applies to illness. Arthur W. Frank, in an extremely valuable analysis, argues that "[t]he *postmodern* experience of illness begins when ill people recognize that more is involved in their experiences than the medical story can tell."[10] In Frank's version, modern
and postmodern denote two distinct, successive styles of living with

illness: a modern style that accepts the authorized medico-scientific narrative and a postmodern style in which patients reclaim power as creators and narrators of their own distinctive stories. There are, however, other equally important styles, features, and themes in the postmodern transformation of illness.

Postmodernism—to offer another fragmentary description in lieu of a definition—indicates a world that we recognize as inescapably "constructed." It is constructed not so much with cement and steel, like the modernist skyscraper, as with images and representations. Its main power tools are television, cinema, and the computer screen. The endless images they generate have grown so potent that representations sometimes take on an independent life and supplant whatever they supposedly depict or refer to.[11] The modernist real world—a bold new venture built with the products of mills, factories, and machine shops—dissolves into the computer-simulated postmodern universe of visual images. This simulated postmodern world is a place where life often seems less real (less sharp and full) than its representations on TV and where increasingly—as when a talking cartoon dog sells life insurance—there is nothing outside the image: an unprecedented state of affairs that sociologist Jean Baudrillard describes through his coinage *hyperreal*. "The real," as he puts its somewhat cryptically, "is no longer real."[12]

The concept of a media-generated hyperreal world is crucial enough for an understanding of postmodern illness that it deserves a brief, if homely, illustration—drawn from a football game I attended at the Louisiana Superdome. American professional football is a modernist invention that for many years was played on outdoor fields before twenty or thirty thousand spectators. Today professional football has not just moved mostly indoors. The game I watched was televised for a huge national audience. More important, the action unfolding on the field was continuously interrupted for TV commercials, during which players milled about aimlessly and motorized camera platforms rolled along the sidelines. It soon became clear that the interior of the Superdome was a kind of sport-centered movie set. What happened there was not the final product: the real thing. In fact, the actual game on the field was far less substantial and certainly far less gripping than the game I imagined being broadcast—with the addition of color commentary, close-ups, and play-by-play announcers—to millions of spectators watching at home. Which game was real? The postmodern answer: neither. Postmodernism makes us aware that we have entered an era when flesh-and-blood encounters (like my trip to the Superdome) have been shaped by contact with a realm of images that in some cases decisively transcends them. The indeterminate shadowland in between the image and the material event is home to the distinctively postmodern experience of the hyperreal.

The postmodern world is a place where 90 percent of teenagers across the globe recognize the Chicago Bulls. The Chicago Bulls, in turn, are far more than the players on a midwestern professional basketball team. The name, like the team, is a commodity marketed relentlessly on television, whence it escapes into popular culture and is appropriated by groups as diverse as urban gangs and high-fashion models, who return the image for circulation bearing ever new layers of constructed meaning or implication. Postmodernism in this familiar sense evokes the franchised, déjà vu, simulated reality where shopping malls in Pittsburgh and Los Angeles contain identical stores, where a Las Vegas casino reproduces the skyline of New York City, where the latest Hollywood action film opens simultaneously in Mozambique and Munich. It is the world of consumer capitalism, late-night talk shows, sound-bite politics, satellite weather reports, gay-pride marches, e-mail, and virtual libraries (which contain no books), to name a few postwar innovations. The attendant changes in our sensibilities and understanding have had a significant impact on the experience of illness.

Like a concise definition, an extended discussion of postmodernism—one that takes into account the highest order of philosophical and scholarly debate—is not necessary as we begin to examine changes in the contemporary experience of illness. The facets of postmodernism that have nothing to do with illness simply lie outside our focus. Relevant features that we have not discussed thus far will emerge as we examine specific contemporary illnesses. An immediate plunge into the individual experience of illness, however, is also premature, because it fails to recognize the changed social context in which postmodern illness occurs. The best approach at the start, resisting the attractions of pure theory and of unmediated experience, will be to explore a few specific ways in which the postmodern world has begun to change human perception. Sometimes a single life, if sufficiently lucid, can serve as a lens to bring diffuse and complex social forces into sharper focus.

A POSTMODERN LIFE

Andy Warhol, born Andrew Warhola in 1928 to an impoverished immigrant family in Pittsburgh, for a time cultivated a public image that associated him directly with the chic, drugs-and-sex, club-hopping lifestyle of the super rich, whose occasional deaths from heroin overdose simply contributed to a macabre glamour. His albino-chalk skin—which during the 1960s (in what he called his "degenerate period") he accentuated with an unvarying costume of black leather jacket, tight black jeans, high-heeled black boots, and frazzled silver-white wig—lent him an unhealthy air, as if he emerged only at night, pallid, wasted, strung out on artificial stimulants. In truth, while he invited misjudgments that reinforced his counterculture image, Warhol rarely touched alcohol, declined drugs, exercised regularly, and maintained long periods of celibacy. His chief excess, in addition to an almost compulsive drive to collect things, was the prescription diet pill Obetrol, which he used to maintain a stylishly trim figure. His unexpected death in 1986, at age fifty-eight, of complications following surgery to remove a badly infected gallbladder was an aberration in his otherwise fashionable, dramatic life.

Although Warhol died in a way that surely no one expected, his place of death—the hospital—follows the pattern of postmodern dying. In 1900, at the beginning of the modern period, almost everyone died at home, surrounded by family, perhaps in the presence of the

family doctor. Today we die not only away from home but also enfolded securely within the multibillion-dollar business of hospital
medicine. Postmodern death occurs amid nurses, interns, specialists,
tubes, computers, and life-support equipment, assembled at great
cost. The only thing truly uncommon about Andy Warhol's death is
its mystery: people seldom die from gallbladder surgery.

There were allegations of hospital neglect and staff error—although malpractice suits (another new trend in postmodern medicine) did not materialize.[13] Allegations, of course, do not equal proof.
Yet, as medicine has grown vastly more complicated in its reliance on
drugs and technology, the opportunities for mistakes have multiplied. Medical error is a serious public health problem: autopsy studies have found rates of fatal missed diagnosis—that is, missed diagnosis resulting in death—as high as 35 to 40 percent. A hospital stay
now exposes patients to infections native only to hospitals—so-
called nosocomial infections, which kill over sixty thousand Americans annually, many of them elderly.[14] (There is even a *Journal of Hospital Infection.*) In fact, iatrogenic illness—the medical euphemism for
illness caused by physicians or medical procedures—has become
such a serious problem that people often fear hospitals and doctors
more than they fear dying. In its hospital setting and its unresolved
allegations of medical neglect, the death of Andy Warhol is as postmodern as his multiple portraits of Elvis Presley.

Warhol matters here because he illustrates so vividly some distinctive features of postmodern experience that as they were transforming culture were simultaneously transforming medicine and illness.
He is among the first truly postmodern artists, even more popular in
the 1990s than during his lifetime, a figure whose life and art (he consciously blurred the line) both shaped and expressed crucial features
of the postmodern era. Warhol, in effect, leaves us in no doubt that
the postmodern era, despite its continuities with the modernist past,
confronts us with a new experience of the world.

His early career clearly reveals an eagerness to depart from modernist models. Unlike the great modern painters who endured years

of bohemian poverty and neglect for the sake of their art, trading sketches for drinks in Paris cafés, Warhol left for New York City immediately after college to work as a commercial artist. His drawings proved so successful—he specialized in women's shoes—that he soon earned upwards of sixty thousand dollars a year, an immense figure in the 1950s. This background in commerce would almost automatically disqualify him from participating in the defiantly nonmercantile and antibourgeois world of modernist art. It was only the advent of pop art in the early 1960s—with its appropriation of slick commercial images from comic books and advertisements—that pushed Warhol to explore his postponed ambitions as a painter. The streamlined, Americanized name he adopted was simply one more sign of his break with the past. What truly signaled his transformation into a postmodern artist, gaining him instant notoriety, was the 1962 exhibition in which he first showed his large-scale paintings of Campbell's soup cans.

What might Warhol's soup cans tell us, indirectly, about illness? They reflect the emergence of a new, postmodern, postindustrial consumer-culture economy in which no aspect of life would be left untouched by the power of images, including the life of the body.[15] Of course, the colorful, oversized replicas of ordinary soup cans sparked instant controversy—the postmodern artist continues the modernist tradition of creating art that questions the boundaries of art—but it is clear that Warhol's subject was not a random choice. One year earlier he had completed (although not exhibited) an equally provocative six-foot, black-and-white painting of a Coke bottle. In these early works he followed the lead of Jasper Johns and Roy Lichtenstein, whose celebrated paintings of flags and comic strip panels were likewise nourished by a background in commerce. Yet Warhol brought to pop art—the short-lived movement he quickly distanced himself from—something unique: an uncanny grasp of what constitutes a distinctive imagery of postwar America. The commodities he chose to paint were, of course, fixtures of everyday life, but it took Warhol to transform them into visible signs of a new order. Postmodern experi-

ence cannot be disentangled from the spell of the commodified artifacts he held up for our gaze. He showed us that art, too, had become
another commodity in the circular marketplace of images.

Maybe the surest sign of his distance from the immediate past was
Warhol's (incomplete) disdain for the prized modernist value of originality. In fact, he chose subjects and techniques that seem to efface
the sense of an origin. He copied from photographic slides projected
onto canvas; he used stencils, offset printing techniques, rubber
stamps, and wood blocks.[16] "Usually, all I need," as he explained his
art, "is tracing paper and a good light."[17] His silkscreens preeminently used the techniques of mass production to erode any clear distinction between copy and original. It was an art that consisted entirely of copies. If his soup cans and Brillo boxes retain a link with the
shock value of modernist experiments, they shock through their apparent commercial banality, through an explicit violation of hallowed
modernist standards of high seriousness. Their emotionless, simplified depiction of everyday objects seems a gesture of anti-art or at the
very least a deliberate turning away from the themes and ambitions
of the great modernist painters. Indeed, his work helps establish a
pattern basic to postmodern painting, which one theorist calls a new
form of art whose pictorial techniques embody "a skepticism as to
the possibility of high art."[18] The pioneering abstract expressionist
painter Willem de Kooning, a veteran of the battles to create a modernist aesthetic, knew Warhol's work and despised it.

For a sense of what appalled de Kooning and for an illustration of
the difference between modernist and postmodern outlooks, we
might briefly compare two famous works—Warhol's *Marilyn (Three
Times)* (1962) and Picasso's *Portrait of a Young Woman* (1936). The comparison helps illuminate changes that reshape postmodern culture,
including the culture of medicine and illness.[19]

The two works, although separated by a mere twenty-five years,
reflect not just different styles but different worlds. Warhol's banal
commercial subjects, his depthless pictorial surface, his mechanized
techniques are all regularly attacked by proponents of modernism as
an almost evil capitulation to popular taste.[20] Not only did Warhol

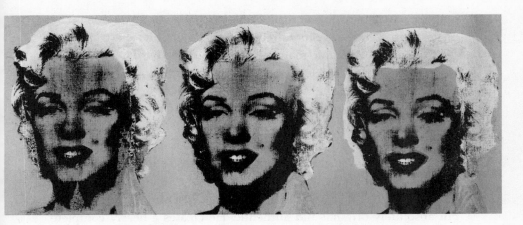

Figure 1. Andy Warhol, *Marilyn (Three Times)*, 1962, synthetic polymer paint and silkscreen on canvas. Copyright © 1997 Andy Warhol Foundation for the Visual Arts / ARS, New York. Reproduced by permission.

not invent or even reconstruct the image he presents, he based *Marilyn (Three Times)* directly on a 1953 Hollywood publicity photo (figure 1). The triple repetition of the image helps emphasize its status as a mere reproduction. This is not an in-depth analysis of character, as in modernist portraiture, but a superficial pose (pure cheesecake) emptied of feeling or insight. The deliberate tawdriness of the surface—rose-colored flesh, yellow hair, unmodulated blue background—creates an art that appears devoted to excluding any complication. Yet, of course, much is going on.

Warhol's choices require us to acknowledge a world where reality is increasingly manipulated and defined—constituted—by the power of mass-produced commercial images. One archetype of this new postmodern world of the hyperreal is of course Marilyn Monroe—not the flesh-and-blood woman born Norma Jean Mortenson but the world-famous Hollywood icon, a carefully crafted public image that later absorbed the tragic unhappiness of the real-life actress. If modernism got its news from radio, the postmodern world understands events through the visual technologies of television and film:

nothing now attains to full reality unless we view it on a screen. The image is in some sense more real—more potent and electrifying—than the erotic, dynamic material world it allegedly depicts. "Marilyn's lips weren't kissable," Warhol noted, "but they were very photographable."[21] The slightly blurred line and color in *Marilyn* are no mistake. Warhol said he noticed the effect while viewing an out-of-focus television set.

The difference between Warhol and Picasso is as vivid as the contrast between a TV picture and an X ray. Picasso's modernist experiments explored radically new techniques for representing experience: techniques that reveal something not just strange or shocking but absolutely original and authentic. He creates a nearly complete break with earlier realistic traditions of painting. In his *Portrait* we thus view a young woman (Marie-Thérèse Walter, mother of his daughter Maya) reinvented by the artist as she might appear not to a portrait painter but to the unconscious mind or to a philosopher capable of grasping deep structural truths (figure 2). The portrait also conveys a disquieting bleakness—the desiccated heart and bleached bones set immobile against a barren seascape—as if suggesting the strains and ambiguities that developed in their relationship as Picasso began to turn his attentions to Walter's eventual successor, Dora Maar.[22] From the alchemy of personal emotion and revolutionary style, Picasso creates an image that (like much of his work) destabilizes the spectator's ordinary point of reference. Even viewers familiar with cubist experiments may feel that they have never seen anything quite like this before.

Warhol's portraits, by contrast, depend on the celebrity that certain images achieve when circulated endlessly through the mass media, as in his versions of such famous contemporaries as Elvis Presley, James Dean, Mick Jagger, and Chairman Mao. Typically, his genius lies less in creating original images than in discovering already existing images whose power he absorbs. He often borrowed photographic images directly from magazines or newspapers, adding a splash of color or the accidental variations of the silkscreen process. The postmodern age of electronic reproduction had found in

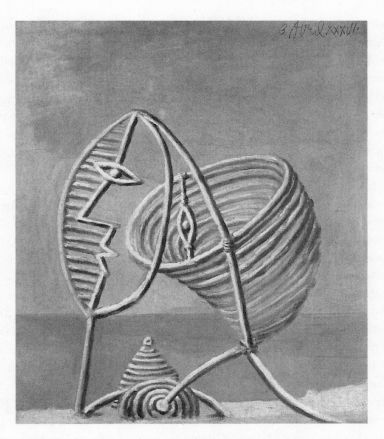

Figure 2. Pablo Picasso, *Portrait of a Young Woman*, 1936, oil on
canvas. Courtesy Musée Picasso, Paris. © Photo RMN—
Gérard Blot.

Andy Warhol its pop Michelangelo. It had also found a return to the
narrative impulse deliberately excluded from much modernist art
and wholly eliminated in such non-narrative styles as abstract ex-
pressionism. Unlike Picasso's *Portrait*, which defies traditional storytelling, Warhol's portraits often depend on a public knowledge and
tabloid-style gossip. Even his silkscreened electric chair tells a story,
albeit mute, implicit, and open-ended. Many of his visual images

gain impact and mystery through their power to tap into a pool of fragmentary, inarticulate narrative, much as his cows and flowers evoke the lost literary world of the pastoral. His portrait of Marilyn cannot help but evoke a memory of her stardom, glamorous failed marriages, abortive affairs, and suicide, with its allegations of murder and cover-up. It is not surprising, considering the link between his images and such unconventional narrative structures, that Warhol soon turned to directing and producing improvised, fragmented, experimental feature-length films.

Like much postmodern art, contemporary medicine situates us in a world where visual images reproducing fragments of the body (X rays, CT scans, MRIs) connect with implicit narrative contexts.[23] The question is how far medicine can recognize a role for narrative beyond continuous retellings of the authorized biomedical story about tissue damage and organic dysfunction. Warhol confronts us with fragmentary, ambiguous, open-ended, unconventional visual-narrative structures that capture a truth about the complex, changing, technological environment within which we play out the new drama of postmodern illness.

The ascendancy of Warhol also tells us much about changes in postmodern ideas of self and subjectivity that ultimately underlie the experience of illness. Tacitly, he announced the official demise of that most celebrated of modernist icons, the tortured artist, a solitary genius driven to create by angst, demons, alcohol, sex, and metaphysics. Art was no longer the expression of a complex interior soul. Souls or selves increasingly lost their former quality of inwardness, as if an individual were no longer felt to possess absolutely unique and hidden powers awaiting art or religion to call them forth. Selves were now, like Warhol's paintings, all surface and exterior, constituted less by some mysterious inner spirit than by an amalgamation of overt, public, cultural discourses, such as the image-saturated discourse of television, film, advertising, and commerce. Personal identity in mass culture now seemed merged with the personae of various relentlessly marketed rock groups, sports teams, manufacturers, and fashion designers, whose logos people began to wear on their clothing, like name tags. The New York building where Warhol created his silkscreens and planned his movies was called The Factory—the nickname an ironic rejoinder to the modernist cult of the lone, original, unfettered, antibourgeois artist. "I think everybody," Warhol said in his deadpan style, "should be a machine." Including artists.

As his detractors failed to understand, Warhol had managed to find the pulse of a complicated new era, including its self-reflexive ironies. (He thus created a famous persona for himself as a man almost devoid of personality: a kind of albino of the spirit.) From his childhood fixation on Shirley Temple and Greta Garbo, he sensed the power embodied in celebrities to tap into our fascination with larger-than-life, mass-produced, public images. His work acknowledges a world where reality cannot be distinguished from the images that increasingly constitute and reshape it: soap boxes, soup cans, soft drinks, celebrity photos—the currency of a new order. Although success has made his work so familiar that it seems less daring, early viewers recognized that the impact of Warhol—like the impact of Picasso—was nothing short of revolutionary. "It was as if, in a dark, grey atmosphere, someone had kicked open the door of a blast furnace," recalled an American art critic who in 1965 had attended the first Warhol show in Paris. "The future breathed from the walls like raw ozone." [24] *Marilyn (Three Times)*, we should observe, does not glorify the soft, breathy, vulnerable, blond movie star familiar in Hollywood films. Warhol applies swatches of loud color to the features of a particularly austere photo so as to create a garish, hard, almost virile figure, Monroe as she might appear if played by a maladroit female impersonator. The postmodern world of surfaces and public images is not without perplexities as once stable categories such as gender and sexuality come under pressure from discourses and images ordinarily either suppressed or located at the margins of culture: images (like Warhol's own somewhat ambiguously coded homosexuality) that undermine not only the categories but also, perhaps more important, the stability that such categories formerly seemed to assure. [25]

Postmodern illness is born out of the culture that Warhol captured and shaped so boldly. The changes in our culture have in effect trans-

formed the experience of illness. The power to make us sick or well
inheres not only in microbes and medications but in images and stories. (Powerful images often convey a compressed and nonlinear, if
never entirely graspable, story.) Warhol's Coke bottle is more than an
improbable object for an artist to paint, as opposed to a mountain or
a still life. It is not, strictly speaking, an object, not a material thing.
Nor is it even an image in the sense of visual data received upon the
retina. Once invented and put into circulation, the Coke bottle hovers
above the imperfect realm of matter like the postmodern version of a
Platonic idea. In effect, the form of an ideal Coke bottle gets molded
into chunks of hot glass in factories around the world and delivered
to consumers by an invisible army of engineers, technicians, advertisers, artists, and assembly-line workers. Beyond its flaglike power to
represent an entire country and culture, what proves significant
about the Coke bottle as a postmodern cultural icon is both its omni-
presence (due in part to its status as a masterpiece of commercial design) and its utter nonuniqueness: it stands at the opposite pole from
the original and singular modernist artwork. Every container is
merely one interchangeable unit in an unending identical series. The
image has swallowed up reality until the two become indistinguishable. This is the ambiguous space in which postmodern life (including sickness and health) gets redefined through the play of cultural
images.

The postmodern world that Warhol both shapes and reflects is a
space where we recognize with startling intensity, as if for the first
time, how thoroughly human life gets reconstructed through the
power of culture. The power of culture at its most obvious and reductive level he evokes in a silkscreen filled entirely with images of dol-
lar bills: art, like everything else, is caught up in a consumer economy based on hyperreal images; banknotes—printed images as
money—become the true subject of every painting. In Warhol's art
the traditional opposition between nature and culture has simply
dropped away as cultural forces leave no sanctuary untouched. Culture as it circulates through the popular media has created an unprecedented state in which human biology is now under the mesmer-

izing influence—sometimes the complete control—of the same market forces that bring us Prozac, Nike, Planet Hollywood, and the art of Andy Warhol. Warhol, as an artist at home in this shifty terrain, is a perfect guide to help us recognize the neon crossroads of postmodern illness, where biology meets the mass-produced, mass-marketed images and artifacts of late-capitalist consumer culture. It is a crossroads where illness is redefined through its contact with culture and where culture, in helping to redefine illness, undermines the once firm and traditional Cartesian distinction between illness and disease.

DESTABILIZING DISEASE AND ILLNESS

What doctors mean by *disease* and *illness* is not exactly what patients mean.[26] Contemporary medical textbooks define *disease* as an objectively verified disorder of bodily functions or systems, characterized by a recognizable cause and by an identifiable group of signs and symptoms. *Illness*, by contrast, is used inside medicine to indicate the patient's subjective experience, which may or may not indicate the presence of disease. For example, tests show that many patients with chronic low back pain suffer from lumbar disk disease, but so do 70 percent of people without low back pain. Lumbar disk disease, then, sometimes produces the chronic illness we call low back pain, but many people have the disease without the illness. At this level of analysis, the distinction between disease and illness is useful in preventing confusion. The two concepts have now become so encrusted with additional layers of meaning, however, that they prove not so much useful tools as awkward and antiquated carriers of what are now highly questionable assumptions.

The main assumption underlying the traditional distinction between disease and illness is that knowledge falls into two broad categories, objective and subjective. Every medical student in the United States memorizes this distinction on arrival in medical school. Moreover, in its respect for scientific rigor, medicine gives greatest value to knowledge that can be verified as objective. Thus disease as objective and illness as subjective are categories that convey a powerfully divided sense of worth. What the patient reports is subjective (and untrustworthy), what the lab reports is objective (and true). Numbers are objective (and serious), stories are subjective (and trivial). Doctors are the authorities on disease, while patients remain the more or less unreliable narrators of their own unruly illnesses. The distribution of power within the traditional doctor/patient couple is tellingly one-sided. One knows, the other feels; one prescribes, the other complies; one is paid, the other pays. Although this sharp division has begun to blur under the pressure of postmodern innovations such as the ubiquitous malpractice suit, the old conceptual infrastructure that sustained it is still, confusingly, in place. The distinction between disease and illness, in any case, is not as innocent as it looks.

Perhaps the traditional differences in the understanding of disease and illness are merely a reflection of the truism—which has far-reaching and mostly ignored implications—that doctors and patients view the world from different perspectives. For the patient, illness is always a lived experience, while a patient's report of illness indicates to doctors the likelihood of a medical problem requiring biological explanations of disease.[27] This inescapable degree of separation between doctor and patient must not, however, be interpreted as confirming a rigid split between objective and subjective knowledge. The split between objective and subjective knowledge, while based in common sense, is far from clear. So-called objective statistics and lab reports are meaningful only so far as fallible human beings produce and interpret them, and interpreters differ. As happens too often, accidents occur, tests may be improperly conducted, or doctors receive faulty data. Although doctors like to regard themselves as objective, the objectivity of medicine is a myth fostered as much by patients as by doctors. In practice, as doctors know, anomalies pop up to complicate every norm. Diagnosis and treatment often go forward in the absence of conclusive facts. "Lesions and signs do not always match," Kathryn Montgomery Hunter writes, "nor do signs and test results. Even lesions and test results sometimes may not correspond."[28] Objectivity remains a valued goal, but the daily practice of medicine is shot through with subjective decision making and ambiguous data.

Similar ambiguities undermine the traditional distinction between disease and illness. The recent lively academic discussion concerning definitions of disease, talk that seldom penetrates into the clinic, most often leaves room for nonbiological, extraphysiological, and social circumstances.[29] Borderline cases and changing social attitudes push back the limits of even roomy definitions. We now view alcoholism as a disease, for example, but it is often next to impossible to diagnose individual heavy drinkers with an objectively verified disorder.[30] Is drug addiction a disease? What about chronic pain? Doctors in one clinic will offer a diagnosis of reflex sympathetic dystrophy— continuous post-trauma burning pain in a limb or extremity without significant nerve damage or observable lesions—while doctors in another clinic think the category is a sham.[31] The ambiguous status of Gulf War syndrome (a multisymptomatic affliction of American troops who served in the 1991 war in Iraq) concerns institutional politics as much as science. Patients who suffer from an unverified illness are no less sick than patients whose disease matches the textbook. Sometimes they are worse: not only ill but also frustrated, disabled, worried, out of work, and out of hope. The traditional biomedical distinction between disease and illness, seemingly clear and reasonable, fits imperfectly in a world that is often opaque and irrational, where the logical and the biological often fail to coincide. Its most unfortunate side effect lies in forcing us to employ a language whose assumptions implicitly validate the medical profession and devalue the patient.

The term *postmodern illness* implies a shift, incomplete and ongoing, in which the patient, no longer merely a bundle of symptoms reported by an unreliable, subjective ego, emerges at moments as a valued participant in the medical process of diagnosis and treatment. In this shift *disease* and *illness* also undergo change. While continuing to convey their traditional biomedical meanings, they increasingly carry as a tacit subtext an awareness of how these artificial distinctions

limit understanding and create unnecessary, harmful distance between patients and doctors. We are coming to see that disease and illness are not oppositions rooted in the nature of things, like fire and
ice, but socially constructed categories with somewhat porous and
imperfect application to the array of maladies, disorders, syndromes,
and conditions—some quite new and mysterious—that patients today ask doctors to care for.[32] A study of postmodern illness needs to
acknowledge and explore the changes that destabilize traditional
medical usage in ways commensurate with the changing postmodern
world.

Postmodern illness, as I use the phrase, encompasses both the patient's experience and whatever biological condition initiates or accompanies it. In effect, it conflates two concepts that medicine normally prefers to keep separate. The traditional division between
disease and illness, however, while it makes good sense to a scientist
tracking the AIDS virus under an electron microscope, simply cannot
stand up to the complication of postmodern ailments and understandings. From a postmodern point of view, AIDS is never simply
about the science of a microbe.[33] People infected with the human immunodeficiency virus (HIV) live within cultures that directly affect
their health: cultures marked in the developed world, for example,
by homophobia, government funding, gay rights activists, research
grants, racism, pharmaceutical companies, addicts, and blood transfusions. Outside the lab, microbes follow the terrain of cultural
geopolitics. Life-extending multiple drug therapies available to a U.S.
citizen in San Diego are unavailable—because they cost too much—
to a patient in Port-au-Prince or Kinshasa. HIV was not simply discovered, like a comet, but slowly put together as a legitimate diagnosis through a process of social consensus that included debate among
international laboratories, sometimes stormy annual conferences,
peer-reviewed journals, grant proposals, and the exclusion of contrary views deemed extreme, incorrect, or merely annoying. From a
postmodern perspective, doctors and medical researchers are never
wholly objective, despite even heroic efforts to achieve verifiable results, much as patients are never wholly subjective, despite evidence

that we know the world as filtered through our individual egos. What underlies these changed assumptions, assumptions that desta-bilize a traditional biomedical reading of disease and illness, is a new understanding of culture.

THE CULTURE OF ILLNESS

The language we are learning to speak in the postmodern country of the ill gives a prominent place to the idea of culture. An awareness that both doctor and patient stand within a cultural context is what modifies both the objectivity valued in medicine and the subjectivity native to the patient's experience. Objective judgment, after all, is fi-nally a cultural artifact, not everywhere defined or valued equally— sometimes not even possible, as in the inherently uncertain realm of subatomic physics. Similarly, the sick person is not a mere subjective monad locked within an individual ego, an untrustworthy prisoner of consciousness, but, like physicians, an actor within a widely shared, intersubjective culture. Culture, of course, is always a plural-ized concept: the social basis of health differs widely across groups, nations, and continents.[34] Yet, no matter how rich or plural the possi-ble diversity, a shared, intersubjective culture is what creates the be-havior that sociologist Talcott Parsons identified as "the sick role": a way of being (when we are ill) assigned to us usually without our knowledge.[35] Illnesses, in the manner of sick roles, differ across time and space. Despite presumably identical processes of cell biology, the experience of cancer—including such transpersonal measures as in-cidence and mortality rates—is different on an impoverished reser-vation in Montana than inside the Beverly Hills compounds of the rich and famous.[36] Western nations sharing many basic cultural simi-larities—England, France, Germany, and the United States—reveal distinctive variations in the medical treatment they offer and in how they understand health and sickness.[37] Illness, in short, is never wholly personal, subjective, and idiosyncratic, nor is disease wholly objective, factual, and universal, but both take on their specific, malleable, historical shapes through the mediations of culture. William James, the modernist father of postmodern pragmatist philosophy and the only major American philosopher with a degree in medicine, put it this way: "[h]uman motives sharpen all our questions, human satisfactions lurk in all our answers, all our formulas have a human twist."[38]

The rediscovery of culture might be called a precondition of postmodern thought.[39] Although postmodernism takes almost as doctrine the rejection of claims that knowledge can be grounded in anything like an absolute, essentialist, universal, or (God help us) metaphysical basis for thought, a belief in the importance of culture is as close to providing a foundation as postmodernism is ever likely to come.[40] Beyond disputes about the definition of culture, countless issues are open to debate, including such chicken-and-egg controversies as whether culture is the source of all representations or rather the product of representations. It seems clear that cultural texts and contexts maintain an interaction complex enough to justify Stephen Greenblatt's concept of a "poetics of culture."[41] No one, despite the inevitable arguments, can doubt the impact of culture on everyday life. It shapes us like the force of gravity. In fact, the postmodern era has so vastly extended the domain of culture that it now includes the realm traditionally considered its opposite: nature. You cannot hike into the remotest uninhabited wilderness today without inhaling particles of human civilization. The concept of wilderness is itself a cultural construction, of course. Even wild nature in all its sheer materiality—from floods to mud slides—now reveals the shaping or meddling hand of humankind.

Culture, in its tamer versions, usually takes the tangible shapes created by various interrelated symbol systems, systems that are also cultural creations, like the codes governing Parisian fashion or the choreographed moves of kung fu. Scholars have noted that postmodern culture achieves a certain uniqueness by placing closely together elements borrowed from widely disparate symbol systems, like the Pachelbel D-Minor Canon played behind a television ad for luxury cars. Postmodern culture typically leaps across space and time when, for example, an Anasazi pot is displayed in a Victorian hotel refurbished in contemporary Denver. Its eclectic, rootless style is international, postcolonial, affluent, underwritten by a late-capitalist consumer economy that transforms local markets into connections in a global network. As Jean-François Lyotard observes, "one listens to reggae, watches a western, eats McDonald's food for lunch and local cuisine for dinner, wears Paris perfume in Tokyo and 'retro' clothes in Hong Kong."[42] Not all, however, is affluence and jet-set travel. In contrast to the modernist focus on Europe, postmodernism engages the voices of far-flung and often oppressed groups, from women in the developing world to Chinese political dissidents. African Americans, for example, infuse postmodern culture with fragments of contemporary black experience, such as the persona of the risk-taking, high-flying, impromptu performer: Michael Jordan hanging above the rim, Martin Luther King Jr. marching toward the police lines, the latest hip-hop artist testing the edge.[43] Electronic technologies, meanwhile, connect people and data formerly dispersed and isolated across the globe. Participants in an Internet support group for cancer patients illustrate just one more way in which postmodern culture has changed the experience of illness.[44]

An awareness of the role that culture plays in the experience of illness unavoidably invokes questions and texts lying far outside the ordinary range of medical knowledge. We must explore, for example, not only laboratory data and epidemiological research but also novels, television programs, films, advertising, bodybuilders, and obscenity laws. The disparate texts and activities that represent the domain of culture cannot be off-limits to a study of postmodern illness. The result, from a biomedical point of view, is something close to intellectual chaos: the controlled experiment from hell and "normal science" run amok. From a postmodern point of view, however, it is only by opening the clinic and research laboratory to an increasing number of messy cultural variables that medicine, which is scientific but not strictly speaking a science, will begin to understand what most patients already know or strongly suspect about the changed arena of contemporary illness.

CULTURE, ILLNESS, AND FREEDOM

There is a tendency in current scholarship to understand culture as a kind of oppressive force that leaves individuals no option but to choose among the limited roles that society, coercively, has scripted for them. Teens, for example, have no option but to choose among the culturally scripted roles of smoker or nonsmoker, drug user or nonuser. Their freedom consists only in a particular style of choice, or in a personal navigation between hotly promoted extremes from abstinence to promiscuity. In postmodern culture, we seem to have similarly little choice when we fall ill except to enter (or risk remaining outside) the culture of medicine. Yet, if we leave aside momentarily the medical horror stories of patients steamrollered by incompetent doctors or by callous insurance companies, the degree of personal freedom available seems quite extraordinary when compared with the vision of culture as an oppressive, coercive force that narrows choice to a selection among a few inadequate predetermined scripts. Consider the last months of Anatole Broyard.

Broyard died of prostate cancer in 1990, and in the fourteen months before his death he wrote a series of remarkable meditations that reveal how far he chose to resist and to reformulate the traditional scripts of dying. Writing at age sixty-nine, he had lived through the transition from modern to postmodern, and he fully understood how postmodern medicine had extended the modern redefinition of death. "[T]he real narrative of dying now is that you die in a machine," he wrote. The story of his own dying not only shows how he resisted the mechanized death perfected by postmodern medicine but also explores illness and dying from a point outside the traditions of religious thought. "Once we had a narrative of heaven and hell," he wrote, perhaps alluding to the "grand narratives" that Lyotard contends have lost their credibility in postmodern times, "but now we make our own narratives."[45] Broyard's personal narrative of dying, composed from a point beyond religion and biomedicine, is neither irreligious nor unscientific. He rediscovers the soul as a resource in resisting illness ("Soul is the part of you that you summon up in emergencies" [40]), and he regularly consults doctors, although with a critical and idiosyncratic eye, looking for (but not finding) a specialist who recognizes that doctors too are storytellers (53). Medicine alone, however, will not do. "Technical explanations flatten the story of illness," he writes in his journal (66). In choosing to create his own narrative as opposed to the culturally predetermined biomedical story of organ failure and platelet counts, Broyard takes the path that Arthur W. Frank finds typical and distinctive of the postmodern experience of illness.

As book critic for the *New York Times* and an editor for the *New York Times Book Review*, Broyard is disposed to value the power of narrative. He fills his own story with references to writers (Tolstoy, Philip Roth, Norman Cousins, Oliver Sacks), as if his own illness makes better sense when seen through the lens of books. More is at stake, however, than the habits of a literary man. He emphasizes that narrative contains or releases therapeutic powers. A sick person, he contends, can make a story out of illness as a way of trying "to detoxify it." In seeking to detoxify his own illness, Broyard experiments with inventing "mininarratives" and exploring the resources of metaphor: "I saw my illness as a visit to a disturbed country, rather like contemporary China. I imagined it as a love affair with a demented woman who demanded things I had never done before" (21–22). Not all of us, of course, would take comfort in Broyard's particular metaphors, but his point is that we must each become the authors of our own narratives. No one else's will do. Actual writing is not required: some of the best narratives remain oral. Nor is narrative alone enough. Broyard says that he has begun to take tap dancing lessons as a preparation for writing. Why tap dancing? It's something "I've always wanted to do" (25). This illness is constructed as a story that begins with a rejection of self-denial and with an embrace of desire, no matter how odd or unbecoming. He creates the miniature bildungsroman of a distinctively postmodern self determined to expand rather than shrink under the advance of a life-threatening illness.

"I'm making my own narrative here and now" (42), Broyard insists as he works on an essay titled "The Patient Examines the Doc-

tor." The reversal of roles in his title typifies the reversals that characterize the narrative he creates. The traditional role of the patient emphasizes passivity and suffering. (*Patient*, like *passive*, comes from the
Latin root "to suffer.") Broyard instead wrests comedy from the dark
moment when, finally unhooked from a urethral catheter and able to
urinate again, he sprints from his hospital bed toward the bathroom,
only to fall short, splashing the floor with a mixture of blood and
urine. "Illness is not all tragedy," he observes. "Much of it is funny"
(46). Funny, of course, if your narrative belongs among the mixed
genres that leave room for comedy. The determination lies not in the
events—blood and urine are neither inherently comic nor serious—
but in the narrative perspective through which individuals rewrite
their own illnesses.

The narrative reversals that allow Broyard to find comedy in situations custom-made for pathos or tragedy extend to the portrait of his
literary colleagues hovering over him in solemn vigil. "The way my
friends have rallied around me is wonderful," he begins, setting us
up for the reversal that follows: " . . . all these witty men suddenly
saying pious, inspirational things" (5). It is one of Broyard's most
startling traits that he finds his cancer somehow bracing and even, as
he calls it, intoxicating. Nietzsche famously wrote that what does not
kill us makes us stronger. Broyard knows that his prostate cancer will
kill him—the only question is when—but instead of demoralizing
him it calls forth a blaze of intensified energy. His is a narrative
aware of its own ironies, in which the patient paradoxically experiences the opposite of a decline in his vital powers. "A dangerous illness," Broyard writes, "fills you with adrenaline and makes you feel
very smart" (6).

Impudence is a key concept for Broyard as he constructs his
Blakean narrative of delight as unrestricted energy. (Like Blake, who
associates illness with thwarted or stifled impulses, Broyard says that
a "sick person's best medicine is desire" [63].) He tells the story of a
dying fifteen-year-old boy who asked his father to arrange him on
the hospital bed in an unspecified "impudent" position. "I'd like my

writing to be impudent" (24), Broyard concurs. Sharing the postmodern taste for confession, he does not hesitate to explore both his memories of erotic pleasure and his fears of medically induced impotence. Sexuality has only a minor place, if any, in the biomedical account of illness, but Broyard creates a counternarrative in which health and sex are closely linked. "My urologist, who is quite famous," he begins, in another of his sly openings that set us up for a surprise, "wanted to cut off my testicles. ... " He continues, "[b]ut I felt that this would be losing the battle right at the beginning. Speaking as a surgeon, he said that it was the surest, quickest, neatest solution. Too neat, I said, picturing myself with no balls. I knew that such a solution would depress me, and I was sure that depression is bad medicine" (26). The narrative that Broyard composes is no exercise in wishful thinking or literary distraction. He shapes his medical treatment to the story he constructs of a defiant jester-hero who proceeds through illness with his full power and integrity undiminished.

Broyard's narrative gives shape not only to his own experience but also to the characters around him. He clearly enjoys the superstar status of the handsome, tennis-playing Cambridge urologist he sought out—as a patient, he says he wants a doctor loaded with "magic"— and he also enjoys putting the clipped biomedical account in its subordinate place. The doctor's preference for the surest, quickest, neatest solution does not necessarily create the best story, from a patient's point of view. Broyard's verbal prowess in retelling the vignette about his rescued testicles gives him the upper hand over the fabled urologist, whose "solution" is exposed as therapeutically inept, even if surgically indicated. Broyard draws the phrase "bad medicine" (to describe the depression of being surgically castrated) from the discourse assigned by Hollywood film writers to the backward and patronized Indian, the ignoble savage, but he reverses its spin in order to give an ironic demotion to his superstar white rational urologist, who is implicitly corrected and taken to school by his wild (ballsy) patient. Had the doctor bothered to learn his patient's story he would have known how much an erotic life meant to this sixty-nine-year-old man-of-letters. "When the cancer threatened my sexuality," Broyard observes in yet another reversal, "my mind became immediately erect" (27).

It is appealing to linger over Broyard's self-conscious narrative construction of his illness—illness rewritten as personal liberation—because the details reveal a man who meets death on his own terms. Illness brings out the poet in him, makes him more daring, and accentuates his humor, his insight, his love of life. He writes of critical illness as a great permission or absolution: "All your life you think you have to hold back your craziness," he writes, "but when you're sick you can let it out in all its garish colors" (23). The crucial point is not that illness allows Broyard to explore the intoxicating freedom that he experiences only after the diagnosis of cancer. What matters most—since other patients will have quite different experiences—is his insistence that illness offers the patient an opportunity to employ the full resources of narrative reconstruction. "The patient," he insists, "has to start by treating his illness not as a disaster, an occasion for depression or panic, but as a narrative, a story. Stories are antibodies against illness and pain" (20). The storyteller—according to Arthur W. Frank (another cancer patient who turned his experience into narrative)—is the new figure of the postmodern patient: no longer a victim of disease, not the object of medicine, but a person struggling to recover and to reshape the voice that illness so often takes from us.

Broyard's quirky, courageous, impudent narrative (the description he prefers is "irresponsible" [67]) offers one final insight concerning the stories that characterize postmodern illness. The experience of postmodern illness, no matter how offbeat or even poetically deranged, is always framed by the culture in which it occurs. It is his struggle *against* what he perceives as the dehumanizing pressures of biomedicine that shapes Broyard's story. The freedom of postmodern patients in effect is necessarily limited: defined by an inability to move wholly outside the legacy of modern culture and the primacy it grants to the (scientific) story of medicine. Thus, even in offering us a scandalous and bracing vision of the patient as a narrative free spirit,

Broyard's story defines freedom as the opposite of something that he recognizes in the surrounding biomedical culture as confining, mechanical, and ultimately life denying. Every reversal in his prose and in his behavior is the sign of a need to assert his own story *against* the stories already circulating within the dominant culture. No doubt his ultimate reversal—the pattern underlying every other resistance mobilized in creating his own narrative of illness—lies in a fact we learn from Henry Louis Gates Jr. (chair of the Department of Afro-American Studies at Harvard University). Broyard, according to Gates, was born black and spent his lifetime as a "virtuoso of ambiguity and equivocation" deliberately choosing to pass for white.[46]

We simply do not know what narrative of illness Broyard might have created in a culture less dominated by modern biomedicine, even as we cannot know what life he would have chosen in a culture less divided and structured by racism. Significantly, in Broyard's narrative the biological details of his cancer receive almost no discussion. It is as if to overcome the automatic medical emphasis on illness as strictly an episode in human biology—a matter of cell counts and medications—that he needs to assert almost an opposite conviction: what really matters about his cancer is its disconnection from mere biological events. The cancer of Anatole Broyard will take whatever significance he chooses to give it. "Any meaning of illness," he insists in opposition to a purely scientific and biological view, "is better than none" (65). Narrative, of course, is among the most common and most powerful instruments we possess to confer meaning upon experience.[47] In creating a personal account of illness in which biology figures only by indirection as a noticeable absence or visibly repressed power, like a parent excluded from a wedding, Broyard undertakes to rewrite the narrative that medicine would impose on him. His aim, he says, is to transform his illness into a "mere character" in his own intellectual and spiritual autobiography (62). It is an impossible, heroic task—illness, like race, always escapes our individual control—but Broyard's struggle against the limits of biomedicine aptly illustrates the paradoxes, promise, and imperfect solutions that go to make up postmodern illness.

chapter two

What Is Postmodern Illness?

So long as we feel well, we do not exist. More

exactly: we do not know that we exist.

E. M. CIORAN,
The Fall into Time (1964)

The search for postmodern illness begins with a curious fact: almost every era seems marked by a distinctive illness that defines or deeply influences it. Although nearly vanished today, bubonic plague dominated the Middle Ages, constituting not only a horribly painful death but also a social catastrophe comparable to the havoc of World War II. Some twenty-five million people, one-fourth the population of Europe, perished between 1346 and 1350 in the Black Plague. A disaster so widespread turns even the survivors into victims. Carts piled high with corpses rumbled through the streets. Macabre images of death—worm-eaten flesh, dancing skeletons, eyeless skulls—decorated taverns and churchyards, overflowing even into the margins of hand-copied books. In Provence, Catalonia, Aragon, Switzerland, southern Germany, and the Rhineland, Jews were murdered and their houses burned by Christians fearful that Jews had brought on the plague by poisoning wells and springs.[1] People lived in dread of the fatal symptoms. Any passing headache or chill might foretell the swift transition to vomiting, giddiness, delirium, diarrhea, burning fever, and the telltale, deadly, swollen lymphatic knots in the groin and armpits that Boccaccio described being as large as eggs. In the case of bubonic plague, illness was far more than a passing threat: all the familiar landmarks of human life in fourteenth-century Europe, from piety to promiscuity, altered because of the presence and fear of the Black Plague. What illness, if any, helps give the postmodern era its particular character?

Comparison of illness in the postmodern era with illness in the preceding fifty years highlights some clear differences.[2] Illness in 1900, for example, was much more likely to kill. At the beginning of the century, about 28 people per 1,000 died each year in the United States, but the death rate began to decline markedly in the 1960s and is now around 10 people per 100,000.[3] The causes of death differ too. Adults in the modern era died of pneumonia, influenza, tuberculosis, typhoid fever, and dysentery; today adults die from cancer, heart disease, and stroke. The infectious diseases that (before the clinical introduction of penicillin in 1944) terrified patients in the modern era have been replaced in the postmodern era by chronic, gradually debilitating illnesses such as arthritis, diabetes, and multiple sclerosis. The explanations for such changes are not always clear.

Historian Thomas McKeown, in a painstaking study of the history of disease since the time of the prehuman Australopithecus, came to the conclusion that the most common causes of sickness and death in every era are determined by "the prevailing conditions of life."[4] The vast changes in living conditions that occurred as masses of displaced rural poor crowded into cities, for example, determined the common causes of illness during the Industrial Revolution. Certainly improvements in sanitation, in nutrition, and in the general standard of living did as much as antibiotics to influence the course of illness during the modern period, and McKeown's research suggests that the changing conditions of postmodern life will shape contemporary illness. Indeed, the changes in postmodern illness are as distinctive as the changes in postmodern life and warfare that left hundreds of oil wells ablaze after the Persian Gulf War. (The fires were fueled not just by oil but by the hugely expanded Western appetite for fossil fuels.) Increased affluence and longevity in the developed world have confronted nations with a growing host of so-called lifestyle illnesses associated with high-fat diets, cigarette smoke, stressful jobs, disintegrating families, and a couch-potato mentality. The workplace has become for many people a building that hermetically seals in recycled air containing petrochemical residues from furnishings and supplies. We live amid electronic appliances, spend four hours a day watching television, and eat meat produced on industrial farms where animals never see the sun. The prevailing conditions of postmodern life have changed significantly in ways that might well affect human health. Still, while we can identify with confidence some broad changes in the conditions of life across the twentieth century, such differences constitute merely a starting point in the search for postmodern illness.

HISTORY AND THE SILENCE OF THE ORGANS

Illness always seems to tell us more about a person or an era than health does, although it is not clear why. French surgeon René Leriche wrote in 1936 that health is "life lived in the silence of the organs."[5] Perhaps a well-being so complete wholly escapes attention. In contrast to illness, health runs the risk of appearing inherently shallow: a mute version of the unexamined life. Once the organs break their silence, we experience both our bodies and our world anew, in the manner of Adam and Eve abruptly cast out from paradise. Now, because our muscles ache, we are conscious of the effort required to walk and sit up, just as a broken bone suddenly reminds us that arms and legs employ an inner architecture of calcified connective tissue. Illness contains the same power that medieval theologians attributed to evil in precipitating a fall from timelessness into time. Illness forces us to leave the world where bodies are almost innocent of the need to seek assistance. As German philosopher Hans-Georg Gadamer puts it, illness is always "a social state of affairs."[6]

As a social state of affairs, illness involves not only the hospitals and doctors from whom we seek assistance but also cultural practices and shared meanings. Bubonic plague, for example, depends on a bacterium carried by a flea that is carried by a rat.[7] The spread of bubonic plague thus owes much to altered urban living conditions in the Middle Ages that brought rats and people into closer contact, as well as to the development of the medieval shipping industry that sent rat-infested vessels on a circuit from Constantinople to Italy and northern Europe. Moreover, the infected patient presented far more than a medical problem. All afflictions, according to medieval doctrine, came from God and were subject to various religious interpretations—as punishments for sin, trials of faith, or even, paradoxically, signs of divine favor. Thus the plague-crazed flagellants who whipped themselves through the streets in atonement offered a spectacle as rich in spiritual meaning as any medieval morality play performed on the cathedral steps. They gave a flesh-and-blood embodiment to the dominant values of their time and (like the medieval lepers wearing bells and confined to colonies outside the city) stood as monuments to the power of illness to define an entire era.

Subsequent eras highlight different illnesses, but the power of certain maladies to mark an entire era proves remarkably constant. In the Renaissance, with plague reduced to an intermittent threat, doctors witnessed the rise of a new epidemic illness that went by the somewhat misleading name of *melancholy*. This affliction was no pleasing Keatsian opiate but a stupefying total lethargy akin to derangement—suicidal madness, as Dürer depicted it—doubtless something similar to the disease we call depression. Melancholy had long been recognized within Galenic medicine as a basic human character type, caused by a dominance of the bodily humor called bile, and it was often attributed, in astrological thinking, to the ascendancy of the planet Saturn. The melancholic character was not ill but merely somber, although people born under the sign of Saturn supposedly inherited artistic gifts and even genius that might at times turn dangerous. It was only in the Renaissance that melancholy suddenly intensified its threat. An entire era (not just individuals born under the wrong planet) seemed at risk from, even redefined by, their new relation to illness.

Any explanation for such shifting patterns demands an awareness that illness is a social state, open to historical change. Thus several hundred years after the rise of melancholy in the Renaissance, the Enlightenment highlighted two very different illnesses, syphilis and gout, which also had long histories. Syphilis had afflicted Europeans at least since the time of Columbus, and gout is an ancient variety of congenital arthritis.[8] Enlightenment culture in effect transformed these two venerable afflictions into powerful contemporary signs within the emerging system of middle-class values. Doctors and moralists (often indistinguishable) linked gout directly to the dissipated lifestyles of the aristocracy, while syphilis did double duty in its association with both aristocratic immorality and urban poverty. In Ben Franklin's frugal new world of virtue and godly toil, syphilis and gout were more than biological conditions; they were markers of a rejected social order.

Changing times, with their altered living conditions, thrust new maladies into prominence. Nineteenth-century Europe was haunted by tuberculosis. Although an ancient affliction, it took on the features of this new historical era, in which sufferers were associated with values and anxieties specific to nineteenth-century culture. The familiar symptoms of pale skin, hectic flush, emaciated limbs, and wracking cough coincided with the stereotypical characteristics of artists, waifs, bohemians, and assorted romantic spirits, many of whom, like Keats and Chopin, died of TB. Its wasting symptoms slowly pared away the flesh (hence the popular name "consumption"), seeming to leave behind pure spirit, in effect confirming Romantic convictions that suffering refined the soul. TB effectively relaunched the Christian myth of illness as a spiritual force. Nineteenth-century writers who died of the disease (including Charlotte Brontë, Robert Louis Stevenson, Elizabeth Barrett Browning, Balzac, Chekov, and De

Quincey) leave no doubt why the public associated TB with creativity and the artistic temperament. Frail, expiring heroines—Marguerite in *Camille* (1852), Violetta in *La Traviata* (1853), Mimi in *La Bohème* (1897)—heightened the romantic aura of the disease by linking TB with the Keatsian triad of beauty, death, and hopeless love.[9] The commonness of TB as it spread across Europe and America soon added an opposite imagery: it changed from being an affliction of artists and poets into a disease of middle-class burghers drained by commerce and bourgeois tedium. Tuberculosis was, in short, a lifestyle, a parable, a theater of illness complete with tacit rules, recurrent images, and complex social meanings that came to dominate the imagination of an entire century.

The astonishing rise of biomedical research beginning in the mid–nineteenth century served to explode numerous myths surrounding illness, as when Robert Koch in 1882 announced that he had isolated the tubercle bacillus, making the cause and course of TB a matter of scientific record. When Nobel Prize–winner Selman A. Waksman demonstrated in 1943 that the once fatal bacillus could be eradicated with streptomycin, any lingering cultural mythology surrounding TB quickly vanished. The power of TB to convey elaborate social meanings declined in tandem with the rapid decline in cases worldwide, exposing the once fearful killer as just another infectious illness treatable with antibiotics. With tuberculosis declining and deprived of mythic force, another ancient and poorly understood illness, a new focus for public fear, emerged as if to take its place, expressing the values and anxieties of yet another distinctive historical period. Almost simultaneously with the decline of TB, cancer arose as the most feared killer—the representative or distinctive illness—of the modern era.

Like TB, cancer also generated a potent cultural mythology. As Susan Sontag has shown in her brilliant study *Illness as Metaphor* (1978), the cultural images and ideas surrounding cancer developed, oddly, almost a reverse version of the cultural myths earlier associated with TB. The distinctive mythic and metaphoric force attributed to cancer seemed in part directed by anatomy. That TB attacked the lungs over

90 percent of the time enhanced its associations with breath, spirit, and soul. Cancer, by contrast, locates fleshy tumors almost any-where—not only in the lungs but also in the most stolid strongholds of matter: bones, blood, stomach, ovaries, prostate, pancreas. Its metastatic spread to other organs and tissues gives it the ominous, sci-fi power to take over an entire body. In taking over the body and in filling it with tumors, cancer, as Sontag observed, seemed to force out spirit, transforming the patient into a being who—in direct op-position to the mythology of TB—is all flesh. Patients suffering from cancer in the modern era ran (and still run) a risk of feeling implicitly de-spiritualized, reduced by their disease to mere matter, at the mercy of renegade cells reproducing nonstop like a runaway produc-tion line. In a process that biomedicine only augments with its focus on cells and organs, the tumor in effect replaces the person, the per-son in effect becomes the tumor. It is just such a process of biomedical reduction that Anatole Broyard sought to limit and oppose with his impudent narrative of erotic intoxication, transforming his cancer into the occasion for an almost poetic and romantic rediscovery of the spirit.

Plague, melancholy, gout, syphilis, tuberculosis, and cancer are not the only illnesses that possess the power to define or represent an entire era, but there is no need to proceed further. Here they serve to frame the questions at the heart of this book. What is distinctive about illness today? How does illness in the postmodern era differ from illness as it was understood and experienced in the recent past? Which particular malady now constitutes the distinctive postmodern illness?

IN SEARCH OF POSTMODERN ILLNESS

A search for the distinctive or representative postmodern illness quickly turns up a number of fascinating candidates. Even long shots can, on reflection, stake quite reasonable claims. Multiple personality disorder (MPD), while known for several centuries, reemerged as a celebrated disorder only after 1970. Although a statistically rare and disputed diagnosis, it seems a perfect metaphor to describe our stressed-out era in which the self—reduced by some theorists to a babble of competing discourses—is pulled in a dozen directions by the various pressures and options of postmodern life.[10] Any serious illness threatens to break down or alter identities, which must then be reclaimed and reframed, but the postmodern self (notoriously many-sided, contradictory, inconsistent) seems especially vulnerable to illness and its power of fragmentation. Only in the postmodern era have we begun to appreciate the threat to selfhood posed by Alzheimer's disease as it gradually erases the patient's personality and personal history—leaving behind what or whom? Alzheimer's disease erodes the self while MPD dramatically splinters it, but in both cases the focus of damage is less the body than the person.

Clinicians often explain multiple personality disorder by invoking the psychological process of dissociation, in which extreme trauma initiates a split in the personality, as if survival required the invention of an alternative self to whom the trauma occurred. In its more philosophical dimensions, MPD revives enduring questions about how our human identity depends upon our memories of our own past, without which we cannot know who we are.[11] An illness as traumatic as MPD—splitting, multiplying, and dissociating the self—lends nostalgic charm to the modernist cliché of an adolescent or midlife crisis, which implies selves homogeneous and solid enough to suffer breakdown, selves unlike the pliant, wispy postmodern men and women in the novels of Ann Tyler, who do not so much fall apart in the face of trauma as simply drift on. An everyday postmodern self, unlike the modernist self-made man or the Jazz Age flapper all brass and style, resembles nothing so much as a slowly rising column of cigarette smoke.

We can say securely that MPD is not the representative postmodern illness. It remains on the fringes of public awareness, less terrifying than sad and uncommon, thrust into the headlines at intervals by bizarre courtroom dramas.[12] Elaine Showalter, professor of English at Princeton University, goes so far as to argue that MPD is a media-driven current version of nineteenth-century hysteria.[13] Her argument, while controversial, introduces an important point. Postmodern illness often involves a crucial element of ambiguity about whether the disorder really exists.

This ambiguity, extending from the causes to the very existence of certain postmodern illnesses, is central to the experience of chronic fatigue syndrome (CFS), another of Showalter's prime contemporary hysterias. Although the clinical evidence about CFS remains inconclusive, patients report symptoms so varying and so hard to link with an organic cause that some doctors—privately if not openly—see the disorder as belonging to the long history of psychosomatic illnesses, like another long-exploded nineteenth-century diagnosis called "spinal irritation." Lining up on the opposite side are advocates for patients suffering from CFS and doctors both with and without a special interest in its treatment.[14] The facts remain murky. So too with Gulf War syndrome. Five years after the 1991 Persian Gulf War against Iraq, some 5,000 to 80,000 veterans (from a total force numbering 700,000) remain ill with vague symptoms that so far "defy diagnosis." Did they contract delayed chronic illnesses from exposure to unknown microbes or to a variety of known and suspected toxins?[15] Or are their symptoms, while undoubtedly real and troubling, due (as Showalter believes) to hysteria and war neurosis? Again the advocates square off in an unsettled debate. Among similarly contested current diagnoses we should also count multiple chemical sensitivity, attention deficit disorder, and male menopause. A limbo of uncertainty, in short, awaits the numerous patients who suffer from conditions that puzzle mainstream biomedicine, and such uncertainty—amplified by the popular media in their zeal for debate—is central to the experience of postmodern illness.[16]

When such disputed conditions eventually emerge from limbo, either confirmed or debunked according to the standards of biomedical science, another one seems to pop up and take its place. For Showalter, this uncanny quality of popping up on cue illustrates the emotional, media-driven basis of what she calls contemporary "hysterias." With logic equal to Showalter's, however, we might see the

procession of strange and novel illnesses as related to the unprecedented "technological upheaval" of the contemporary world (including the steady fallout of additives, synthetics, and petrochemical
fogs) to which historian Mirko D. Grmek attributes the emergence of
AIDS.[17] In effect, specific postmodern illnesses come and go, but the
ambiguity and uncertainty remain.

AIDS is in many ways a mirror of postmodern uncertainties.[18]
There is, most important, no cure. The human immunodeficiency
virus (HIV) that causes AIDS has a long latency period, symptoms
vary, function is unpredictable, and experimental therapies abound.
Its once irreversible power to kill (now slowed by drugs) and its association with changing sexual behavior and gender roles give it a
prime claim as the master illness of our time.[19] Grmek argues that an
epidemic such as AIDS could not have occurred before the mingling
of races, before the liberalization of sexual mores, and, above all, before medicine had controlled serious infectious diseases and introduced both intravenous injections and blood transfusions: in short,
before the postmodern era.[20] Even the AIDS Memorial Quilt expresses a distinctive sensibility. (Now immense and still growing, it
defies the concept of a finished artwork and is impossible to experience in a single viewing: we do not so much view it as move within
it.) Unknown before 1980, AIDS certainly has a chronological claim
as postmodern. It has already killed over eight million people worldwide, and thirty million people are infected with HIV.[21] Moreover,
AIDS is the main cause of death in the United States among adults
between the ages of twenty-four and forty-four, making it the most
potent epidemic since the modernist outbreak of poliomyelitis, which
reached its peak in the United States between 1942 and 1953. Vaccines produced by Jonas E. Salk and Albert B. Sabin put an end to polio, but there is no vaccine against AIDS. The most effective current
treatment consists of expensive multiple drug therapies that at best
promise to transform HIV into a chronic fatal disease whose sufferers
survive up to several decades.

AIDS could be called, in good postmodern style, a metadisease: instead of attacking a specific organ it attacks the immune system re-

sponsible for protecting us from multiple illnesses. Not only is it a
new disease but it reflects a way of thinking about disease unknown
before the mid–twentieth century (as Grmek says, it is "not a disease
in the old sense").[22] Eerily, the period famous for inventing systems
thinking in electronics and communications now finds itself vulnerable to an infectious disease that attacks a crucial and complex human
system, while the transmission of AIDS by semen and blood—fluids
strongly associated with sexual activity and IV drug abuse—marks a
chilling turn in the 1960s sex-and-drug revolution so important to
postmodern self-exploration. Yet, despite its social significance and
its devastating impact, especially in the gay community, AIDS causes
far fewer deaths each year than either cancer, stroke, or heart disease.
Its greatest threat presently lies in the developing nations—above all,
in east Asia and in central and East Africa. The continuous recent attention to AIDS in the developed world (directly related to current
political, social, and economic pressures) may greatly exaggerate
dangers that the disease poses to people who live outside specific urban coastal centers and who avoid high-risk behaviors. There are
other strong candidates, moreover, for the role of distinctive postmodern illness.

Statisticians remind us that today the number one killer of adults
in Western industrial nations is heart disease. Despite all our biomedical progress, we now die most often because our hearts give out.
There are complicated reasons for the prevalence of heart disease. We
live longer, putting increased strain on the heart. Research has wiped
out many infectious diseases that used to kill people before their
hearts did. High-fat diets have clogged our arteries with heart-
damaging cholesterol. It is doubtless sheer coincidence that the rise
of coronary disease also coincides with the postmodern emphasis on
corporate downsizing, welfare cutbacks, and Me-Generation pursuits
of personal wealth that make a "good heart" seem old-fashioned. Yet,
heart disease is certainly one price we pay for overbusy and affluent
lives in which only 20 percent of the adult population gets sufficient
daily exercise. As undeniably the most lethal illness facing adults in
the West, heart disease stands as one prominent measure of what

postmodern civilization, for all its doctors and high-tech labs, cannot overcome.

Meanwhile, one result of the women's movement—another unmistakable sign of the times—is a new emphasis on illnesses, such as osteoporosis and breast cancer, that especially affect women. *The Harvard Guide to Women's Health* (1996) is representative of many publications that address a medical subject in effect reinvented in the postmodern era.[23] Formerly neglected within a patriarchal health care system in which most doctors were male, women's illnesses have begun to claim increased attention that parallels a new social and political emphasis on equal rights. (Entering classes of medical students now enroll about equal numbers of males and females.) We hear more daily about illnesses such as anorexia for which women are the main or exclusive population at risk. Doctors meanwhile have begun to recognize the high risk that women face for conditions such as heart disease that were previously regarded as afflicting mostly men. Certainly, the rapid entry of women into the workforce—nearly three-quarters of all women in the United States work outside the home—marks a huge difference between modern and postmodern life, and no doubt the added burden on many women (who hold full-time jobs as well as shouldering the bulk of housework and child-rearing duties) helps explain their special risk for conditions ranging from malnutrition to chronic pain. Women's afflictions remain so diverse and ill-defined, however, that they prove hard to consolidate into a tangible candidate for distinctive postmodern illness. The recent increase in medical attention, while promising, is not yet enough to overcome centuries of neglect.

Depression, by contrast, seems an obvious candidate for defining postmodern illness, and many people are unaware that women prove twice as likely as men to suffer from depression. One in four women will undergo a serious clinical depression in her lifetime, and 70 percent of all antidepressants are prescribed for women. Yet, depression strikes across a wide and perhaps underreported segment of postmodern society, including children and the elderly. Major depression in the United States occurs in some 2 percent to 4 percent of the community, in 5 percent to 10 percent of primary care patients, and in 10 percent to 14 percent of medical inpatients.[24] Its stature in contemporary life is reflected in the best-seller by psychiatrist Peter D. Kramer, *Listening to Prozac* (1993), which takes its title from the new antidepressive drug (a selective serotonin-reuptake inhibitor) that has replaced tranquilizers in the mythology of popular medication. Whatever else it entails, depression involves a biochemical imbalance in the brain. That it also runs in families suggests a susceptibility scripted in the genes. Yet this complex disorder with a likely genetic component is peculiarly prevalent in the late twentieth century—eleven million cases annually in the United States alone—and seemingly responsive (if only in what triggers it) to the surrounding culture. People born since 1960 face three to ten times greater risk of depression than their grandparents did, and the average age of onset has steadily dropped from the early thirties to the early twenties.[25] Depression might be imagined as the reverse of everything our culture admires: it cancels our romance with speed, reducing the sufferer to a near comatose immobility, creating a pleasureless, profitless gloom that drags down anything lighthearted or joyous. It is as if in a single illness the frantic do-it-all, have-it-all lifestyle of postmodernism crashes to a halt.

Dr. Kramer's decision to name his best-seller after a popular drug used to treat depression introduces us to another postmodern trend. People have long been fascinated by their own illnesses, but illness has recently emerged from the obscurity of medical treatises and private diaries to acquire something like celebrity status. The commerce between illness and celebrity passes in two directions. Specific diseases (like AIDS) achieve almost independent fame, which they impart by proxy to various little-known sufferers, while famous celebrities deliberately associate themselves with specific diseases as spokespersons or fund-raisers. Disease and fame seem somehow mutually contagious. Each year a cluster of illnesses and disorders, from muscular dystrophy to multiple sclerosis, reclaims its annual allotment of TV time, promoted (the term is not too harsh) by well-meaning movie stars and athletes. Hardly any major disease these days goes without its telethon, marathon, benefit, banquet, or street fair. One retired baseball player advertised ointment for hemorrhoids—confirming the unspoken rule of postmodern confession that nothing is unmentionable. (A nonfiction memoir of childhood incest with her father currently puts one recent author atop the *New York Times* book list.) Dyslexia, aphasia, and autism burst into prominence attached to the autobiographical tales of entertainers, actors, and assorted media bigwigs. Alcoholism and drug addiction, often glamorized by Hollywood in films and in private life, have recently become vehicles for ghostwritten books by fading stars, hyped by the same publicity firms that manage their careers.

Celebrities are not alone in the postmodern authorship of illness. Memoirs about living with illness are a hot property, and a new subgenre has emerged (so-called pathographies) in which ordinary people describe their illnesses with an ardor that previous generations reserved for love and war.[26] Writers such as William Styron and Reynolds Price transform these autobiographies of illness into powerful contemporary documents, while in lesser hands the enterprise may be therapeutic or even lifesaving, as the ill write their way to a new self-understanding. In any case the subgenre lends specific illnesses both wider understanding and new prominence. Public awareness changed decisively, for example, when former president Ronald Reagan announced that he suffered from Alzheimer's disease: his announcement generated an answering chorus of talk shows, dramas, and TV documentaries. The demographics of a rapidly graying U.S. population mean that we will hear far more than in the past about illnesses of advancing age, from prostate cancer to senile dementia. New candidates for representative postmodern illness are even now waiting in the wings.

The most common contemporary medical problem—and hence a serious issue in any discussion of postmodern illness—is pain. One prominent researcher went so far as to describe it as "the greatest health problem of our age."[27] Most people regard pain as a symptom, not an illness, and thus it constitutes a crucial redirection of postmodern thought that doctors now treat chronic pain less as a symptom than as a diagnosis. Over one thousand pain clinics have opened in U.S. cities since the 1960s. Depending on definitions and on the population studied, each year anywhere between 7 and 56 percent of Americans suffer from back pain alone.[28] Migraines, toothaches, tendonitis, and irritable bowel syndrome are just a few of the pains for which patients seek medical help. Indeed, pain is the most common symptom that brings patients to doctors, and pain relief is big business for drug companies and advertisers. You cannot get through the nightly news without seeing a commercial for analgesics. (In the advertising business these commercials even have their own insider name: piggy-spots.) It could be argued that what really distinguishes the postmodern era is our obsession with pain. Or, perhaps obsession is the malady that best characterizes the postmodern era of fan clubs, collectors, sex addicts, workaholics, and stalkers.

The search for a defining or representative postmodern illness, in short, quickly encounters an overabundance of candidates. The source of such abundance may lie finally in our cultural fixation on health. People in every era, of course, have sought remedies for what ails them, from Roman baths to Chinese herbs. Yet never before have average citizens been at the mercy of electronic media desperate to fill airtime with the latest medical information; never have people faced the daily deluge of health-related advertising subsidized by hospitals, insurance carriers, and huge international pharmaceutical companies. Every major newspaper hires a health reporter. Each new issue of *Nature, Science,* and the *New England Journal of Medicine* gets prereleased to TV networks that scan it for breaking stories on health, no matter how small the study or how preliminary the data. It is tempting, if ultimately erroneous, to identify the distinctive postmodern illness as a culturewide hypochondria that takes the form of health worship. In upper-income brackets, the pursuit of fitness—often a quest to keep age and illness at bay—has all but replaced concern for religious salvation. In an ironic turn, the quest seems to generate ever new ailments, from tennis elbow to runner's knee.

Unfortunately, the threats to health are real and hard to avoid: allergies among health care workers from latex gloves, incurable asbestosis among custodial workers from school and office heating systems, hepatitis B among teenagers frequenting amateur tattoo studios.[29] Who can forget mad cow disease? Indeed, illness has become a quasi-public performance played out before an audience of support groups, e-mail lists, and paramedical legions. Michel Foucault described sexuality (long associated with health and increasingly medicalized in the postmodern world) not through analyzing behavior but by analyzing what, in different eras, we say and cannot say about sex.[30] Like sexuality, health and illness today are wrapped up in new ways of talking and writing—a discourse that extends far beyond doctors and patients to include alternative healers, personal trainers, eastern mystics, organic farmers, wellness counselors, acupuncturists, nutritionists, and music thanatologists, among others. Whatever else it includes, postmodern illness is the immersion in a unique, extensive, and almost inescapable domain of language. If you do not speak the lingo, it resembles an incomprehensible jabber.

The abundance of candidates might suggest that what proves truly distinctive about the postmodern age is the *absence* of a defining or representative illness. *Lack*, a favorite postmodern term, is what we find wherever we turn: a plenitude of emptiness. The paradox of lack, while inviting as an intellectual exploration, simply cannot withstand such granite presences as depression, heart disease, drug addiction, breast cancer, and AIDS. Doubtless, the abundant varieties of contemporary illness can leave us feeling overwhelmed: some call it the disease-of-the-month syndrome. The media-driven proliferation of illnesses, however, assumes significance only in the context of wider cultural changes. Health care now accounts for one-eighth of the gross national product of the United States, so that illness seems to proliferate in a direct ratio to the percentage of national wealth spent on resisting it. Perhaps the more we are willing to spend as a culture on well-being, the more illness we will uncover. Medical insurance systems that focus on treating symptoms—rather than on promoting health—may finally create a kind of inadvertent sorcerer's apprentice effect: the faster they try to sweep away the evidence of illness, the longer and faster they must keep on sweeping.

BODIES, SPIRITS, AND MACHINES

It is an axiom of postmodern life that, just as each new subgroup spawns its own magazine, every fresh idea generates a conference, and every conference generates a follow-up conference. Sometimes, for variety, they are called symposiums. In the era of duplicate knowledge, almost no academic discipline outside medicine has managed to avoid holding a conference on the body. (Medicine, which has turned conferences into a mixture of education, tax break, and publicity machine, deals not with the body as a cultural and theoretical category but only with actual bodies.) There is good reason to be skeptical. Thus, a crescendo of disbelief should have greeted recent flyers announcing that the University of New Mexico School of Medicine would host a two-day conference in Albuquerque on the topic "spirituality in health care." Even the organizers expected only a small audience. Astonished, they had to turn away applicants when registrations hit eight hundred and were still rising. An understanding of postmodern illness has to include whatever it was that was going on in Albuquerque.

An interest in the spiritual dimensions of healing represents an important trend within postmodern culture. Healing, in this case, is a process distinct from cure, in the sense that people can gain a sense of peace and wholeness even in the grip of incurable disease. Wholeness is a key concept. The words *health* and *healing* both come from the Old English term *hal* (whole): the *wassail* preserved in Christmas carols derives from the Middle English toast *waes hoeil* (be well) drunk at Christmastide from the wine-filled wassail bowl. Health, healing, wholeness, and wellness thus are knit together in an ancient unity that holds great appeal for postmodern proponents of alternative or complementary medicine. Individuals and even corporations now promote the pursuit of this new goal called wellness—not just good health, which may be a stroke of luck, but a lifestyle attentive to diet and exercise, programmed for maximum, interconnected mental, physical, and spiritual satisfaction.[31] Journalist Bill Moyers investigates contemporary trends—almost any topic he touches, once Moyerized, enters instantly into the mainstream—and it constitutes a cultural landmark that in 1993 he aired a popular television series about health (accompanied by the inevitable coffee table book) with the title *Healing and the Mind*. The last two interviews in the book, which accurately reflect the focus of the entire broadcast, are titled "Healing" and "Wholeness."[32] Illness in the postmodern age is understood as fragmentation, and what we seek from the process of healing is to be made whole.

The New Mexico conference on spirituality offered a forum for discussing how healing and wholeness involve far more than medications. Speakers included national figures such as physicians Dean Ornish and Larry Dossey. Ornish has done pioneering work in combining meditation, stress-reduction exercises, group therapy, walking, and a vegetarian diet to reverse serious heart disease, while Dossey is best known for books on the health benefits of prayer. Such nontraditional topics, although unusual in medical education, now command a growing academic audience. Two years before the conference an interdisciplinary group at Harvard University—studying relations among mind, brain, and behavior—held an invitational workshop on the topic of placebos.[33] The placebo effect, an unpopular topic within medicine, refers to the benefit of medically inert substances such as sugar pills in relieving pain and other symptoms. Even a white coat or other medical insignia can trigger the placebo effect. Although the percentage of people who respond to placebos varies from zero to one hundred percent depending on circumstances, there is no doubt placebos work: they can even grow hair.[34] Ultimately, the placebo effect—while it can be reproduced in laboratory animals through classical behaviorist conditioning—depends in humans on the power of belief to initiate biological processes. When patients believe that it is medically effective, a sugar pill can relieve pain as effectively as morphine. Prayer might be described as belief multiplied by infinity, and thus (in some circumstances and for some people) it ought to contain a power at least as useful as the placebo for alleviating symptoms and improving health. Traditional biomedicine has little to say on prayer and placebos, and the New Mexico conference on spirituality stood so far outside the mainstream that—despite official ties to the School of Medicine—it took place only through vigorous efforts from the relatively unthreatening and marginal Office of Continuing Medical Education.

The conference was not about postmodernism: it *was* postmodern. As such, it had little interest in origins, but participants might have liked to know that the English words *health, healing,* and *wholeness* all ultimately derive from a Sanskrit root (*kevalin*) that refers to "a soul freed from matter."[35] In medieval Christian theology, the Latin word for *salvation* is *salus*, which means "health." Health in Native American culture always involves a right relationship with the spirit world. Chinese healers invoke the invisible flow of energy (*chi*) through bodily meridians in a process that the mind adjusts by means of disciplines such as t'ai chi. Only under the influence of positivist science during the nineteenth century were mind, soul, and spirit dissociated from matters of human health and illness. So secular or literal is biomedicine today that the single entry for *healing* in the huge database known as Index Medicus refers to "wound closure." It is easy to argue, nostalgically, that we have lost something once considered valuable. But are minds and spirits still of value to medicine? Few people in the New Mexico audience were prepared to hear Robert G. Jahn, dean emeritus of the School of Engineering and Applied Science at Princeton University, explain what he had found.

Robert Jahn was the star of the conference, according to one physician who described the impact of his talk. What Jahn described was the work he oversees as director of the Princeton Engineering Anomalies Research (PEAR) program. PEAR was established in 1979 with the sole purpose of bringing rigorous scientific study to the interaction of human consciousness with "random physical processes"—or, simply put, the influence of the mind on machines. Operators sit in front of machines that have been equipped with numerous fail-safe features to guarantee the impossibility of human tampering. During a seventeen-year period, in fifty million experimental trials, over one hundred different operators sat in front of the machines using their own personal strategies in an effort to influence the randomized strings of information that the machines are programmed to create. The unavoidable conclusion of Jahn's research? Human consciousness can alter the mechanical output of information. The influence of mind extends not just to bodies—much as stress can alter the immune response—but even to the operation of machines.

How this happens is a matter for conjecture. Jahn proposes that the human operator and the machine come to constitute a single interactive system. In a single interactive system, what he calls a "resonant bond" develops that will introduce order into otherwise random physical processes and thus create results markedly different from results produced by an isolated machine. What especially fascinates Jahn in all this weird science is its implication for human health, as the bond that he conjectures between mind and machine seems a likely model for the demonstrable bond between mind and body. As he puts it: "Through an amazing array of hard-wired, soft-wired, and—in all likelihood—wireless connectors and activators, the mind and body have elaborate options for guiding, protecting, and providing for each other to the higher welfare of the whole."[36] Jahn's research does not mean that you can stop a speeding locomotive with your mind, but it helps to make sense out of apparent anomalies like the placebo effect and acupuncture. What most impressed the physician who called him the star of the conference was that these startling claims for the power of mind came not from a mystic New Age oracle but from a respected Princeton professor of aerospace sciences. He seemed to have the facts.

Postmodernism is relentlessly interdisciplinary, and the knowledge gained from collaborations among disparate fields of study is changing how we think about mind, body, emotion, health, and illness. Evidence such as Jahn's disconcerting research has led to various private and public avenues of support for the new subfield known as complementary or alternative medicine. The once arcane subfield has grown prominent enough recently in the United States to merit a formal address at the National Institutes of Health—the Office of Alternative Medicine, established in 1992.[37] Here researchers receive help as they pursue a variety of nontraditional approaches to illness and health, from acupuncture and macrobiotic diet to visual imaging, therapeutic touch, and the manipulation of electromagnetic fields, including many techniques based on a principle of mind-body interactions. As a near grab bag of promising and bizarre therapies, the concept of alternative medicine aptly illustrates what postmodern theory calls the logic of the supplement. From a postmodern perspective, alternative medicine constitutes an indigestible leftover generated through the binary thinking endemic to Western rationalism: a residue in excess of what the biomedical model can accommodate or explain. It simply will not fit within a Cartesian system that resolutely opposes science to superstition, knowledge to error, fact to conjecture, and body to mind. Inexplicably, techniques of alternative medicine at times work quite well. As in the case of Chinese acupuncture, they may suggest the relevance of an entirely non-Western way of understanding. Despite its office at NIH, however, alternative medicine holds a marginal place in U.S. medicine, tolerated mainly because patients like it, and its lack of strong scientific credentials dooms it, so far, to the role of an optional add-on to standard biomedical therapies. ("If drugs don't work, let's try meditation.") Patients and physicians who pursue an eclectic course of adding on a few alternative therapies probably do not recognize—although some surely suspect—that the supplement in effect undermines the oppositions on which biomedicine has established its superiority. Alternative medicine is neither a rival capable of fully supplanting biomedicine nor a collection of optional therapies perfectly consistent with business as usual in the health care industry: it is an approach to illness that implicitly and uneasily calls into question the adequacy of the biomedical model.

A BIOCULTURAL MODEL

The most disorienting challenge to traditional thinking posed by developments in the postmodern era is the perception that illness is no longer a purely biological state—no longer a brute fact of nature—

but rather something in part created or interpenetrated by culture. This idea, while almost a commonplace among sociologists and anthropologists, meets rocklike resistance among doctors and patients committed to the biomedical model that has dominated Western medicine for the past 150 years. Like Andy Warhol, postmodern illness calls long-standing assumptions into doubt. It upsets established patterns of thinking not only about disease but also about the relationship between bodies and minds. No wonder many people resist. Resistance, however, while it confirms that ideas about illness are today deeply in dispute, cannot ultimately stop the coming changes. The basic argument I want to develop—my response to the question of what is distinctive about postmodern illness—can be put quite simply. *Postmodern illness is fundamentally biocultural—always biological and always cultural—situated at the crossroads of biology and culture.*

The claim that postmodern illness is fundamentally biocultural meets resistance particularly because many patients prefer that their illnesses have a strictly biological cause. The only alternative, they erroneously believe, is to consider their illnesses as purely psychological and mental. After a lifetime of tormenting, unexplained symptoms, Alice James (the talented, invalid sister of William James and Henry James) felt actual relief when she was diagnosed with cancer. Cancer was a firm, organic diagnosis: physical illness. Many patients today feel similarly desperate for a diagnosis of organic disease when their illness disappoints expectations generated by the biomedical model. Chronic pain patients often insist that doctors must have "missed" some hidden physical cause—as sometimes happens, through error or through the limits of current diagnostic instruments—but ongoing tissue damage is not required for chronic pain. What both patients and doctors cannot help overlooking, inevitably, is whatever the biomedical model tells or encourages them to ignore, including the role of culture in illness.

A biocultural view of illness does not require abandoning all the marvelous drugs and procedures based on the biomedical model. Research sparked by the biomedical model constitutes a supreme achievement of the recent past and remains a powerful force. Moreover, the practice of medicine, even within the biomedical tradition, is not monolithic. Hospitals and clinics are often divided by conflicts that have little to do with science.[38] Various subspecialties have quite distinctive outlooks: surgeons do not see eye to eye with psychiatrists, internists sometimes quarrel with orthopedists. Family practice, while well within traditional biomedicine, pays considerable attention to psychosocial dimensions of illness.[39] Still, Western medicine for over a century has worked to perfect a dominant scientific discourse based on viewing disease as the product of biological and chemical mechanisms within the body—a view for which the biomedical model provides a convenient shorthand—and this traditional biomedical model remains, despite resistance, slippage, and some outright defections, entrenched as the ruling paradigm of contemporary Western medicine.

The continuing power of the biomedical model throughout the postmodern era is demonstrated, indirectly, by a bold critique that appeared in 1977. In "The Need for a New Medical Model: A Challenge for Biomedicine," author George L. Engel, then professor of psychiatry and medicine at the University of Rochester, began from the observation that the science-based biomedical model is "now the dominant model of disease in the Western world."[40] He proceeded to criticize it both as reductive (shrinking biological phenomena to a language of chemistry and physics) and as dualistic (disconnecting body from mind). He also pointed out that the success of the biomedical model in treating breakdowns in the "mechanisms" of disease has not come without a price: bodies were modeled on machines, and healing was defined as the application of corrective drugs or surgeries.[41] It was a price people willingly paid in exchange for benefits unattainable by earlier medicine. Indeed, the biomedical model proved so successful in supplanting its rivals that Engel described it as not only the dominant scientific model of disease but also the dominant folk model. In effect, almost everybody took (or mistook) it for truth.

Postmodern illness occurs within the distinctive context in which we are coming to recognize the limits of the biomedical model, without knowing exactly what will replace it. A growing number of patients can sense what the biomedical vision of the body as a machine requires us to ignore, exclude, and falsify. For Engel, its focus on abstract patterns of organic disease means that the biomedical model cannot deal effectively with concrete social and psychological influences on illness, with illness as, in his words, "a human experience." He proposed, in opposition to the biomedical model, an approach that recognizes the interplay between a biology of disease and the pervasive influences on illness that come from minds and from social experience. To this new alternative model he gave the awkward but influential name of "biopsychosocial."[42]

Engel's biopsychosocial approach has much in common with the postmodern vision I am calling biocultural. Yet, while sympathetic to its underlying principles, I resist adopting Engel's term here for three reasons. First, its influence today is indirect at best, marginal at worst. Although a few medical schools make a biopsychosocial approach central to their teaching, elsewhere it is not so much opposed as treated with indifference or institutional cynicism. Lip service is the rule. Second, business as usual in crowded hospitals and clinics usually means drugs and surgery. There is little time for extensive psychosocial therapies, and the financial disincentives are strong. "Capitation fees"—fixed annual fees paid to doctors per patient—actively discourage focus on complex, nonbiological dimensions of illness. Third, and most important, the 1977 model that Engel called biopsychosocial needs significant revision in order to extend and enrich its understanding of cultural processes with the benefits of two decades of postmodern thinking.

This new thinking, which sometimes goes by the name of poststructuralism, has revitalized disciplines in the human sciences by emphasizing what has been called the social construction of reality— a concept that refers to the ways in which the world we inhabit is framed and in large part created by the forces of human culture, including language, myth, and ideology.[43] Social forces, in effect, always reconfigure the contexts of human life. Truth, within this poststructuralist vision, is plural and contingent: it is truth (with a

lowercase *t*) situated within history, limited by the outlook of specific
disciplines, shaped by the interests of dominant groups, perplexed
by the inherent indeterminacy of language, caught up in a flow of social power: uncertain, temporary, ironic.[44] One crucial outcome of
this new thinking is a vastly extended interest in culture. Anthropologists now study not only indigenous tribes but also surgeons in
Houston, historians write about the social impact of fire and ice,
philosophers think about film, linguists discuss gender, and literary
critics trace the politics of colonial discourse. No matter how hard to
define, culture in such boundary-crossing enterprises is not separate
from family dynamics or science or medicine but rather constitutes
the all-encompassing medium to which they contribute and within
which they unfold. Everything from wigs and wilderness to professional wrestling and cosmetic surgery can now be understood as a
social text: the world, in short, is textual; and, as a famous poststructuralist dictum puts it, there is nothing outside the text.[45]

Postmodern analysis, stripped of its most debatable claims,
demonstrates how human life is socially constructed and how people
as well as institutions exist only within the context of cultural systems that govern the flow of knowledge and power. It shows that historical systems tend to distribute knowledge and power through social discourses: the discourses of science, say, or of sexuality. It shows
that such power operates often diffused not through traditional hierarchies but through an invisible network of familiar institutions and
everyday practices that shape how we think, feel, and view the
world. A few of the institutions and practices crucial in shaping how
we understand ourselves and our bodies would include money,
films, police, fast food, beauty pageants, prisons, and encyclope-
dias—to which we must add, of course, medical techniques, theories,
and textbooks. Medicine makes a powerful contribution to contemporary culture and to the postmodern fashioning of the self.

This new understanding of culture has weighty implications for
illness. We must recognize that maladies, while always biological, are
also in part cultural artifacts, in the same way that medicine is a cultural artifact as it operates through discourses that distribute social

power across institutions and individual lives.[46] The psyche of the patient is inseparable from the social forces and symbol systems that constitute human culture, so that selfhood, like illness, is a biocultural construction.[47] This very postmodern idea makes no sense to some psychiatrists and to many nonpsychiatrists who see it as denying the everyday flow of consciousness in which our thoughts, feelings, and selves appear distinctly our own. There is no denial, however. Instead, postmodernism reconceives the inner life of consciousness as in large part generated through the social operations of power.[48] Of course, an adequate account of selfhood cannot rest on cultural analysis alone but must integrate both cultural and biological analyses. The crucial point is that individual psyches express possibilities not only available within a specific culture but also generated by cultural forces, and culture thus becomes a mirror in which we can recognize the forces that shape individual psyches. From a postmodern perspective, the psychological is always cultural, just as the personal is always political.[49] Even such intrinsically biological stages of human development as puberty, menarche, menopause, and old age are saturated with the meanings that specific cultures assign. The significance thus attributed to culture does not deny that each person builds up a unique identity. Rather, it dissuades us from making a fetish of individual differences and prevents us from mistaking the uniqueness of each person for something impenetrably internal and private. It lets us see, ultimately, in what ways the personal experience of illness is always mediated by cultural forces.

Postmodern illness is biocultural in the specific sense that we now recognize how human biology engages in a continuous commerce with the forces of human culture. Although some maladies originate in the mind, minds operate only in the context of cultures and produce symptoms only through biological processes. Even psychogenic pain produced in a laboratory experiment is always biological and always cultural. More often, our illnesses arise from innumerable interactions with an environment where the social and the biological constantly intermingle: home, for example, to the female *Anopheles* mosquito, whose malarial range and impact we regularly alter by human activities. Postmodern illness, in brief, is an outlook that understands a specific malady, whatever its particular causes, as created in the convergences between biology and culture.

There will be critics who claim (in the ultimate move toward debunking it) that a biocultural model is nothing new. Certainly, in its intellectual lineage, a biocultural model has links to medical traditions stretching back to the ancient Greeks. (From a postmodern perspective skeptical of claims to an absolute, unprecedented moment of origin, it could not be otherwise.) In championing a rational, empirical, biological medicine distinct from magic and religion, Hippocrates saw one cause of disease in environmental forces such as diet and work. Aristotle explored various "nonnatural" (nonbiological) causes of illness, including climate. Renaissance theorists argued that personal habits like excessive study could cause illness by unbalancing bodily fluids, and eighteenth-century doctors traced specific illnesses to the influence of what we call lifestyle. Crucial differences, however, separate such premodern foreshadowings from a postmodern biocultural outlook.

The postmodern world is in many ways—including its vastly increased human population—unique. Earlier medical traditions, even when receptive to nonbiological influences, existed within cultures where alchemy and phrenology were respected explanatory systems, where doctors routinely bled patients to death, where toothache and grief were listed among the regular causes of death. We have inherited, by contrast, a culture in which scientific biomedicine has almost burned away the memory of its prescientific ancestors. Nothing in the history of medicine mirrors our transitional moment when a new understanding of the links between biology and culture is calling the all-powerful biomedical model into question. We can see that TB in the nineteenth century and bubonic plague in the Middle Ages illustrate convergences between biology and culture, but this insight is a gift of contemporary historians. Keats, Chaucer, and Hippocrates could not understand their illnesses as, in our sense, biocultural. Moreover, civilization had not yet accelerated its impact and clutter to the unthinkable degree that it could raise the temperature of the planet, directly influencing health. Now researchers clone large animals in the laboratory, and even Mars bears on its surface the marks of human culture. Postmodern illness belongs to this new, if far from innocent, time.

The incompleteness of our transition to a biocultural outlook, of course, creates uncertainty and confusion. Postmodernism implies uncertainty—it comes after modernism, but is unsure where it is headed. While popular imagery based on modernist biomedicine viewed the body as a machinelike carapace or well-fortified castle, fending off external threats from hostile bacteria and viruses, postmodern culture shows us something quite different with its vision of selves and bodies newly vulnerable to the workings of our own immune systems.[50] It is questioning the nature of the self that falls ill, the self that is now increasingly fragile and incohesive, the site of contradictory social discourses, like a radio program overlaid with sound from other stations. It is altering the character of illness as chronic ailments and ambiguous syndromes confront patients with radical doubt about their health. It is changing the relation between doctor and patient as litigation, group practice, and insurance companies fracture an earlier trust. Along with astonishing gains in drug therapies, laser surgery, genetic testing, and emergency medicine, it is giving us epidemics of alcoholism, obesity, chronic pain, and heart disease, as well as terrible new illnesses inseparable from our own sexuality and aging. Most important, it is exposing flaws in the reigning positivist biomedical model of disease. It is telling us that only by recognizing the convergences between biology and various cultural forces—forces as remote from the purview of modernist biomedicine as the ozone layer—can we come to understand the distinctive features of illness in the postmodern world.

chapter three

The White Noise of Health

White noise: . . . a steady, unvarying, unobtrusive

sound, as an electronically produced drone or the

sound of rain, used to mask or obliterate

unwanted sounds.

The Random House Dictionary
of the English Language

On 26 April 1986, in the Ukrainian town of Chernobyl, reactor number four in an aging and poorly designed nuclear power plant blew up. Fire in the graphite moderators produced radioactive gases and aerosols that over the next ten days contaminated thirty-five hundred square miles. The world learned about the accident only when Western scientists detected a radioactive cloud drifting over northern Europe. After initial silence and then volleys of denial from officials in what was then the Soviet Union, teams of engineers and construction workers at great peril soon encased the entire reactor in a thick concrete shroud. Although the drifting cloud of radiation suddenly reminded us that an event occurring in the remotest Ukraine might have a direct and devastating impact on human health across the globe, the irony of Chernobyl is that, once decently covered, the infamous site has mostly slipped from public memory, registering as just one more local technocratic foul-up, like the fatal gases released at Bhopal or the massive tide of petroleum that the *Exxon Valdez* released into Prince William Sound. We hear about Chernobyl now only on anniversaries—in reports belonging to the genre of "x"-years-later stories that are a staple of postmodern journalism—in between which there seems to be no occasion for additional thought.

Chernobyl, a disquieting signature of our age, is a prime example of postmodern environmental damage. Unlike the atomic explosions in August 1945 over Hiroshima and Nagasaki that revealed the devastating force discovered and unlocked by modernist science, postmodern devastation is usually less visible and less violent, although consequences may be equally dire. Radiation exposure killed some 250 people almost immediately following the Chernobyl accident, but indirect casualties are impossible to determine. Some 400,000 to 600,000 civilian and military workers have engaged in multiyear cleanup operations at Chernobyl, with limited use of protective clothing. The U.S. Department of Energy has predicted up to twenty-eight thousand fatal cancers from the Chernobyl releases. In Byelorussia, which borders on the Ukraine, congenital abnormalities increased 70 percent within four years; thyroid cancers and leukemia shot up; hypertension soared; and animal studies showed severe depression of the immune system. Not surprisingly, the International Atomic Energy Agency found that most villagers living in contaminated areas wanted to move away.[1] Can anyone, however, really succeed in moving away from the threats to health posed by postmodern environmental damage?

The magnification of scale at Chernobyl, while horrible, permits us to recognize a crucial, distinctive feature of the postmodern era: human enterprise has reshaped and perhaps irreversibly damaged the environment during the last fifty years of the twentieth century. *Environment*, in effect, is not a synonym for *nature*, that is, if we define nature as everything untouched by culture. For postmodern thinkers, nature is now simply another social construction, and environment proves an especially useful new concept because it expressly encompasses the transformation of the natural world by culture.[2] It includes cities and garbage dumps, bays polluted with human waste, air thick with the emissions from automobiles and manufacturing processes, water tainted with the chemical runoff from industrial farms. It includes—in its widest application—not only human artifacts such as strip malls and landfills but also human populations and the social structures that shape human beings and their activities, from families, tribes, and nations to unions, armies, and multinational corporations. Illness too must now be included among the artifacts of culture: both a product and a component of our reconfigured environment.

Illness today is often environmental illness. The proliferating maladies now dependent on our relationship to the environment provide perfect illustrations of the biocultural character of postmodern illness. Further, in recognizing the connections between illness and the environment reshaped by human enterprise, we begin to recover something of the biocultural heritage that modernist medicine mostly rejected or ignored in pursuing a science focused on the interior of the body. Medicine is still slow to recognize and to address the complicated and far-flung environmental sources of contemporary illness. Medical writing, in fact, usually employs the term *environment* in a restricted sense to denote the specific surroundings of a patient that reinforce dysfunctional behavior. The wider, even global contexts of environmental damage and its links to public health have not found a place within biomedical curricula that focus attention on internal organs—heart, liver, brain—and on bodily systems. Postmodern illness is in one sense an opportunity for medicine to recover the wisdom of its own past.

EARLY ENVIRONMENTAL MEDICINE

Beliefs in the relation between human health and the environment have a long history. The ancient Greek physicians of the Hippocratic school taught that human health is directly influenced by air, water, food, climate, topography, and even the direction of the prevailing winds. The second-century Greek anatomist and physician Galen, whose writings formed the basis of European medicine through the Renaissance, also called attention to links between the external and internal worlds. His theory—tracing health to an equilibrium among the four internal fluids (called humors) supposed to dominate human life—recognized that heat and cold, for example, could unbalance the body in ways that dispose a person to illness. Even astrology, a system that retained its intellectual power from ancient Mesopotamia through the beginning of the seventeenth century, sees our health or illness as largely determined by the position of stars and planets. This long-standing belief in the influence of the environment on illness is fossilized in everyday speech. The word *flu*—imported into England in 1743—derives from the Italian *influenza*, which conveys the view that epidemic illnesses can be traced to the "influence" of fetid air from swamps, bogs, and urban miasmic locales. Similar beliefs about the influence of the environment on human illness held sway well into the twentieth century before positivist medicine dismissed them as superstitions. Patients suffering from the wet, wracking coughs of tuberculosis were advised to seek mountain or desert climates, where their symptoms would improve with sunshine and dry air.

Several hundred years ago, writers began to observe links between illness and specific occupations. A pioneering treatise in this new field—later called industrial medicine—is Bernardino Ramazzini's *The Diseases of Tradesmen* (1700). Professor of medicine at the University of Modena, Ramazzini studied over fifty types of workers, from ragpickers and street sweepers to printers and masons, observing the specific hazards they faced, especially from chemicals, dust, metals, and abrasives. His work inspired similar studies of other occupational hazards, such as the skin diseases of workers in the silk trade.

What Ramazzini and his immediate followers had no reason to address was the larger context of widespread environmental damage that can erode the health of whole populations. For example, no one in the nineteenth century understood that the famous pea-soup fogs of London—the source of numerous respiratory illnesses—were a recent invention, caused by burning soft coal for heat. Population is another environmental force that Ramazzini did not need to consider in analyzing the diseases of tradesmen. World population in 1650, when Ramazzini was born, stood at a mere 500 million, a figure that had stayed relatively stable for centuries. Although Europeans had long been responsible for changes in the local landscape—the barren heaths and moors of England were created by human deforestation before the Middle Ages—the pace of change had been slow. With the Industrial Revolution, all across Europe populations begin to grow rapidly, with an inescapable impact on health. Expanding cities with no effective sanitation were a nightmare of disease. In London, until the first sewage system was designed in the early nineteenth century, human waste was thrown into the street. (The eighteenth-century fashion for snuff had a side benefit in blocking out the stench of civilized life.) By 1850, world population in the two hundred years since the birth of Bernardo Ramazzini had jumped two-thousand-fold, to one billion people. Scientists insist that such rapid jumps in population—the first huge increase followed the invention of agriculture—are due not to biological rhythms but to the impact on cultural forces of biology.

The urban poor in this world of rapidly growing population worked back-breaking days in dismal factories, raising their families in tenements infested with disease-bearing rodents. Exposure to toxins increased in step with the increase in commerce and international trade. The phrase "mad as a hatter" entered the English language in the nineteenth century, most likely referring to the odd tremors and twitches of workers who contracted mercury poisoning in the manufacture of hats.[3] The novels of Dickens and Zola dramatize ways in which nineteenth-century industrial growth ruined the lives and destroyed the health of the working poor. Even legislators finally got the message, but laws to improve working conditions and prohibit child labor were not enough to protect health.

By 1930 world population had doubled again. It had doubled once more by 1975, to a staggering four billion people. The postmodern world, which holds twice as many people as its modernist predecessor, is a unique place simply by virtue of this unprecedented accumulation of human beings.

The complex links connecting environment and illness are illustrated by two unrelated conditions that together suggest how major changes in culture directly affect human health: black lung disease and malaria. The vast increase in human population brought a huge increase in the production of material goods, and black lung disease (now vanished from medical dictionaries) made its brief appearance during the mid–twentieth century, when the bituminous coal industry of southern Appalachia achieved national importance. With the advent of mechanized mining, introduced in the 1930s, the workforce shrank while dust levels greatly multiplied. The new technology of power hammers, grinders, and sandblasters exposed workers to fine silica dust that lodged in the lungs and produced debilitating silicosis.[4] By the late 1960s, as workers aged and jobs continued to disappear, earlier vague references to "miner's asthma" (as doctors hired by the mining companies dismissively called it) gave way to a unionized "black lung movement" designed to secure financial benefits for miners who had spent years inhaling the lethal thick black dust.[5] It is hard to find a clearer example of the multileveled social construction of illness in which biology and culture are inseparably joined.

Malaria, like black lung disease, is an illness shaped or reshaped by the recent quantum leaps in population and technology. An ancient infection that even as late as 1950 was estimated to kill a million people annually in India alone, malaria regularly terrorized populations throughout the wet, humid regions of Africa, Central and South America, Southeast Asia, and the Mediterranean.[6] Malarial infections among workers, for example, delayed one of the great engineering feats of the modern era, the fifty-one-mile Panama Canal, and the canal owes its completion in 1914 to bacteriologists Walter Reed and Ronald Ross, who proved that malaria is transmitted by the bite of the *Anopheles* mosquito. In 1955 a global program to eradicate malaria began under the leadership of the World Health Organization, with impressive results. For over two decades, African health planners assumed that all fevers in small children were malarial, and they taught mothers to treat feverish children immediately with the antimalarial drug chloroquine. The incidence of malaria in Africa dropped precipitously.

The history of malaria shows how human alterations of the environment change the nature and patterns of illness. World Health Organization programs to treat children with chloroquine have inadvertently created new, chloroquine-resistant strains of the malaria sporozoan. So resourceful is the malaria parasite that it has evolved strains resistant to multiple drugs, resistant, in fact, to every drug that science has invented.[7] In regions with prolonged rainy seasons, trying to eradicate mosquitoes is like trying to eradicate rain. As human activities such as war, trade, and migration put large groups of people on the move, especially between rural and urban areas, infected individuals carry the evolved strains into regions where the local populations have no acquired immunity. In Brazil, hospitalizations for malaria rose from nearly zero in 1960 to almost 300,000 twenty years later, and they doubled again by 1988 to 600,000. In 1990, 1 million African children died from malaria, and malaria killed another 2.5 million people worldwide. Malaria, as these statistics confirm, is now one of the most lethal diseases of the postmodern era. The comeback of the malaria parasite is rarely mentioned in the hyperbole about high-tech, computer-age, biomedical wonders, probably because the disease mostly affects people in developing countries. This silence and isolation will change. The huge jump in world population during the postmodern era—from some two billion in 1950 to a predicted ten billion in 2025—comes almost entirely in the developing world (see figure 3), and this vast new market for goods and services will bring diseases of the southern hemisphere into far closer contact with the increasingly mobile populations of the north.

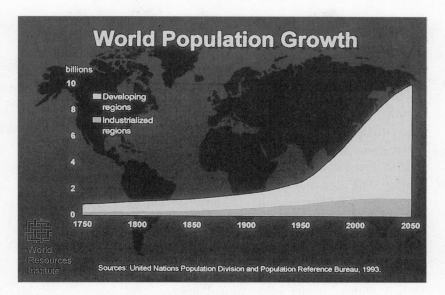

Figure 3. World Population Growth. Courtesy World Resources Institute, Washington, D.C.

Affluence and access to technology multiply the damage any population inflicts upon the environment, so that one American has the impact of fifty Bangladeshis.[8] What will happen when the entire population of China drives sport-utility vehicles? Who can predict the cascading environmental damage set in motion when Africa trades in its savannas for housing developments? We have not seen the end of maladies created or re-created by human alteration of the natural world.

NATURE AND HUMAN HEALTH

"Nature," wrote Henry David Thoreau in the mid–nineteenth century, "is another word for health."[9] Today, Thoreau's one-word prescription to cure the ills of his increasingly sedentary, citified fellow countrymen rings rather hollow. Nature is just not what it was. Even while Thoreau was urging his contemporaries to restore their health by returning to nature, nature was changing in ways that neither the early settlers nor the indigenous tribes before them (both of whom transformed the land) would recognize.[10] And we keep changing the natural world. Many reputable scientists argue that by burning enormous quantities of fossil fuels and filling the atmosphere with greenhouse gases, we change the climate of the earth, triggering a series of related disasters from floods and hurricanes to outbreaks of tropical disease. The idea of a distinctively postmodern illness—biocultural at the core—finds premonitions almost everywhere in the effects of human changes to the environment, whether they take the form of increased skin cancer from ozone depletion over Australia, the poisoning of inner-city children from lead-based paints, the outbreaks of Hanta virus as rodents multiply in the newly populous southwestern United States, or the international epidemic of human allergies linked to the worldwide increase in the use of diesel fuel.[11] The emergence of obscure maladies such as Legionnaires' disease (communicated by a bacterium found in various damp locales, including the ventilation systems of airtight convention hotels) illustrates how, as we alter our environment, we suffer the illnesses that we simultaneously construct or reconstruct. In this sense, nature is no longer the cure for but the streamlined, fuel-injected carrier of affliction.

The paranoia common to contemporary life is not enough to explain why so many people attribute almost every bodily ill to contamination of their air, water, and food. In the United States, pollution has almost replaced germs as the all-purpose, postmodern explanation for bad health. The paranoia may be justified. Scientists have provided strong evidence for the role of environment in illness, and the facts are clear. The chemical assault we face today accelerated greatly in the aftermath of World War II, when businesses that formerly produced bombs, tanks, and combat aircraft retooled to supply the expanding automotive, agricultural, and petrochemical industries. The accelerated change and its resulting damage went mostly unnoticed until Rachel Carson in *Silent Spring* (1962) first informed a wide audience about how our addiction to fossil fuels put birds, fish, and the entire natural world in jeopardy. It would be misleading, however, to suggest that the link between illness and environmental damage reveals a straightforward cause-and-effect mechanism similar to the causal mechanisms of the biomedical model. As science is showing, the relationship between health and environment is often far more complex than a direct causal bond linking polluted streams and dying fish to human disease.

The complexity of relations between illness and environment is visible in the strange history of sickle-cell anemia. Sickle-cell disease is a genetically inherited disorder, often lethal in children, that arose from a random mutation of the hemoglobin molecule. That sickle-cell disease originated in India and Africa during the introduction of agriculture some four thousand years ago is far more than a mere antiquarian detail. India and Africa were then especially afflicted by malaria.[12] Sickle cell is a recessive trait, and thus children who inherit only one gene for sickle cell will carry the trait but not develop symptoms of the disease. (Under unusual circumstances, children with only one gene for sickle cell will develop the disease, but in a milder and usually not fatal form.) The payoff to all this genetic history: possessing a single gene for sickle-cell disease confers protection against malaria.

The connection between malaria and sickle-cell disease, then, offers a powerful illustration of how human illness may develop and persist through complicated interrelations among genes and the environment. Because the environment in Africa included the malaria sporozoan, and because children with a single sickle-cell gene were protected from death by malaria, the laws of genetics ensured that the trait for sickle-cell disease would thrive. Protection against malaria, unfortunately, came at a cost. A child who inherited two sickle-cell genes from parents who either had the disease or were carriers would, unavoidably, contract sickle-cell anemia. Today one in twelve black Americans carries a gene for sickle hemoglobin, and one in every four hundred black newborns in the United States has sickle-cell anemia or a related disease.[13] The illnesses today seem unconnected to the environment—but only because we remain blind to their biocultural history.

In less complicated versions, the links between illness and the environment, happily, are now becoming clearer. Specialized publications such as the *Journal of Environmental Health* (begun in 1963) have encouraged research, and their growth parallels the development of several new health care specialties, including an entire area called environmental medicine.[14] In a subfield of environmental medicine, specialists in occupational health deal with the relation between injuries, afflictions, and the changing workplaces that relentlessly grind out fresh ailments. Emergent new postmodern afflictions such as repetitive stress injuries and carpal tunnel syndrome—the hazards of cashiers and keyboard operators—suggest how far machines and electronic appliances have come to constitute our immediate environment. We are beginning to recognize that illness today simply cannot be disjoined from our newly engineered cultural landscape of dams, superhighways, air conditioners, advertising, jet planes, television, and fast food. It is said that Japan had no incidence of arteriosclerosis until the traditional diet of rice, fish, and vegetables gave way to a Western smorgasbord of steak, pizza, and French fries.

Many puzzles remain. Few environmental illnesses reveal their origin with anything so measurable as a radioactive cloud. Some origins no doubt lie concealed in a complex mix of personal genetic predispositions and multiple environmental forces, including microbes that seem to come out of nowhere as we destroy tropical rain forests and warm the atmosphere. Why should the genetic alleles for Tay-Sachs disease—a lethal brain defect in young children—be ten times more common among east European Jews than among the rest of the population? Why is the prevalence of cystic fibrosis five to ten times greater among northern Europeans than among Asians and Africans?[15] Like the history of sickle-cell disease, the histories of these diseases may need to account for deeply hidden environmental facts. Meanwhile, many common ills—from whiplash injuries and gunshot wounds to alcoholism, heart disease, and hospital infections—are so obviously embedded in our new culturally constructed environment that the puzzle is mainly how to prevent them. Cholera in the United States, for example, has increased 500 percent since the 1980s as Americans have increased their travel to developing nations.[16] Like malaria, tuberculosis has revived because our overuse of medications permits the bacillus to develop drug-resistant strains. An awareness of the interconnections that link human maladies to the environment does not guarantee that we can solve the problems it teaches us to recognize.

Postmodern illness, because of its complicated links to the culturally constructed environment, ultimately demands that we rethink the sources of medical knowledge. Laboratory tests and scientific studies cannot reveal everything that doctors need to know. The social, cultural, and personal dimensions of illness must be understood through other means, and one neglected but useful resource is narrative. Narrative, we might say, constitutes a mode of understanding appropriate for situations too variable and too untidy for laboratory analysis. Further, storytellers thrive at the margins of power, casting a skeptical eye on contemporary culture, and their somewhat independent status permits them to offer impassioned critiques, visionary alternatives, and an outsider's objectivity. Narrative may also require readers to confront self-consciously the ways in which their culture has taught them to think about illness, to imagine ways in which they might experience a healthier relation to the earth. The United Nations reports that fourteen million children die annually from causes related to environmental degradation.[17] For the children, if not for ourselves, we need to hear from voices silenced or overwhelmed by the prevailing biomedical discourse of science, policy analysis, and cost containment. We need a knowledge that comes with narrative.

AIRBORNE TOXIC EVENTS

Don DeLillo's award-winning postmodern novel *White Noise* (1985) contains in its central section the chilling description of a black cloud of chemical toxins that passes one evening over a small college town, tracked by helicopters and spotlights: "The enormous dark mass moved like some death ship in a Norse legend, escorted across the night by armored creatures with spiral wings."[18] This account by DeLillo's first-person narrator, Jack Gladney, evokes a mythic resonance, but it is a mundane and very contemporary myth, a myth of bungled technology and domestic terror, which includes a new understanding of death. According to Gladney, death now comes in two varieties, natural and artificial (283). The ominous black cloud— "[p]acked with chlorides, benzenes, phenols, hydrocarbons" (127)— constitutes a vivid image of the new postmodern threat of artificial death. The threat is not just new but, like fate for an earlier culture, foreseen and accepted as inescapable. As Gladney's middle-class family drives to a designated evacuation center seeking refuge, they discover in effect that there is nowhere to go except home.

The central disaster in *White Noise,* which the authorities in their Orwellian newspeak dub "The Airborne Toxic Event," is the result of an industrial accident—but also as wrapped up in fate as any catastrophe in Norse myth. Like the nuclear meltdown at Chernobyl, like the *Exxon Valdez* oil spill, it was predetermined by the inherently unstable relations among humans, technology, and the (once) natural world. Toxic black clouds will continue to appear in the postmodern world because all the preconditions for their appearance have already been met.

Medicine in the novel is not so much an antidote for disaster as a part of the complicated, interlocking systems that produce it. Jack Gladney's direct exposure to the black cloud of Nyodene D—described as a mixture of by-products from the manufacture of an insecticide—keeps him making regular, if ineffectual, visits to his doctor, while his wife, Babette, remains so obsessed with dying that she seeks out an untested experimental drug, Dylar, engineered for the express purpose of removing the fear of death. Dylar, of course, is a fraud, no more potent than Jack Gladney's doctor in staving off death. "Death is in the air" (151), as one speaker puts it, not referring to the black cloud. Dylar is an emblem of our efforts to find an artificial cure to protect us from the threats of artificial death ubiquitous in the artificial new postmodern environment.

White Noise is a complex, double-edged study of cultural change. While the Gladneys (Jack, Babette, and their four children) seem to represent a typical American family living in an idyllic college town, they provide a snapshot of the loose and shifting confederations that constitute the postmodern household. This is Jack's fourth marriage, Babette's third, and the permutations of kinship grow dizzying. As scholar Thomas J. Ferraro observes: "Each adult lives with a third or fourth spouse, a son from a previous marriage, a daughter from a different previous marriage, a stepson from one of the latest spouse's previous marriages, and a stepdaughter from another of that spouse's previous marriages. Every child lives with one progenitor, that parent's current mate, one half-sibling of the opposite sex whose other parent lives elsewhere, a combination of stepsister and stepbrother who are only half-siblings to one another." [19] The surprise is that this cobbled-together unit functions rather smoothly. Various characters describe the child-centered Gladney home—in opposition to the rather moribund campus—as strangely magical, a place where masses of information and data whiz through the air like radio waves ("extrasensory flashes and floating nuances of being" [34]). What makes the novel difficult to grasp—despite its accessible language and minimalist plot—is DeLillo's evenhanded depiction of postmodern culture as both frightening in its technological-consumerist emptiness and also wondrous in the strange, new possibilities it opens up. He allows free play to opposite and seemingly incompatible tendencies: on one hand, intricate new technologies as common as automatic teller machines put us in contact with remote and mysterious pools of data; on the other hand, disasters loom so massive that they cannot be the work of individuals but only the unanticipated consequence of intersecting technological systems run amok.[20]

"We didn't grow up with all these shifting facts and attitudes," says Babette as she reflects on the uncertainties of postmodern life (171). The dark toxic cloud, the unintended product of a system normally hidden from view, functions in the novel as far more than a specific danger. Drifting indistinctly in the night sky, it represents (beyond one more local foul-up) an intangible and amorphous threat born from the newly shifting relations among humans, technology, and the environment: a threat inescapably enfolded within the fabric of everyday life. *White Noise* reflects a quarter-century advance beyond Carson's *Silent Spring* because it takes for granted the chemical assault to which Carson first called attention. The cloud of Nyodene D reminds us that pesticides are still big business. (On top of several hundred billion pounds of pesticides already released into the global environment during the twentieth century, we add another five to six billion pounds each year.)[21] Yet, DeLillo prefers to let the decentered focus of his novel linger upon more common, innocuous, and almost omnipresent images of contemporary life with their illusion of stability and purpose: the station wagon, the supermarket, the expressway.

"The station wagons arrived at noon"—so runs the first sentence, creating a Norman Rockwell vision of parents and students returning like clockwork to start the academic year at idyllic College-on-the-Hill. As Professor Jack Gladney continues to observe the annual fall rite, DeLillo produces one of the catalogue-like inventories that soon begin to dominate the novel: "The roofs of the station wagons were loaded down with carefully secured suitcases full of light and heavy clothing; with boxes of blankets, boots and shoes, stationery and books, sheets, pillows, quilts; with rolled-up rugs and sleeping bags; with bicycles, skis, rucksacks, English and Western saddles, inflated rafts." All very ordinary—except in the disquieting suggestion that a nearly identical procession of mass-produced consumer goods is simultaneously flowing across every campus in the Western world: "the stereo sets, radios, personal computers; small refrigerators and table ranges; the cartons of phonograph records and cassettes; the hairdryers and styling irons; the tennis rackets, soccer balls, hockey and lacrosse sticks, bows and arrows; the controlled substances, the birth control pills and devices; the junk food still in shopping bags— onion-and-garlic chips, nacho thins, peanut creme patties, Waffelos and Kabooms, fruit chews and toffee popcorn; the Dum-Dum pops, the Mystic mints" (3). What begins as light comic realism in the jumble of typical dormitory stuff comes to assume increasing weight as the novel at length delineates (with an almost poetic attention to detail) the artificial, thing-filled, commodified landscape that constitutes the distinctive postmodern environment.

The supermarket serves DeLillo not as just another contemporary landmark but as a power source or *ur*-metaphor. It is where our commodities come from, where they collect, where they multiply at night like creatures endowed with independent life. The supermarket is the inner sanctum of white noise. It takes something beyond satire, it takes a perception of the marvelous within the ordinary, almost a moment of revelation, to reveal the incessant background music of consumerism. Jack's friend and colleague, Murray Jay Suskind, a champion of the new world of postmodernism, grows almost lyrical as he contemplates the riches latent within an everyday supermarket: "This place recharges us spiritually, it prepares us, it's a gateway or pathway. Look how bright. It's full of psychic data. . . . Everything is concealed in symbolism, hidden by veils of mystery and layers of cultural material. But it is psychic data, absolutely. The doors slide open, they close unbidden. Energy waves, incident radiation. All the letters and numbers are here, all the colors of the spectrum, all the voices and sounds, all the code words and ceremonial phrases" (37–38). Murray regularly lectures Jack on the wonders contained in the magic kingdom opened by technology and consumerism, in which even hospitals begin to resemble supermarkets: "New devices, new techniques every day. Lasers, masers, ultrasound. Give yourself up to it," he tells Jack. "Believe in it. They'll insert you in a gleaming tube, irradiate your body with the basic stuff of the universe. Light, energy, dreams. God's own goodness" (285). Indeed postmodern medicine—with its array of new procedures from angioplasty to radiation therapy—belongs to a realm in which the miraculous has come to seem routine. It is DeLillo's art to show us how everyday systems from medicine to manufacturing are subtly interconnected— the miracles linked with the disasters—and how they affect the people who live in their midst.

The supermarket finds its logical extension not only in the hospital but also in the brain waves of the characters who inhabit the mostly indoors, electronic, consumerist environment of the postmodern novel, where even sex has been repackaged as an incentive for sales or a means of acquiring illegal drugs. Every few pages DeLillo interpenetrates his story with a "sublittoral drone" (168) of brand names and products: Dacron, Orlon, Lycra Spandex; Corolla, Celica, Cressida; cough suppressants, decongestants, antihistamines, pain relievers. The ceaseless litany connects the supermarket directly to its alter ego, the TV set, as fragments of programming drift through the text like flotsam. In the Gladney household, the TV is always on. Electronic images and representations thus begin to assume the force and density once attributed to objects. As her family watches Babette perform on a local cable television show, she seems to them more substantial on the screen than in real life. Even at home, characters tend to view themselves as if they were on camera, living in the shadow of their own images, and they seek to offset the resulting loss of self-possession by surrounding themselves with possessions. The material goods that he buys on a shopping binge are what supply Jack with the one moment when he experiences "fullness of being" (20). In the product-oriented, supermarket-driven age of information, language and selves are subtly reshaped by the technologies of simulation and reproduction. Jack, despite his professorial interests, regularly lapses into the speech patterns of a TV weatherman.

Expressways are as common to the postmodern landscape as the supermarkets and station wagons that they serve, and all for DeLillo maintain a latent connection with violence. "I see contemporary violence," he said in a rare interview, "as a kind of sardonic response to the promise of consumer fulfillment in America."[22] Jack's search for fulfillment includes the consumer's ultimate possession, a home, "in what was once a wooded area with deep ravines." The woods are gone. "There is an expressway beyond the backyard now, well below us," Jack continues, "and at night as we settle into our brass bed the sparse traffic washes past, a remote and steady murmur around our sleep, as of dead souls babbling at the edge of a dream" (4). More white noise. Another image of the natural world engineered for human purposes in such a way that its insistent peril goes unnoticed. The violence we do to nature, in *White Noise*, inevitably recoils against us. Setting out to kill a mysterious Mr. Gray, who has supplied Babette with the death-defying experimental drug Dylar, Jack not only wounds Gray but ends up shooting himself in the hand. Less melodramatic violence takes shape in the final chapter when Wilder—the youngest child of Jack and Babette, their sole comfort against death—rides his plastic tricycle across six lanes of expressway traffic. Wilder miraculously crosses unscathed, but it is obvious that next time the expressway will prevail. The real accident was his escape. Our fate is as "sealed" (a recurring term in the novel) as the certainty of more Chernobyls, although following disaster we also seem capable of readjusting quickly to our comfortable substitutes for nature. DeLillo's final paragraph begins by describing the panic of shoppers lost in the confusion of a supermarket that has rearranged its shelves, but the book concludes reassuringly at the checkout counter ("equipped with holographic scanners") where we wait, alongside the tabloid racks, glancing at familiar headlines that tout "[t]he miracle vitamins, the cures for cancer, the remedies for obesity" (326).

The quest for health is, naturally, an inescapable duty (or fate) in DeLillo's artificial postmodern environment of consumerism, where death is in the air and not even nuns believe in salvation. (DeLillo at one point used as a working title for his novel-in-progress *The American Book of the Dead*.) Babette regularly jogs to control her weight, much as Jack runs through endless diagnostic tests at a high-tech lab with the mortuary name Autumn Harvest Farms. Health, however, is precisely what is missing from this culture of merchandise. "It's all a corporate tie in," Babette observes, far closer to the truth than she knows. "The sunscreen, the marketing, the fear, the disease. You can't have one without the other" (264). This is the environment that human beings have constructed in the short three hundred years since the beginnings of the Industrial Revolution, and it is this environment, more than the occasional black toxic cloud, that sends Jack and

Babette Gladney and the rest of us running anxiously to our doctors. What are the implications for human health and the environment when in the next few decades we double the number of supermarkets, expressways, station wagons, airborne toxic events, and desperate, health-conscious consumers with their corporate sponsors?

BIOPHILIA

Surgeon-writer Richard Selzer in his autobiographical book *Down from Troy: A Doctor Comes of Age* (1992) incorporates into the flow of his life story a long meditation on the architecture of modern hospitals: "Just as I would never again live in a house without wind chimes, I would not call a building a *hospital* that did not have a fountain on the premises. Were I to design a hospital, I would cause it to be built around a large reflecting pool, from the center of which would rise a fountain. Let it be a tall fountain with a powerful upward thrust and, at descending intervals, lateral leaves or petals to catch the fall, breaking it into a thousand secondary and tertiary *cascatelli.* There can be nothing so consolatory to the sick as a fountain." [23] Selzer's wind chimes recall the eolian harp favored by Romantic poets, which uses breezes playing across metal wires to create a natural music, even as his fountain taps into Romantic images of creative, harmonious, healing, restorative nature. He positions his imaginary hospital facing west, so as to catch the irradiation of the fiery sunset. Fire, air, and water, in this artful placement, create a context that transforms mere hospital bricks into the fourth and final element that the ancients believed to make up the universe: earth. "What is brick, after all," Selzer writes, "but the earth taken up, molded and burnt in the fire. Each brick is a fragment of the planet" (93). Selzer constructs his hospital on aesthetic principles that make it a place where patients come to heal—or to die—in "mysterious correspondence" (94) with the natural world. It reflects the vision of a writer who spent his life as a surgeon in buildings constructed on exactly opposite principles, as if the sole purpose of medical architecture were to shut nature out.

Is there a "correspondence" between nature, aesthetics, and health? One study of the importance of windows—conducted at six hospitals—found a "pronounced" preference among patients for "visual contact with nature."[24] In another study, patients whose windows faced a natural setting fared much better than patients whose windows faced a brick wall: they had shorter postoperative hospital stays, received fewer negative evaluations from nurses, and took fewer potent analgesics.[25] Perhaps visual contact with nature is enough to promote healing. Rachel and Stephen Kaplan in *The Experience of Nature: A Psychological Perspective* (1989) argue persuasively that natural settings promote what they call "restorative experiences." Beyond historical taste or cultural bias, our desire to escape to the mountains and seashore—or just to have a room with a view— seems to reflect needs for contact with the natural world that take their origin far back in the history of human evolution.

The so-called biophilia hypothesis, proposed in 1984 by eminent Harvard biologist Edward O. Wilson, holds that the love of nature is not an acquired taste but a built-in human need. Wilson contends that our contemporary response to nature is the product of a long, complex process of genetic and cultural "co-evolution."[26] That is, much as deer, buffalo, and hippopotamus have taken shape through their extended history of interaction with their particular local environments, *Homo sapiens* is the product of millions of years of evolution in which protohuman brains and nervous systems developed in concert with the natural world. Small wonder, despite rockets to the moon, that so many people feel strangely drawn to the savanna-like settings where early hominids evolved the traits and practiced the skills necessary for survival. The biophilia hypothesis further assumes that the ancient human relation to nature extends beyond a need for material sustenance and for conditions that favor survival. It encompasses a need for satisfactions that are aesthetic, intellectual, and even spiritual.

Solid evidence in favor of the biophilia hypothesis comes from psychological studies in human preference and aversion. Ideas of human beauty, it appears, are not wholly fashioned by culture (as much current thinking would claim) but reflect a built-in genetic tendency to prefer faces whose symmetries are linked to advantageous traits such as disease resistance, health, fertility, and youth.[27] The flip side of preference is aversion, and research suggests that—just as monkeys and apes demonstrate a strong natural fear of snakes—humans seem predisposed to avoid settings and objects that constitute a threat to our survival. When was the last moonless night you strolled down a long dark alley?

Most important, the biophilia hypothesis, with its proposal that evolution has predisposed humans to need contact with the natural world, holds crucial implications for our ideas of health and illness. It suggests that if we deprive humans of restorative natural settings and force them to spend their lives in environments not conducive to competent functioning, they will fall prey to aesthetic, cognitive, and spiritual dissatisfactions that frequently coincide with or even create illness. Certainly, it is an accepted fact in real estate that homes with the best views or in the most impressive natural settings command the highest prices, so that we affirm with our checkbooks the value of aesthetically pleasing landscapes. For people in urban slums, the link between landscape and competent functioning works in reverse. Their poor health is at least in part a function of their damaged environments. Three recent studies in the *New England Journal of Medicine* offer much to consider in our relationship to the changing postmodern landscape: air pollution can shorten human lives by up to two years; drive-by shootings are an important cause of early morbidity and mortality among children and adolescents in Los Angeles; and degraded environments show a strong correlation with birth defects.[28] People who live in unpolluted, nonthreatening, aesthetically pleasing natural settings—so the biophilia hypothesis predicts—will enjoy better health than people living in polluted, threatening, ugly, degraded environments. Is this idea really so hard to accept?

It is of course poor people and ethnic minorities who are almost always forced to live in the worst conditions, where human-produced
hazards degrade the environment and subvert health. A community
of desperately poor people, including many children, lives atop Mexico City's main garbage dump, where starvation vies with disease as
the more immediate threat. While poverty almost guarantees exposure to environmental dangers, so too does race. Among children in
American inner cities, bronchial asthma is often caused by an allergic
reaction to proteins in the saliva and feces of cockroaches—insects at
home in the urban decay that so often entraps racial minorities.[29] Life
amid vermin, toxic chemicals, hazardous waste, and the disease-
bearing rubbish of industrial development is a fate that the wealthy
escape and that disproportionately befalls communities of color.[30]

It is hard to summarize our perverse relation to the earth in a single image, but one candidate is regularly overlooked. Worldwide,
some 100 million unexploded land mines have been left behind after
conflicts end, daily crippling civilians, mostly poor and nonwhite, often children. Land mines in Cambodia alone have maimed nearly
thirty thousand people.[31] The agony and bleak futures of children
with their legs blown off are no accident, as *White Noise* reminds us.
Only the identity of the victim is left to chance. Postmodern warfare
has greatly improved our destructive powers, employing high-tech
explosive plastics, for example, invisible to metal detectors. Progress
through international agreements in banning the use of land mines
seems imminent, despite U.S. resistance, but weapons experts will no
doubt invent even more ingenious means of turning the environment
into a source of random injury or death. It is their job.

Land mines (like the chemically defoliated forests of Vietnam)
stand as instructive metaphors for the human-created postmodern
environmental damage all around us. Or consider a nonmilitary image. British researchers have concluded that nearly two-thirds of the
mortalities from sudden infant death syndrome (SIDS) are linked to
tobacco smoke. The risk of SIDS increases 800 percent if a baby is
merely carried into a room where people have been smoking.[32] Land

mines make more noise, but the indoor environment is no less effective as a killing machine.

COMING PLAGUES?

If you really want to scare yourself, you can find plenty of recent evidence that the planet holds enough deadly viruses and bacteria to turn your neighborhood into a charnel house. More important, especially as regards a biocultural view of illness, human activities are intimately related to the recent spread of lethal microbes. As Laurie Garrett explains in *The Coming Plague: Newly Emerging Diseases in a World Out of Balance* (1994), our risk of disease has not increased over the centuries in a direct linear relationship with increases in the human population.[33] At some point, of course, many more people usually means more illness, since disease thrives in crowded quarters and in the havoc created by competition for scarce resources. The relation between population and the risk of disease fluctuates in response to complex biological rhythms that we do not yet fully understand. It remains clear, however, that history is not a record of ever decreasing risk. Cultural forces and human activities can decisively alter the nonlinear relationship between *Homo sapiens* and the world of microbes.

The new or revitalized killer diseases that have recently emerged— with AIDS simply the most dramatic example—confront us with numerous difficulties in understanding our relation to the changed postmodern environment. As we have seen, Legionnaires' disease spreads through a different mechanism (air-conditioning systems work just fine) than does the New Mexico Hanta virus, spread by mice and other rodents. So far the Ebola virus (or "the flesh-eating virus," as the tabloids love to call it) attacks a different population than does the staphylococcal strain responsible for toxic shock syndrome. One indirect source of current illness is, as we have seen, the success of medical research in nearly eradicating various ancient microbial diseases. The mosquito that bites a vaccinated child carries away a microscopic quantity of vaccine: vaccines, in effect, have become part of the environment. In a postmodern health care system where patients overdemand and doctors overprescribe powerful drugs, we spawn new strains of mutant bacteria immune or highly resistant to current antibiotics. Tuberculosis is on the rise among urban heroin addicts in the United States, and malaria constitutes a serious threat to public health in Africa, where it is now the main cause of death. Microbes are not stable targets but organisms capable of quicksilver adaptation to changes in the environment, including changes introduced by the so-called wonder drugs designed to eradicate them.

No disease illustrates more clearly than AIDS the danger that humans face from an environment defined in part by the ever changing microorganisms that inhabit and create it. AIDS would not have attained its present grim status without the intricate interaction between biology and culture. Culture, for example, provided the chief means for spreading the human immunodeficiency virus that causes AIDS—through blood transfusions, contaminated needles used to inject illegal drugs, and unprotected sexual activity. The speed with which HIV spread across the globe required systems of transportation capable of moving people rapidly over vast distances. It also required large centers of population through which a virus can spread efficiently. The postmodern era has witnessed an upsurge of megacities (cities with a population over ten million) unprecedented in the history of the planet. In 1950 New York and London were the earth's only cities with populations over ten million. By the turn of the century there will be at least twenty-four megacities, including Cairo, Buenos Aires, Beijing, Calcutta, Jakarta, Tehran, Bangkok, Manila, Istanbul, and Mexico City.[34] Postmodern microbes are as international as postmodern cuisine.

The postmodern environment is dominated not only by huge cities but also by the cultural life that they support. Megacities as centers of international commerce draw people from all over the earth. They acquire masses of poor people whose hard lives make them magnets for illness and crime. Big-city prostitution, for example, has created ideal conditions for spreading sexually transmitted diseases. A newly mobile workforce facilitated the spread of HIV throughout Africa: workers infected in cities by prostitutes returned on weekends to spread the infection in their local villages. When it arrived in America, HIV found a convenient route of transmission through the social practices of intravenous drug users and of gay males. Indeed, culture shaped the transmission of HIV not only through specific institutions such as gay bathhouses in San Francisco but also through the sexual freedom of gays who felt released from centuries of repression and legal persecution. By 1983, just a few years after it first appeared in the United States, AIDS had killed over twelve hundred Americans, and the numbers soon shot upward.

In short, although AIDS kills because HIV undermines the body's resistance to disease, we cannot understand AIDS solely through research in microbiology. We also need to consider a culture that includes jet planes, prostitutes, politicians, intravenous drug users, bathhouses, and sexual mores favorable to multiple partners, to name only a few important contributing factors. (Of course, HIV is also transmitted by heterosexual partners, as is the rule in Africa; worldwide, 70 to 75 percent of all transmissions occur through heterosexual contact, while in the United States women and minorities comprise the two fastest-growing HIV-positive groups.) Variations in patterns of infection across groups and regions reflect differing cultural practices as much as the adaptability of the virus. Culture even dictates who will benefit from the new multiple drug therapies employing protease inhibitors. With treatment costs running about fifteen thousand dollars each year, Americans will live longer while Africans die sooner, simply because annual expenditures for health care in Malawi, for example, average three dollars per person.[35] Prevention remains the surest course for avoiding AIDS, and it too requires cultural processes, especially education. AIDS, in a classic illustration of how illness is created at the crossroads of biology and culture, shows us how postmodern life forces a reconsideration of the intimate and complex relations between microbes and the humanly reconstructed environment.

CIVILIZATION AND FOLLY

Our health, then, is related to our environments in ways we are just beginning to understand. As we increase our efforts to engineer the landscape to conform with human specifications, we also seem to increase the general level of illness. There are of course conspicuous success stories; some U.S. cities have improved the quality of their air, forests have returned to the northeast, and the drainage of swamps has prevented the breeding of malarial mosquitoes. Yet some successes substitute gains in one region for losses in another. Draining swamps reduces malaria, but the loss of wetlands leads to increased salinity of coastal waters, with corresponding damage to marine ecosystems. Asthma has increased steadily in the twentieth century—doubling in the last two decades—annually affecting some thirteen million Americans and causing nearly five thousand deaths. It now appears that childhood infections protect against asthma, so that medical success in reducing childhood infections may actually fuel the epidemic of asthma.[36] Success at reducing smoke pollution in industrial nations has masked the problem of fine particles (known as PM10 particles) still circulating in the lower atmosphere and linked with respiratory symptoms in children, pneumonia in the elderly, cardiovascular disease, immune system disorders, and premature mortality.[37] More ominous, modest gains for environmental quality in the developed world may be completely offset by accelerating damage in China, India, Africa, South America, and other populous developing regions.

The main point is that, although life expectancy has increased, a high-tech, energy-dependent, consumer lifestyle has not brought the developed world a period of unprecedented health. Historian Roy Porter rightly warns against the facile and long-standing prejudice that equates civilization with the spread of disease.[38] The serious question is not about the health value of civilization but about what kind of civilized society we want. Along with their benefits, unfortunately, affluence, technological development, and biomedical progress

in Western nations have accompanied the rise of new or intensified illnesses. By-products of development have in fact left industrial nations
vulnerable to a growing list of maladies that bodes ill for future generations, and almost any newspaper can provide a survey of bad news
from the front lines:

> Human sperm counts have dropped 50 percent worldwide since
> 1938, according to a Danish study.
>
> A high number of babies with testicular malformations were born to
> mothers who had eaten beef tainted with the chemical fire-retardant
> PBB.[39]

Testicular cancer is rising sharply in the United States and Europe,
with dramatic geographical variations that suggest environmental
causes for the rise. For example, although testicular cancer has risen
300 percent in Denmark since the 1930s, the rate is unchanged in Fin-
land. One possible explanation: Denmark relies heavily on farming
and Danes are regularly exposed to agricultural pesticides, while Fin-
land is nonagricultural.[40]

Some damage reaches humans only indirectly, in the form of lost
resources and diminished opportunity, but the effect on health can be
devastating. In just two decades, industrial overfishing has turned
the once fertile Grand Banks off Newfoundland into a biological
wasteland. The abundant North Atlantic cod (which helped under-
write the early economy of New England, as commemorated in the
name Cape Cod) is now all but wiped out, a loss that not only alters
forever the ecology of the ocean but also eradicates an important
source of protein and twenty thousand local jobs, with their contribution to the welfare of fishing families.[41] How much of our touted
health care system is engaged simply in repairing the damage we do
to fellow humans when, through ignorance or greed, we degrade our
own environment?

Civilization, as the roster of new and revived diseases makes clear,
is not synonymous with health. Traditional hunter-gatherer bands
normally achieve high levels of nutrition without great effort. Small

populations, low density, and limited contact with other groups greatly reduce the opportunity for viruses to take hold; nomadic lifestyles prevent bacterial infections that stem from accumulated waste; general health is good. Only when hunter-gatherers temporarily or permanently relocate to cities does their health deteriorate. As anthropologist Mark Nathan Cohen observes, the influenza virus cannot easily survive outdoors but is quickly transmitted within the houses built by sedentary peoples. Fleas and certain other parasites thrive indoors where their life cycles are not interrupted by continual movement. When humans domesticated animals, the gains (especially in eliminating seasonal hunger) turned out to be a loss for health. "Measles," writes Cohen, "apparently originated as rinderpest among cattle or distemper among dogs; smallpox came from cattle (but possibly from monkeys); influenza from pigs or chickens; the common cold from horses; diphtheria from cattle. Most human respiratory viruses probably arose only after animals were domesticated."[42] Ancient or modern, health has much to do with the environments we inhabit and construct.

The growing recognition that illness is closely linked to our environment raises the urgent need for new thinking. "The natives of the rain," as the sage modernist poet Wallace Stevens put it, "are rainy men."[43] What illnesses are endemic to the postmodern natives of freeways and supermarkets and station wagons? What would change if we shifted from a human-centered perspective to an earth-centered view in which the health of individuals was understood only in the context of healthy or unhealthy ecosystems? Despite some progress, medicine has moved slowly in recognizing how human illness is intimately related not only to earth, sky, and sea but also to the great indoors. One important exception is *Critical Condition: Human Health and the Environment* (1993), written by four physicians, which compares our situation today with the grave peril during the Cold War, when we faced the threat of nuclear annihilation. "The world now faces a similar threat to human health and survival," the authors of *Critical Condition* conclude, "from changes to the global environment—stratospheric ozone depletion, habitat destruction, species extinction, global warming, and the poisoning of air, water, and soil by toxic and radioactive substances."[44]

Although the danger is quite real, a language of apocalypse tends to mask the most significant peril. What threatens us is not the end of the world, not the elimination of all life in a single cataclysmic mushroom cloud, but rather a gradual, unending, cumulative deterioration in the name of progress. In a world grown jaded to disaster, environmental degradation is a particularly insidious foe because we live with its damage every day, because it is a nightmare so familiar it recedes from view like scenes of inner-city blight. There is no single, all-purpose, photogenic villain. The enemies are everywhere and include each hapless or heedless consumer. A language of fright may doubly defeat reform both because it sounds so stale and because it offends our inherent presumption of innocence. How could *we* be the cause of something so awful?

Environment is the unnoticed, inescapable white noise that surrounds and interpenetrates postmodern illness. As *Critical Condition* shows in a sober sequence of tables and statistics, we face an unprecedented threat from environmental changes created and sustained by humans. Optimists who believe that technology will always save us from our errors and blindness might recall that Victor Frankenstein was a student of medicine and science. They might also reflect that no technical breakthrough in the annals of biomedicine has yet solved a problem so basic in its links to our cultural environment as the mounting epidemic of chronic pain.

chapter four

Reinventing Pain

Nature has placed mankind under the governance

of two sovereign masters, *pain* and *pleasure*. It is for

them alone to point out what we ought to do, as

well as to determine what we shall do.

JEREMY BENTHAM,
Principles of Morals and Legislation (1789)

Pain is no doubt as ancient as illness. Unlike carpal tunnel syndrome or repetitive stress injuries, it has presumably accompanied humankind right from the start, playing a crucial role in making us who we are. Jeremy Bentham, the great-grandfather of utilitarian thinking, saw pain (along with pleasure) as a basis not only for morality and law but also for everything we do. In his metaphor, pain holds sway over individual lives much as a sovereign rules a state. It governs us, that is, not only when it appears in full regalia, displaying its power like a king at a banquet, but also when it remains behind the scenes, remote and invisible; its presence is diffused through a thousand daily acts such as the caution we exercise stepping across an icy patch of sidewalk.[1] We would have to rewrite the rules of survival in a painless world. Illness, too, would be completely altered. Among its other functions and burdens central to the experience of illness, pain serves as the most common symptom that brings patients to doctors.

The argument that postmodern illness is somehow distinctive will prove hollow or at least deeply limited unless pain too occupies a distinctive place, while a demonstration that pain holds a distinctive place in the contemporary world will go far toward supporting claims for the unique historical character of postmodern illness. The stakes are high, but not so high as for individual patients who find themselves in the grip of what Bentham called the "sovereign" power of pain. Imagine, given our reliance on the invisible and diffuse presence of pain to regulate our lives, the deep crisis a person must experience when pain, inexplicably, seems to go crazy. The postmodern chronic pain patient lives on the borders of just such an anarchic, irrational world, as if inhabiting a land where sovereign power has fallen into the hands of a tyrant or terrorist. Such intractable pain no longer governs a life, in Bentham's sense, but plunges the sufferer into a frightening chaos from which death may seem a desirable release.

The basis of postmodern medical thinking about pain is a distinction between acute and chronic. We know what to expect from acute pain: it comes and goes, more or less predictably, its stay measured in hours or days or (for severe cases) weeks. Usually a few aspirin tablets will reduce the hurt or send it on its way. Chronic pain, by contrast, lingers, torments, and threatens to stay forever. It can look familiar—taking on the appearance of endless headaches, backaches, and aching joints—or it can adopt bizarre forms such as the "phantom limb" pain felt by amputees in a missing arm or leg. Its differences are so vast that chronic pain generally demands wholly unique therapies: medications effective for acute pain often simply multiply the problems facing chronic pain patients. Almost unknown as a diagnosis in medical writings before the twentieth century, chronic pain now grips so many people in the postmodern era that it is commonly and justifiably described as an epidemic. Such chronic pain can depress the immune system and destroy cancer-fighting cells in animals. It has driven people to suicide. In short, it can kill.[2] Thus, although its antiquity would seem to make pain the preeminent symbol of a timeless and universal affliction, we need to recognize in what ways its changing social and medical history transforms pain into an emblem of the new world of postmodern illness.

THE DIMENSIONS OF CRISIS

"Chronic pain has torn my life apart." So writes a typical chronic pain sufferer.[3] The destructive force of pain is inevitably played out within the privacy of an individual life. Pain is always a subjective, personal experience, and our developing insight into its sharable and intersubjective dimensions can never fully penetrate the mystery of a single human consciousness. Yet we do possess some reliable data that help sketch the magnitude of this new postmodern epidemic. We know, for example, that chronic pain may expand to fill the patient's entire being and create permanent disability. Quality of life measurably plummets. A life filled with intractable pain is not merely arduous and disordered but very likely pathological. Patients suffering from chronic low back pain—the most common form of nonmalignant chronic pain—experience rates of depression three to four times higher than those of the general population.[4] The social costs, moreover, are immense. Figures worked out in the early 1990s showed that pain in the United States alone—experienced in various conditions from headaches to cancer—causes more than 900 million lost workdays each year at a total cost to the economy of some $120 billion.[5]

An accurate sense of the crisis would require us to investigate the human lives behind every statistic, but the figures alone are alarming. For example, some twenty million people in the United States suffer from arthritis and another seven million from low back pain. About 3 percent of Americans experience daily headaches, and 10 percent suffer weekly headaches. Every day one in six Americans is in pain. The National Center for Health Statistics estimated that in 1988 one-quarter of the population experienced moderate to excruciating pain that required major therapy such as opioid narcotics. Nineteen percent of Americans were partially disabled by pain for periods of weeks or months, while another 2 percent were permanently disabled.[6] Low back pain is a consummate postmodern malady. Although impairments of the back and spine are rare in developing countries, where they are perhaps simply unreported or (because only limited help is available) ignored, such impairments are, in the West, the most frequent cause of limited activity in persons under age forty-five; for all ages, they rank behind only heart disease and osteoarthritis as the cause of disability payments to workers.[7]

All this faceless pain produces another measurable reflection in the desperate and often compulsive search for relief. In 1989 Americans spent $1 billion for prescription analgesics and another $2.2 billion for over-the-counter painkillers. Meanwhile, the annual world output of aspirin stands at a staggering thirty thousand tons. This mountain of pills suggests that pain is not receding under the assault of biomedical science but consolidating its position as an immovable force. A postmodern theory of pain will need to suggest why this is so—and the explanation, as we will see, involves changes in culture rather than in biology. Pain is immovable and monolithic—but not homogeneous. Not all pain is the same. There are almost as many different varieties of pain as roses, from the everyday cramp and ache of arthritis to the terrifying sense among sufferers of panic disorder that their chests are about to explode. (Cancer pain in particular has a distinctive profile.) We seem in no danger of running out of pain despite a cornucopia of biomedical publications and overflowing medicine cabinets. As the statistics mount, they add solid weight to Norman Cousins's intuitive claim—based in part on his struggle with a painful spinal ailment finally diagnosed as ankylosing spondilitis— that no form of illiteracy in the United States is more widespread or costly than ignorance about pain: "what it is, what causes it, how to deal with it without panic."[8]

The public ignorance and confusion simply mirror the situation within medicine. No sound education exists even for doctors. A 1988 study of British medical schools revealed that four schools had no teaching about intractable pain and the others averaged just over three hours in five years.[9] John J. Bonica, founding president of the International Association for the Study of Pain, reviewed seventeen top textbooks in medicine, surgery, and oncology looking for a "detailed description of the symptomatic treatment of acute postoperative, post-traumatic, visceral, and cancer pain." How seriously did these textbooks consider pain? They gave it just one-half of one percent of the available space.[10] In a 1989 interview Bonica bluntly described the general situation in medical education, saying, "No medical school has a pain curriculum."[11] We should not expect a quick solution. Writing in 1995 in the *Journal of the American Medical Association*, C. Stratton Hill Jr. observed: "Medical school curricula are woefully lacking in teaching medical students treatment of acute pain and the complexities of chronic pain treatment."[12]

We are left, then, with a large-scale crisis of pain that our systems of public and professional education have so far been unable to address effectively. They are ineffectual partly because, whether through error or silence, they perpetuate the limitations of the standard biomedical model that over the past two centuries we have absorbed into our cultural thinking about pain. So long as we continue to think of pain according to the biomedical model as no more than the result of an electrochemical signal sent along nerve fibers from the site of tissue damage to the brain, we have little recourse as sufferers but to continue the search for drugs and other therapies that block the transmission of pain signals. Such drugs, as everyone can testify who has received novocaine for tooth repairs, prove effective in stopping short-term acute pain, but they are far less effective against chronic pain. What we need—beyond more efficient use of available medications—is a medical community and a general public who understand the postmodern reinvention of pain. Pain can no longer be adequately described or treated on the assumptions of the old biomedical model. It demands a new model that is—under whatever name—biocultural.

THE PARADOX OF DRUGS AND MEANING

Inevitably, headlines about pain focus on the dangers and advantages of drugs. Drugs seem inseparable from our thinking about pain—and for good reasons. Doctors today have at their disposal elaborate and powerful new drug therapies, especially opiates and opiate-like narcotics, which for difficult pain problems associated with cancer, for example, are often prescribed together with traditional anti-inflammatory analgesics and with other medications that possess analgesic side effects, such as tricyclic antidepressants, anticonvulsants, and benzodiazepines. Specialists argue that effective drug therapies can control the pain of terminal cancer in 95 percent of all cases, and oncologists are now taught that there is no standard or ceiling dose of morphine.[13] As long as the side effects are tolerated, the correct dose is the amount of morphine sufficient to relieve the pain. You would think, then, that cancer patients no longer face the prospect of dying in pain. You would be wrong.

The problem of undermedication for pain has been well documented since the pioneering study in 1973 by Richard M. Marks and Edward J. Sachar that demonstrated the failure of physicians to use effective narcotic analgesics for medical inpatients.[14] More than two decades after Marks and Sachar reported their findings, the situation remains more or less unchanged. The U.S. Department of Health and Human Services reported in 1994 that cancer pain goes "frequently undertreated." Authoritative appraisal puts the undertreatment of cancer pain at a consistent 50 percent of cases. Twenty-five percent of cancer patients are estimated to die in severe, unrelieved pain. The dilemma of inadequate pain treatment is not restricted to cancer patients. An extensive study published in 1996 found that, judging by the reports of family members, 50 percent of seriously ill, hospitalized patients died in moderate to severe pain. After alerting hospital staff to the problem and after undertaking measures to provide better communication between doctors and patients, the investigators repeated the study to measure anticipated improvements in the treatment of pain. They found that absolutely nothing had changed.[15]

Patients today unnecessarily suffer and die in severe pain, despite authoritative data warning doctors of the regular tendency to undermedicate. Patients in earlier eras of course also suffered and died in pain. What makes this pain postmodern is the bitter irony that in almost all cases effective medications are available but not used.

What can account for the paradox of undertreated pain? We live in a culture where illegal drug use is a major nationwide crisis responsible for enormous social damage, from the wreckage caused by addicts and criminals to the wasted lives of children. Some medical undertreatment doubtless stems from fears that opiates and opioids will prove addictive, but these fears are in large part groundless. A well-known study puts the rate of addiction among hospital patients at less than one-tenth of one percent.[16] Even if addiction were more than a remote likelihood, what possible reason is there for fearing to addict patients who have only a few days or weeks to live? In the absence of effective medical education, physicians simply reproduce the myths and misinformation about pain that circulate in the general culture. In fact, because clinical teaching about pain is left mostly to interns and residents, misinformation and cultural biases are (in the words of pain specialist C. Stratton Hill Jr.) "systematically transferred from one generation of physicians to another."[17] Zealous and misguided governmental policies that tightly restrict the medical use of opioids simply make a bad situation worse—not only punishing innocent patients but punishing them even on their deathbeds. Pain always relies on biological processes, of course, but it is culture and its myths that dictate whether we will effectively address—or else ignore and misconstrue—the biology of pain.

Patients, absorbing the medical mythology of their culture, are often no less wary of opiates and opioids than are many doctors. This power of culture over illness is easy to recognize in a non-Western example. Children in Japan who refuse to attend school and thus vio-

late an overriding Japanese cultural norm are diagnosed with a condition called "school-refusal syndrome." Similarly, well-informed
Western physicians who prescribe effective doses of opiates and opioids can encounter in patients an aversion to narcotics so deep-seated
in its cultural sources that it could merit inventing a new diagnosis
called "drug-refusal syndrome." Yet it is not just narcotics that arouse
mixed attitudes in setting off fears of addiction within a drug-taking
culture. Pain too has an ambiguous double status. As subjective and
intangible, pain always runs a risk of getting dismissed as unreal
when unconfirmed by tests and biomedical data. Further, in our defiantly material culture, anything erasable by two aspirin tablets
hardly seems serious or substantial. Finally, a persistent puritan ethos
and frontier mentality in the American character can make it seem
godly, or at least manly, to endure pain. Pain builds character. No
pain, no gain. Such cultural platitudes, while usually harmless and
occasionally even helpful, prove deeply injurious when they encourage patients to resist medications proven effective in the treatment of
intractable pain. The pain they experience owes as much to their cultures as to their nervous systems.

This tangled knot of cultural assumptions creates the paradoxical
view reported in one recent survey of the American public: too little
is being done to relieve pain, and we take too many drugs. As often
happens, the public is both confused and correct.[18] The confusion
carries over to questions about the possible meanings of pain. It is a
standard assumption of the biomedical model that pain has no meaning. British gerontologist Ray Tallis expresses the prevailing opinion:
"I have a prejudice against pain," he writes, "believing that, once it
has done its job of warning us of danger, it is meaningless."[19] This
prejudice (as Tallis rightly calls it) represents the victory of science
over earlier explanatory systems such as religion, philosophy, and
folklore that in effect saturated pain with meaning. Pain was regarded, for example, as a sign of original sin, a test of faith, a means
of redemption. It stood for the virtue of difficult choices, the vice of
evil choices, and the common humanity that binds us together in sor-
row.[20] To be sure, pain is meaningless if we view it as merely a prod-

uct of the transmission of an electrochemical signal (what specialists call "nociception"). Pain from this perspective is chiefly a problem in biochemistry, with no more meaning than a dysfunctional alarm bell. Most patients today obligingly accept the official biomedical assumption that their pain is a meaningless shuttle of internal impulses associated with some sort of visible or invisible tissue damage.

Unfortunately, despite the belief that pain is meaningless, patients (as we will soon see) continue to make meanings out of their pain, most often unknowingly, so that their confusion and uncertainty simply deepen as the pain persists. Lives are not only torn apart but also plunged into self-contradiction, chaos, and despair. Stories about emergence from this darkness have the air of an ascent from the underworld.

A WHOLE NEW LIFE

Reynolds Price is a distinguished American postwar novelist. His success has included a lifetime of teaching young writers at Duke University, and as he walked across campus on a late spring day in 1984 a colleague noticed that his gait had oddly changed. The almost invisible shuffle in his step was the first sign of an illness soon diagnosed as spinal cancer. A tumor the size of an eel had worked its way down his spine, leaving no choice but an aggressive course of surgery and radiation. After three surgeries, a surgical repair, and five weeks of burning radiation at the highest possible level, the cancer was under control, but Reynolds Price had forever lost the use of his legs. His slow adjustment to life in a wheelchair was not the worst of his challenges. The combination of surgery and radiation had damaged his central nervous system in such a way that he was left in constant and almost unbearable pain. (Pain caused by damage originating in the central nervous system—as sometimes happens in stroke and multiple sclerosis—is called central pain.) Doctors at the pain clinic in the university hospital put him on a set of drugs, including the synthetic opiate methadone, which had no effect except to cloud his mind. When he sought help from his neurologist, he found what many chronic pain sufferers discover: conventional biomedicine, when drugs prove ineffectual, has little to offer. "Pain," he wrote after meeting with his diagnosing neurologist, "is something they turn from in embarrassed impotence."[21]

The pain in fact had transformed the life of Reynolds Price far more radically than his paraplegia did. Describing his status three full years after his first surgery, he wrote: "The pain was high and all-pervading from neck to feet; it generally peaked in blinding storms late in the day if I was tired. It intensified in conditions of low barometric pressure; and for dozens of other mysterious reasons, by now it had seized frank control of my mind, my moods and my treatment of friends. Patience had ebbed to its lowest reach" (151). It is a nadir that chronic pain patients know too well. The turning point for Price came when— with the guidance of Duke researchers Francis Keefe and Betty Wolfe—he began to work with biofeedback technologies in learning to control his body temperature through focused thought. Soon he could raise the temperature in one hand by eight degrees and relax the tense muscle fibers in his shoulders and neck. Keefe and Wolfe then suggested he proceed to hypnosis, whereupon his progress was even more dramatic. With the guidance of his hypnotherapist, he focused his thought on distancing the pain until, almost miraculously, for the first time in three years he felt like a free man.

It is worth hearing in Price's words the unusual sense in which he can consider himself pain free:

> Within that limited stretch of biofeedback and hypnosis, no more than eight weeks, I'd grown essentially free from pain. Not free from its constant presence in my body—it roars on still, round the clock every day, in my back and legs and across my shoulders—but free from any real notice of it or concern for its presence, not to speak of the dread and the idiot regimen it forced upon me through three long years. And to be true to present reality, I can honestly say that now still, six years after approaching my mind for the help it could give, in an average sixteen-hour day, I'm conscious of being disturbed by pain for maybe a total of a quarter hour—in scattered minutes, here and there, at this job or that. (157)

What vanishes for Price is not the pain but the confusion and chaos that it so often creates. Or, more accurately, when the chaos and confusion vanish, pain loses the power to tear a life apart. Price achieved his breakthrough not with drugs and surgeries, which in fact had aggravated his pain, but by using his mind. His discovery of the mind's role proved pivotal in allowing him to escape a drug-fogged underworld of constant pain and to begin creating a life he calls not only new but (in a word deeply associated with multiple levels of healing) whole.

The terrible journey that Reynolds Price had to make back to wholeness might be illuminated by examining how Western science created the biomedical model upon a rigorous Cartesian split between bodies and minds. Descartes influentially explained pain through the bodily mechanisms now called nociception, and this explanation allowed doctors to dump all the clumsy, contradictory, prescientific baggage that had associated pain with meaning (especially with religious meaning). When pain was thus officially emptied of meaning, the mind was simultaneously recast as a passive spectator of the body's woe, which now conveyed the same simple single message supplied by an alarm bell: something is wrong. It is exactly this reductive biomedical model of pain that Price found he needed to evade and rewrite. "Like most human minds," he explains, "my own was programmed from birth and reinforced in the cradle with the certainty that *Pain means trouble*—a finger's burned, a knife has cut me, stop everything and tend to both the wound and its cause; then the pain will relent" (158–59). It is this minimal level of biomedically reduced and reinforced meaning that we all bring to pain. What Price came to learn was the need to replace the single, programmed, reductive, biomedical meaning with a complicated, paradoxical, personal meaning: *"The harm is done. It cannot be repaired; pain signifies nothing. Begin to ignore it"* (159).

Price's statement that "pain signifies nothing" is very different from the Cartesian view that pain is meaningless. The whole point of Price's life-saving discovery lies in his recognition that the mind does not function as a passive spectator but plays a crucial role in the construction or reconstruction of pain. His personal discovery in fact parallels the breakthrough of researchers and clinicians who have come to insist, in opposition to the biomedical model, that human pain is not a sensation but a perception dependent upon the mind's active ongoing power to make sense of experience. The primacy that biomedicine assigns to nociception dissolves under analysis. Nociception is neither necessary nor sufficient to create pain. As neurosurgeon John D. Loeser writes, in what can be interpreted as a farewell to the biomedical model: "The brain is the organ responsible for all pain." "All sensory phenomena," he adds, "including nociception, can be altered by conscious or unconscious mental processes."[22] The mind's power to alter nociception makes pain far more complex than a one-message Cartesian alarm bell, and awareness of this complex power—which can augment as well as relieve affliction—creates an understanding so remote from standard biomedical lore that it might be said to open up a whole new world of postmodern pain.

POSTMODERN PAIN

The change in thinking about pain currently under way requires not that we wholly abandon everything contained in the biomedical model—which consolidates several centuries of invaluable research about the human nervous system—but rather that we absorb it into a more comprehensive model that I am calling biocultural. This more inclusive perspective entails four specific claims that I have discussed in detail elsewhere:

1. Pain is more than a medical issue and more than a matter of nerves and neurotransmitters.
2. Pain has historical, psychological, and cultural dimensions.
3. Meaning is often fundamental to the experience of pain.
4. Minds and cultures (as makers of meaning) have a powerful influence on the experience of pain, for better or worse.[23]

Doctors wedded to a Cartesian view of pain that splits mind from body—a view implicit in the mechanistic biomedical model—will find these four propositions instantly counterintuitive, if not just plain wrong. Patients well schooled in a culture built upon the bio-medical model tend to resist them as well. Yet, as the experience of Reynolds Price indicates, the gains that come with a biocultural em-phasis on powers of the mind may save the life of patients whom drugs and surgery cannot help.

One advantage of a biocultural model is that it provides a far bet-ter account of chronic pain. Chronic low back pain, for example, of-ten proves impossible to trace to an organic lesion, such as a pro-lapsed (or "slipped") disk. One study examined ten thousand cases of low back injury submitted for compensation in the state of Wash-ington during 1977 and reported that 75 percent of the cases showed no physical findings.[24] As we already saw in chapter one, many adults who complain of back pain have demonstrable lumbar disk disease, but so do 70 percent of adults without complaints. Treatment can be almost as mysterious as the source of pain. An extensive study showed that long-term functioning of patients treated for back pain is similar whether doctors prescribe pain medication and bed rest or emphasize self-care and education.[25] The traditional biomedical model not only justifies countless unnecessary surgeries for back pain but also fails to explain why the strongest signs predicting that a worker will develop chronic back pain have less to do with the anatomy and physiology of the lower back than with job dissatisfac-tion and unsatisfactory social relations in the workplace.[26]

The truth is that we cannot understand chronic pain through an analysis of tissue damage alone. Current research shows how chronic pain sweeps into its domain such nonbiological contributing causes as family conflict, economic stress, and a history of emotional trauma.[27] Such often invisible blows can help transform a local in-jury—a slip in the shower or a whiplash accident—into an in-tractable torment. Sometimes the influences that contribute to chronic pain may arise from a distant past. One study showed that women suffering from irritable bowel syndrome where an organic cause was not clear proved significantly more likely than women with organic inflammatory bowel disease to report a history of severe lifetime sexual victimization.[28] Chronic pain is so resistant to traditional biomedical thinking that patients' charts swell with referrals as they shuttle helplessly from one doctor to the next. Effective treatment in many cases depends not on finding a previously undiscovered leision but on taking the time to find out what the patient is thinking.

What we think about pain matters greatly. Ancient Babylonians attributed their headaches to assaults by malign demons. Few Americans attribute their headaches to demons, but who does not sometimes feel bedeviled by stress? Harvard psychiatrst Arthur Barsky observes that a headache hurts a lot more if you attribute it to a brain tumor instead of to eyestrain.[29] In a science-based, medicalized culture, the thoughts and emotions (such as our fears of a brain tumor) that influence our pain will often be based on scientific-medical lore, even when the science is inadequate or incorrect. The (slowly) dawning awareness of the crucial role that minds, emotions, and cultures play in pain constitutes a quiet revolution destined to alter our experience, much as it changed the life of Reynolds Price. The revolution still has many doubters and opponents, however, so it is important to emphasize the rock-solid evidence that supports it. Six topics merit special attention: scientific redefinition, cross-cultural studies, interethnic studies, psychological studies, studies on pain beliefs, and problems of disability. Together they help indicate the firm new ground on which we are beginning to create a biocultural model of pain.

Definitions provide a useful index of change. At its founding in 1974, the International Association for the Study of Pain (IASP), the main organization of doctors and scientists worldwide, set up a subcommittee on taxonomy. They could not systematically advance scientific knowledge of pain, they reasoned, unless they could agree on what they were studying. There were doubtless major disagreements because the subcommittee took five years to publish its work. The most fascinating thing about the IASP definition is how it loosens up the biomedical model without entirely renouncing it. "Pain," the IASP authors write, "is an unpleasant sensory and emotional experience associated with actual or potential tissue damage, or described in terms of such damage." [30] Cartesian mind-body dualism comes under implicit rebuke in the phrase "sensory *and* emotional" experience, since human emotions are to various degrees reeducated by the processes of cultural learning. The subcommittee moreover associates pain not only with tissue damage—as in the biomedical model—but also with *potential* tissue damage and with experience described even *in terms of* tissue damage. This change demolishes the one-to-one link between pain and tissue damage assumed in the biomedical model—a link under suspicion ever since Henry K. Beecher (in his classic article on World War II battlefield injuries) described soldiers who suffered terrible wounds but experienced little or no pain.[31] The biomedical model builds expectations that pain is a simple report of tissue damage. "The truth is," writes anatomy professor Patrick D. Wall, "that pain is a very poor reporting system." [32] The IASP subcommittee noted explicitly that people often report pain in the absence of any known lesion and that pain cannot be regarded simply as the response to a noxious stimulus.

The most illuminating changes provided by the IASP subcommittee occur in a series of annotations, in which the authors emphasize that pain must be understood as "always subjective." Further, they distinguish sharply between pain and nociception: "Activity induced in the nociceptor and nociceptive pathways by a noxious stimulus," they insist, "is not pain, which is always a psychological state." [33] We should not be surprised that the revolutionary impact of these annotations gets somewhat muted in the one-sentence IASP definition. This is how committees handle controversial issues. It is common practice in the history of science to mask radical change in a traditional language that prevents outright bloodshed.

Because skeptics may persist in thinking that such lexical and conceptual changes are minor, it is useful to reflect upon a summarizing statement by pain specialist Allan I. Basbaum, professor of anatomy and physiology at the University of California, San Francisco, which carries with it the weight of considerable recent research. "Pain," he writes, "is not just a stimulus that is transmitted over specific pathways but rather a complex perception, the nature of which depends not only on the intensity of the stimulus but on the situation in which it is experienced and, most importantly, on the affective or emotional state of the individual. Pain is to somatic stimulation as beauty is to a visual stimulus. It is a very subjective experience."[34] The most important corollary or addition to Basbaum's statement: pain cannot be considered merely or only subjective. As we will see in research concerning its cross-cultural and interethnic dimensions, pain, like beauty, is intersubjective. No matter how deeply biological its place in human evolutionary development, it always involves the contribution of shared cultural forces and values.

It follows, if culture plays a role in pain, that pain should differ across cultures, and several researchers have examined cross-cultural differences in the experience of pain. One group that compared patients with low back pain in the United States and in New Zealand concluded that American patients used more medication, were more likely to receive pretreatment compensation, and experienced greater "emotional and behavioral disruption." A similar comparison of Japanese and American low back pain patients found Japanese patients significantly less impaired in "psychological, social, vocational, and avocational functioning." Still another study comparing low back pain patients in the United States, Japan, Mexico, Colombia, Italy, and New Zealand found that American patients were "clearly most dysfunctional."[35]

The connection between dysfunction and pain is extremely complex and doubtless involves elements of suffering (discussed in chapter seven). We must not oversimplify dysfunction as if it were a mere reaction *to* pain, the response to a stimulus. Rather, pain, as a lived experience, may come to *include* the culturally created and reinforced meaning that a person is dysfunctional. In Lithuania, for example, where drivers do not carry personal-injury insurance, rear-end automobile collisions fail to produce the lingering headaches and in-

tractable neck pains notorious in Western democracies, where in-
sured motorists receive compensation for chronic whiplash or
whiplash syndrome.[36] Norway, by contrast, with a total population
of 4.2 million, has 70,000 people in a patients' organization claiming
chronic disability from whiplash injuries. We are not dealing with a
simple cash-for-injury exchange, an explanation which (among other
failures) maligns sufferers often desperate to get rid of their pain. The
cultural forces at work in reinforcing pain and dysfunction include
not only various insurance programs but also distinctively postmodern developments such as self-help movements, class-action lawsuits, and politically powerful organizations of patients.

The diverse cross-cultural contexts that give pain its changing
character are quite clear when we move far beyond our borders. The
Sakhalin Ainu people of Japan, while they do not suffer whiplash injuries, distinguish among at least three different kinds of headaches:
"deer headaches" (like the light steps of running deer), "bear
headaches" (like the heavy steps of a bear), and "woodpecker
headaches" (which are self-explanatory).[37] Pain here is described primarily through sounds from the natural world of birds and animals,
while headache sufferers in the industrial world typically describe
their pain through images of jackhammers and chain saws. The difference is not merely in description but in experience. A jackhammer
headache no longer inhabits the natural world but belongs to an ur-
banized realm where people feel increasingly powerless, stressed
out, and under assault—feelings that play back into the experience
of pain.

Differences in the experience of pain—extending well beyond differences in descriptive terms—find a clear illustration in research
studying pain within specific ethnic groups. Such interethnic studies
began with Mark Zborowski's pioneering book *People in Pain* (1969),
which looked at American veterans hospitalized after World War II.
The four ethnic groups he studied—Italian Americans, Jewish Americans, Irish Americans, and a group he called "old Americans" (white,
Anglo-Saxon Protestants established in the United States for several
generations)—turned out to experience pain in ways as distinctive as

their respective cuisines. We need to keep in mind two cautions. First, Zborowski's veterans were all males. Differences in biology, as well as in cultural roles, make gender an important variable in the experience of pain: one group of opioids (known as kappa-opioids) produces significantly greater analgesia in women than in men, probably reflecting a gender difference in pain-modulating circuits.[38] Second, Zborowski's stoic Irishmen and hyperverbal Jews look today uncomfortably like cardboard stereotypes. Yet Jewish and Irish immigrants in the 1950s differ significantly from their assimilated grandchildren, raised on MTV and *Terminator II*. The *Nuprin Pain Report* (1985) finds that second- or third-generation Americans are more likely than first-generation Americans to report suffering from headaches, backaches, muscle pains, and stomach pains. Other researchers detect significant variation among ethnic groups in the emotional dimension of pain. Another team concludes that the attitudes, beliefs, and emotional or psychological states associated with specific ethnic groups may affect pain intensity.[39]

The force of such studies increases when we look at research broadly classified as psychological. Ever since the publication of *The Psychology of Pain* (1978), edited by Richard A. Sternbach and now in an expanded second edition, it has become routine to associate chronic pain with negative emotional states such as fear, loss, and anger. The specific relationship between chronic pain and clinical depression has proved elusive enough to generate a small library of studies. (Tricyclic antidepressants are effective in treating a range of chronic pain patients, but it remains unclear if chronic pain causes depression, or if depression leads to chronic pain, or if some other explanation applies.) George L. Engel's classic 1959 study found that "pain-prone" patients tended to be individuals for whom psychological conditions during childhood—often centering on punishment—create a template for adult experiences of pain and suffering. The novels of Sade, backed up by modern studies of sadomasochism, clearly indicate that some people seem compelled to inflict pain or to seek it.[40] It is no surprise to psychologists that people who feel driven toward extreme states of discipline or penance eventually find their way to pain.

The concept of psychogenic pain—pain not generated by an organic lesion—remains controversial, but a study at the Baylor College of Medicine strongly suggests that the mind plays a crucial role not merely in modifying but in creating pain. One hundred paid volunteers were told that the experiment in which they would participate involved an electric stimulator that might produce a headache. Researchers did not tell volunteers that the stimulator was rigged to produce nothing beyond a low humming sound. The result? Fifty percent of the volunteers reported pain.[41] In the absence of a painful stimulus, a perceiving mind is evidently enough to create pain. The power of the mind to generate pain is matched, of course, by a mysterious power to erase it, as we have seen in the placebo effect. The power of minds and cultures certainly underlies the odd condition known as couvade syndrome, in which the male partners of pregnant women experience various discomforts of pregnancy, including abdominal pain.[42] In the indigenous cultures where couvade is an accepted social practice, husbands often take to their beds and groan while their wives give birth in the fields.

The psychology of pain, while radiating in many directions, always leads us back to a concern with mind and meaning. Consider the malady now called somatization disorder. It is defined by multiple symptoms untraceable to an organic cause, the most common of which is pain. As women vastly outnumber men among its sufferers, some suspect that somatization disorder is merely the postmodern name for hysteria, which disappeared as a diagnosis at the beginning of the twentieth century. The origin of such pain may be impossible to determine, but professor of psychiatry G. Richard Smith, in his book-length study of somatization disorder, cites research showing that a large percentage of women with pelvic or abdominal pain report childhood incidents of sexual abuse. Psychological processes that aggravate pain can even be triggered by a medical diagnosis: patients diagnosed with arthritis reported significantly less pain than patients diagnosed with the still somewhat ambiguous condition known as myofascial disorder. Certainly, pain originating in demonstrable tissue damage can be exacerbated by events that are largely mental and emotional. For example, what psychologists call "negative cognitions," especially anger and punishing responses from family members, have been shown to increase pain in a state as undeniably organic as chronic spinal cord injury.[43]

Most psychologists agree that chronic pain always involves learning. They disagree on what exactly is learned—behaviors, beliefs, or a combination of both.[44] These disagreements would matter less if they did not affect clinical treatment. Strict behaviorists argue that the only valid aim of treatment is to change pain behaviors; when pain behaviors cease, there is no longer a medical problem. Cognitive psychologists counter that harmful beliefs about pain, if ignored, will eventually produce more somatic distress; the absence of pain behavior does not mean an absence of problems. Many treatment programs today pragmatically combine behaviorist and cognitive therapies. Cognitive therapies allow the development of coping strategies effective precisely because they fit the individual's style of thought. Behaviorist techniques break down bad habits and build up positive patterns of function. Donald S. Ciccone and Roy C. Grzesiak suggest the existence of a common ground when they argue that behaviorist techniques prove effective largely because patients develop (even if unknowingly) "new thinking skills."[45] Presumably, the development of new thinking skills through behaviorist techniques of therapy can also, in turn, lead to additional and unforeseen changes in behavior.

Pain beliefs, as researchers call them, are now explored statistically through several sophisticated instruments, including the Pain Beliefs Questionnaire.[46] These instruments are not trouble free. The Pain Beliefs Questionnaire, for example, includes items perpetuating the cultural myth that pain comes in two distinct flavors, mental and physical, whereas a biocultural questionnaire would assume that body and mind are always intermingled in the experience of pain. At Georgetown University, psychologist David A. Williams examines what he calls "core beliefs" about pain, which involve issues of self-blame, cause, and duration. Core beliefs, he argues, predict pain intensity.[47] The understandings that patients bring to chronic pain also center on the need to assign responsibility and to protect their personal identities—since prolonged pain can weaken and threaten their belief in who they are (another instance of the postmodern self under in-creased pressure).[48] Researcher Mark Jensen finds better functioning in patients who believe they have some control over their pain, who believe in the value of medical services, who believe that family members care for them, and who believe that they are not severely disabled.[49] Another study of 100 patients shows that pain beliefs cor-relate directly with treatment outcomes.[50]

Beliefs about pain prove especially important in the specific cul-tural subclass of dysfunction known as disability. As specialists in-sist, disability is not synonymous with impairment. Jim Abbot has played major league baseball despite being born without a right hand. He is impaired but not disabled. Disability is a malleable con-cept invented by Western social welfare systems to provide financial help for people officially pronounced unable to work. Inadvertently, it also offers people new and possibly damaging ways to think about their pain. In Sweden between 1952 and 1982, for example, disability status for rheumatoid arthritis (which is relatively easy to diagnose) showed no increase, whereas disability status for the more ambigu-ous and indefinite category of back injury increased almost 3,800 per-cent.[51] Perhaps Swedes endured a freakish, inexplicable thirty-year eruption of injuries to the back—a kind of miracle, like the total ab-sence of whiplash injuries in Lithuania. It seems far more likely, how-ever, that the creation of disability status with its attendant cash pay-ments has encouraged many people with back pain to believe they are disabled.

Indeed, through the invention of disability status, culture now reg-ulates pain in ways that may well increase, prolong, or even create it. As agents of the state, doctors are required not only to treat pain but also to judge whether it merits compensation—a dual role that can easily turn countertherapeutic.[52] How do you cure a patient you have already certified as disabled? A patient who receives continuing cash payments for disability has a powerful disincentive to recover. Al-though experts reject the view that pain patients with pending legal claims exhibit "compensation neurosis," legal claims for compensa-tion and disability status complicate and often impede treatment.[53] A controversial proposal included in a 1995 IASP report entitled *Back Pain in the Workplace* (edited by the distinguished pain specialist Wilbert E. Fordyce) argued for offering injured workers who show no evidence of overt damage or disease six weeks of rehabilitation and wage replacement on a "temporary disability basis"—after which they would be declared unemployed, not disabled.[54] Behind this pro-posal—a measure some IASP members protested as unscientific, heartless, and extreme—lay an unspoken awareness of the impact of culture upon pain.

There is no doubt that postmodern pain includes the radically new cultural meaning that it can be certified as disabling and exchanged for cash. This immense change—as important as the earlier use of pain to inflict legal punishment—means that we must carefully dis-tinguish whether we are talking about a person in pain, a pain pa-tient, or a claimant.[55] Each cultural status implies a different relation to pain: not everyone with pain seeks medical help, and not everyone who seeks medical help has a financial claim pending. The experi-ence of people with pain who enter the embrace of medicine or of law will differ from the experience of people who do not. No matter how hard we try, it may be hard to let go of pain that brings with it an otherwise inaccessible benefit, as when a spouse discovers that complaints of pain inspire tenderness in a long-remote mate. Effec-tive therapies to address such pain must also address the unsus-pected cultural meanings it may embody.

THE MULTIPLE VOICES OF PAIN

Once we challenge the biomedical notion that pain is meaningless, almost everywhere we look we find examples of pain saturated with meaning. An engineer at a radio station explained how pain had wrecked the marriage of her elderly parents. The wife interpreted pain as a symptom of serious illness, while her husband interpreted it as a normal sign of aging. The husband regarded his wife as a hypochondriac and a nag for worrying about their pain; the wife regarded her husband as a fool for dismissing his pain and a brute for dismissing hers. The war of conflicting pain beliefs dragged on with no end in sight. Their conflict indicates how meanings can remain almost invisible to the people who make or accept them. It also reminds us that the meanings we attribute to pain will likely change over a lifetime.

We know little, unfortunately, about pain in the elderly and about the pain of children, although researchers are beginning to explore these previously disregarded groups. Recent years have seen an attack on the long-standing medical myth—which is to say, incorrect belief—that infants do not feel pain. Most research into pain beliefs looks at people in the midlife, middle-class range, so that we simply do not know what beliefs circulate in minority groups or at the periphery. Teenagers are likely to absorb beliefs about pain expressed in films or in the lyrics to popular songs, where love "hurts so good" and self-mutilation is a badge of honor. The acceleration in teenage suicide has multiple causes, but this vulnerable group is certainly the recipient of innumerable mixed messages about pain and receives no direct education about how to deal with them.

The triumph of the biomedical model has blinded us not only to the pain beliefs explicitly dramatized in songs and films but also to the meanings implicit in such potent cultural arenas as sports and the arts. Athletes are repeatedly praised by the media for overcoming extreme pain, like the astonishing Olympic gymnast from Japan who completed his dismount with a broken leg. Yet such praise and its implicit meanings (to overcome pain is heroic) leave a difficult legacy for chronic pain patients, who cannot surmount their affliction in a supreme moment of glory but must live with it, unpraised and often unobserved, day after day. The sports credo "No pain, no gain" also implies an invisible meaning (pain is good for you), a meaning whose influence can only be debilitating to, say, a patient whose fibromyalgia disrupts her dreams of a career as a concert pianist. Obstetricians regularly tell expectant mothers that the pain of childbirth is "good pain." A professional ballerina comes to regard her bloody toes as a sign of luck, much as some cultures employ pain in rites of initiation designed to signify the passage to adulthood. Urban street gangs, however, also use pain as a rite of passage that signals the initiation of prospective members, and marine paratroopers have been videotaped pounding flight pins into the flesh of their newly graduated comrades. Even the ancient arts of body piercing and tattoo arrive in the postmodern United States bearing invisible and sometimes impenetrable meanings. The hottest fashion model in Paris, circa 1995, was twenty-one-year-old Eve Salvail, whose closely shaved head sported a large serpentine dragon tattoo. Why the tattoo? asked a reporter for *Women's Wear Daily*. Ms. Salvail replied: "It symbolizes pain."[56]

The importance of recognizing how pain inhabits a culture that infuses it with meaning lies in allowing us to reappraise possibly damaging beliefs that we have accepted, most often unknowingly. Among our most unshakable assumptions, for example, is the belief that pain comes in two varieties: mental and physical. This assumption has a commonsense logic, in that a headache clearly differs from a heartache. It also finds ready support in ordinary language, where the adjective "painful" can refer to a broken arm or a loss at chess. "This hurts me more than it hurts you," says the cartoon father as he spanks his son, employing the word *hurt* in two very different senses. A metaphorical language of hurt, however, does *not* justify a philosophical or medical distinction between mental and physical pain. Such language reminds us instead that pain is always inseparable from the cultural contexts—including especially the linguistic contexts—within which we come to understand it. When in everyday talk we distinguish so-called mental pain from physical pain, we are not reflecting carefully about the nature of pain but affirming an intuitive and accurate belief that pain can flow from emotional or psychological sources, even that pain *is* an emotion, although with profound inconsistency we reject this wisdom whenever we fear that people may misinterpret our pain (and dismiss it) as merely or wholly psychological.[57] The confusion within this everyday, inconsistent usage is precisely the confusion of a postmodern culture in which the Cartesian-based biomedical model (with its focus on tissue damage) is losing some of its force—while we remain unsure what alternative model or outlook has sufficient explanatory power to replace it.

The danger in everyday talk about "mental pain" is that the wisdom behind such usage ultimately collapses in the face of the biomedical model, with its implication that real pain is always physical. In the absence of an organic lesion or physical injury, many people find the reality of their pain much in doubt. "Mental pain" becomes another name for "no pain." Like the Victorian women whose pain was dismissed as merely hysterical, many patients today go through a demoralizing experience with doctors who conclude that the pain is not real because they cannot discover an organic lesion. The Cartesian split between mental pain and physical pain thus leads inexorably, when a confirming lesion is not found, to the dismissive comment "It's all in your head." In the grip of this false but almost unshakable distinction, real pain means physical pain, pain anchored in visible tissue damage, understood according to the biomedical model as a meaningless shuttle of electrochemical impulses. Anything else is considered mental or unreal. This Cartesian medicine is simply incorrect and out of touch with current research. Pain is always in your head, no matter what causes it. It could not possibly be anywhere else. Doctors who suggest that certain pain is imaginary or unreal or merely "mental" are just wrong. They are as out of date as scientists who believe in unicorns.

A biocultural model tells us that pain is always biological and always cultural. Pain cannot exist without employing neurotransmitters, cellular receptors, and the biological circuits associated with memory, emotion, and consciousness. It also cannot exist in humans—with the possible exception of newborn infants—unmodified by the conscious and nonconscious learning that comes through culture. Maybe the eventual triumph of a biocultural model will allow us not only to understand the mind-body connections always implicit in pain but also to respect non-Western beliefs that (through spiritual discipline or elevated consciousness) we might feel another person's pain. In any event, the task ahead goes far beyond educating doctors and patients about effective drug therapies. We must come to recognize both the complex meanings that pain can assume and the harm implicit in the erroneous belief that pain is meaningless. Pain always wraps itself in the meanings we create or accept, even when the meaning is reduced to the impoverished, modernist, biomedical belief that pain has no meaning. The relevant postmodern question is whether the beliefs and meanings that we bring to pain are accurate, positive, and helpful—or, as too often happens, inaccurate, negative, and damaging.

Postmodern illness, in moving us (however awkwardly and imperfectly) beyond the biomedical model, raises the unresolved question of who in our culture will be authorized to speak about pain. The biomedical model gave doctors the sole authorized voice. Will a biocultural model allow us to hear voices currently silent, subjugated, or forced to the margins of public discussion? One tentative answer comes from a community health center in Australia. There chronic pain patients create poems and prose pieces about their experience, some of which appeared in a slim collection entitled *People with Pain Speak Out* (1990). The radical assumption behind this collection is that the patient's voice has validity. Chronic pain often pushes sufferers into a silence so weary, resigned, defeated that the mere act of speaking or writing for a public audience no doubt has therapeutic value. The collection also demonstrates that by listening to what patients say about their pain—about what it *means* to them—caregivers can gain crucial information. Here, for example, is a poem written by chronic pain patient Janet Boyd:

A Snowball

Pain is like a snowball engulfing all in its path.
My path.
A snowball of pain careering out of control,
Boring down, planing off my sanity.
The swirling whiteness of pain blotting out
My attempts to live normally.
The crushing weight of the unfettered snowball
Leaves me fighting for survival.[58]

What do we learn about the meaning of pain for Janet Boyd? Pain has expanded to fill her consciousness: it has usurped the everyday world and left only a world of pain. She feels out of control. Pain even threatens to push her into the counterworld of madness. Normalcy is gone. The meanings and acts that daily sustain her have been blotted out by a crushing weight. Her very survival is at risk. A doctor who does not learn this information about Janet Boyd will be in a poor position to offer the help she clearly needs.

The history of persistent medical undertreatment for pain reveals cultural forces more complicated than the failure to listen to the patient. Listening, however, is a good, low-tech contribution toward an eventual remedy. Doctors who average seven minutes per patient simply lack the tools and time necessary to hear what chronic pain patients could tell them. (In my experience, nurses are better listeners, but their voices, like those of the patients, may go unheeded because of medical politics.) Medicine of course cannot ignore the pressures for effective time management. Yet, it is crucial to know whether doctors do not listen because they are too busy or because they believe listening is unimportant. If they do believe that listening is important in treating pain patients, then various inventive options are available to help elicit the meanings at play, including collaboration with anthropologists and historians. Such collaborations in the past would have revealed, for example, that prominent nineteenth-century doctors believed blacks did not feel pain; that sensitivity to pain differed by social class, with aristocrats believed to possess delicate and sensitive nervous systems that left them prey to debilitating afflictions, unlike the coarse laboring masses; that, ever since Plato described the womb as an animal roaming free within the body, women's pain has been interpreted within patriarchal cultures built upon myths about male power and female weakness. Listening is a good start toward replacing ignorance with knowledge.

Today such collaboration could show us in badly needed detail how postmodern pain is shaped by the culture and institutions of our own time and place: television, sports, cinema, popular music, advertising, welfare, and a massive new cost-conscious, government-regulated, opiophobic health care bureaucracy. It could allow us to recognize the complex ways in which postmodern pain, rather than affirming the single doctrine of meaninglessness implicit in the modernist biomedical model, is inherently polyphonic. We could begin to hear the voices formerly silenced not only by pain but also by the neglect of a biomedical culture in which complaints of pain (subjective and unverifiable) simply do not matter.

Nonetheless, acceptance of a new biocultural model will not come easy. Ronald Melzack—coauthor in the middle 1960s of the bold "gate-control" theory of pain, which focused chiefly on the modulation of nociceptive impulses in the spine—now works with quadriplegics who have suffered complete, verified severing of the spinal cord. No nociceptive impulses from the periphery can reach the cortex, yet these patients still feel pain. For Melzack, the challenge of pain has shifted from the spinal cord to the brain's neuromatrix of interconnections, and he is not surprised that researchers shy away from this complex region. "It is difficult," he understates, "to deal with such problems as consciousness, awareness of one's own body, and the brain's capacity to create perceptions, memories, and every other aspect of cognitive activity."[59] Consciousness and cognitive activity open onto the changing historical field of culture, where the influences that modulate pain can mount exponentially. Difficulties, however, are preferable to errors and illusions. Pain did not die with the discovery of surgical anesthesia in the mid–nineteenth century, despite predictions of its imminent demise. Responsible references to its contemporary epidemic status suggest that, if anything, pain has surely multiplied. The discovery of additional wonder drugs may be far less urgent today, at least for cultures already awash with analgesics, than the dissemination of a postmodern understanding that pain is invariably biocultural—saturated in emotion, memory, and consciousness—and inseparably linked to the individual meanings we make of it.

chapter five

Utopian Bodies

The appeal of Utopianism arises, I believe, from

the failure to realise that we cannot make heaven

on earth. What we can do instead is, I believe, to

make life a little less terrible and a little less unjust

in every generation. A good deal can be achieved

in this way.

KARL POPPER,
"Utopia and Violence" (1948)

Utopian thought is deeply historical. Each era invents its own versions of paradise on earth, and these paradises—while often visionary depictions of nowhere—correspond closely to the changing cultures that invent them. The famous utopian republic of Plato embodies fourth-century Athenian assumptions about reason, justice, and civic life, much as the utopian island of Thomas More embodies Renaissance and Christian ideas of moral virtue. Socialist utopias belong to the post-Marxian world of political economics, just as feminism and popular versions of science fiction help to shape the distinctive utopias of the late twentieth century. Western fantasies of perfection, in short, while recurrent and perhaps ineradicable, are not timeless but grounded in the historical desires of people in particular places and times.

The postmodern era confronts us with new versions of utopia that express the historical desires of our own place and time.[1] Postmodernism is normally described as inherently heterogeneous, marked by the absence of a single dominant style or mode of thought. It introduces a late-capitalist profusion that echoes previous styles, splinters unified discourses, decenters orthodox beliefs, validates marginal positions, endlessly deferring full knowledge, adding supplement on supplement. The utopias generated by such a fractured and slippery discourse prove both new and unusual: proposals include the expansive view from Chicago's Sears Tower, the wide-open spaces of the American West, the instant communication offered by the Internet.[2] Although a few specific material or metaphorical dreamscapes hold persistent appeal, like the beaches of Tahiti, there is no single dominant postmodern utopia, but rather an excess of utopias, utopias as diverse as the annual accumulation of grand prizes, a cinematic jumble of utopian thought that generates even its own nightmarish opposites in a series of toxic, robotic, futuristic totalitarian dystopias. Put a bit differently, postmodern utopia is not so much nowhere as anywhere.[3]

The construction of postmodern utopias, while widely diverse, seems especially consistent and significant in what it rejects. Earlier utopias from Plato to H. G. Wells usually centered on the idea of community. From theory to practice, whether in monasteries or in communes, utopia was always configured as a social space: its perfection depended on people living together in civic harmony. Modernist utopias continued this civic thrust, imagining various fulfillments of the promise contained in the radical new social movements that deeply influenced modern literature and art.[4] In the postmodern era, with the exception of a few bizarre cults, the social nature of utopia profoundly changes. The electronic global village gives us both instant communication and a vanishing sense of community. Neighbors watch the same TV shows but do not know one another's names. In the United States, families change houses every few years in a mobility that increases in parallel with the divorce rate and the number of predatory urban gangs. The unprecedented loss of communal feeling is so complete that a number of postmodern utopias reject not only the ideal of a harmonious social or political order but also the very concept of a community. They reject even the standard utopian fiction of a world perfected in the distant future. The future is now. With the sphere of social life imploded, with politics reduced to fund-raising and the clash of special-interest groups, utopia in the postmodern era has, in effect, transferred its location to the solitary, private, individual body. The impact of this cultural shift on the biology of health and illness is something that medicine has not yet begun to consider.

UTOPIA NOW

The fabrication of an individual utopia is hardly unprecedented. John Milton in *Paradise Lost* (1665), writing from the viewpoint of ultra-Protestant concern for personal salvation, foretold that Adam and Eve could achieve a "paradise within" far happier than Eden. The Miltonic paradise within, however, is not a solitary condition but rather a state so profoundly interconnected that it joins each individual human soul, beyond linear time and space, to the central events of Christian history (Nativity, Crucifixion, Resurrection) and ultimately to God. By contrast, the insistently private and secular postmodern utopias reflect a belief that the only valid remaining space of perfection lies, ready at hand, in our own individual flesh: a paradise of curves and muscle.

The individual, malleable, postmodern flesh constitutes in every sense a new body. It dispenses with any reference to shared civic and moral virtues, thereby marking a decisive break with the body depicted in ancient Greek art, which was always the body as contained within and reflecting both the democratic state and the moral-aesthetic realm of ideal form. Unlike the colossal, godlike figures celebrated in Renaissance sculpture and painting, utopian bodies in the postmodern era are disengaged from any discourse about mind or spirit (such as the philosophical discussions that permeated Italian

Neoplatonism). Postmodern bodies are reinvented strictly as objects of vision. The glossy commercial photograph is their ultimate expression. Self and body have become identical, so that paradise on earth now requires simply the glowing, gym-fit look revered in Hollywood as a perfect ten.[5] Most important in constituting a break with previous utopian thought, the new, postmodern body is ultimately self-created. As fashion writer Holly Brubach observes, only with the recent advent of exercise as a cosmetic science have people had the option of transforming their bodies into a facsimile of their own ideal vision.[6]

Not all ideals have equal value, and there are dangers latent in any model of perfection. The main danger in the postmodern relocation of utopia does not lie in trends toward unrestrained pleasure seeking and carnal excess. The need for low-fat diets, safe sex, and unending workouts have placed new constraints on postmodern pleasure. The postmodern body, moreover, no matter how secular, is strangely dematerialized, like the perfect smile of a movie star or like the simulcast pictures of rock musicians flashed above the concert stage on huge TV monitors, mere electrons sprayed across a screen, disappearing at the flick of a switch. This is the body redefined as pure surface: what two influential postmodern thinkers call "the body without organs."[7] Such bodies resemble harmless props, like the life-size cardboard sex objects displayed in video stores, but ultimately they possess a significant culturewide influence. There are dangers implicit in our fixation on these images of bodily perfection—not least of which is their power to lull us into fantasies of a consumer paradise where perfect happiness requires only purchasing the right exercise equipment and diet supplements. Perhaps the gravest danger in the proliferating images of postmodern utopian bodies lies in the confusion they create about the nature of health and illness.

Utopias have often focused on health and illness.[8] Utopian writers use metaphors of illness to describe the imperfect, corrupt, actual world, while ideal communities usually boast a race untainted or untroubled by ills of the flesh. Plato's republic has no need for doctors; More's tour around the island of Utopia reveals a well-organized system of medical care; Swift's hyperrational horses in *Gulliver's Travels* (1726) never get sick, weaken only in advanced age, and die after graceful public good-byes. Cosimo Noto's utopian novel *The Ideal City* (1903), which links technological progress with enlightened politics, includes a long section entitled "The Achievements of Medical Science under a Socialistic Administration." Here again traditional utopias make health a benefit shared by almost all members of a society. Collective utopian politics and the exercise of utopian virtues are what promote a healthy way of life, so that good health in utopia is not a happy accident, like mild climate, but a universal by-product of wise social practices, the summarizing metaphor of an ideal state.

One measure of change in the postmodern era is the degree to which utopian thought—in emphasizing the solitary, secular, individual body—has expanded the role of health from by-product or metaphor to highest good. Health no longer refers, via metaphor, to the ideal social state that generates it but instead signifies the perfection of a single private self. Further, good health is not exactly the issue. What matters is that the individual body *appear* healthy. Image, for the body without organs, is everything. The average family lives in a realm of pictures (created with the favored postmodern technologies of camera and videotape) where they cannot avoid versions of the same concatenated subliminal message: the healthy-looking body is the beautiful body; the beautiful body is the healthy-looking body; health and beauty are the source of erotic pleasure. The opposite of health, beauty, and eroticism, of course, is illness.[9] Thus, actual illnesses that accompany the attainment of perfect form—including the side effects of anabolic steroids, diet pills, silicon injections, and skin-cutting, bone-breaking cosmetic regimens—must be concealed and denied. Ultimately, the outcome is a massive cultural paradox. At the moment when larger-than-life, utopian images of individual bodily health, like the Times Square electronic billboards portraying muscular supermodels stripped down to their underwear, dominate popular thought, the well-being of the general population is threatened as never before by new epidemic maladies. In effect, our robust and visible fantasies of physical perfection—hard bodies glowing with the appearance of youth, health, and sex—seem linked indirectly but inescapably to the landscape of contemporary illness. How could this be?

BUILDING THE PERFECT BODY

The psychopathology of utopian desire—although nowhere given a separate entry among the recognized diagnostic categories—seems to strike women especially hard, but no gender is immune from the difficulties that attend the quest for bodily perfection. (Gay males, for example, play their own variations on this theme.) In the late 1980s Samuel Wilson Fussell, a young man just out of college, found himself in New York City—alone, disoriented, frightened—and the book he wrote about his experience, *Muscle: Confessions of an Unlikely Bodybuilder* (1991), tells the story of his quest to create a utopian body. The path he pursued, bodybuilding, is of course linked with numerous postmodern cultural activities that focus on external appearance, from beauty pageants to cosmetic surgery. The most frequently performed cosmetic surgery around 1990, for example, was the technique called liposuction, in which specialists vacuum fat cells from beneath the skin. Breast implants, face-lifts, and nose jobs rank close behind.[10] These manipulations of the body reflect culturewide commitments to ideals of youth and beauty that cross lines of gender, since both women and men live in an age when the body is regarded as a malleable substance awaiting the imprint of utopian fantasies. Half of America's weight-machine users are women, and men now account for nearly one-quarter of all cosmetic surgery procedures.[11] In the early decades of the twentieth century, bodybuilding existed on the fringes of American culture, a freakish pastime pursued in dank, disreputable gyms; but within the last few years it has been reinvented (much like tattooing) as a quintessential postmodern popular art that cuts across race, class, and gender. It offers a vivid arena for examining how bodies may now be completely reshaped in accordance with the obscure promptings of utopian desire.[12]

The desire for a well-muscled body, while prompted and inces-
santly reinforced by postmodern advertising, is more than an artifact
of contemporary fantasies. George Hersey, in *The Evolution of Allure*
(1996), observes that from a biological point of view sexual selection
is based on specific features—bright plumage in certain male birds,
say—and argues that one way members of any species gain a genetic
advantage is by "augmenting" those specific features, as in male
birds with brighter colors.[13] Successful "augmentations" become part
of the physiology of the species. Arguably, large muscles in men at
some point in human prehistory played a role in sexual selection,
and even now well-chiseled male physiques play prominently in media displays of sexual attraction. It is an axiom of Darwinian theory
that we cannot directly inherit large muscles, but we can inherit
genes that make the acquisition of large muscles easier or harder. We
may also inherit or rapidly develop a drive to augment the features
that we believe give us a sexual advantage. Sam Fussell's daily workouts in the gym (if Hersey is correct) connect with a deeper biocultural history than the average bodybuilder would suspect. Ironically,
compulsive bodybuilding for Fussell leads not to sexual advantage
but to suspended libido and impaired performance. The one sexual
encounter that he describes (with a female bodybuilder) is notable
for its absence of erotic zest. *Muscle* is not a primer about attracting
sexual partners but a description of how biology and culture combine, in this case, to produce a state indistinguishable from illness.

The explicit motive behind Fussell's plunge into the subculture of
bodybuilding was less sexual desire than fear. The violence of urban
life in the United States so frightened him as he walked the streets of
New York City that he decided to protect himself by building up a set
of husky muscles. Yet there were less explicit motives too. His parents
had just gone through a messy divorce, splitting up "bitterly and publicly."[14] Amid his disorientation at the sudden breakup of his family,
the obsessive routines and daily dedication required by bodybuilding
offered at least an illusion of control. The visible changes in his body,
moreover, did exactly what he had hoped: coworkers and strangers
began to treat him with wary deference. The guide and model for his

deliberate act of self-creation is a book at the heart of popular culture, *Arnold: The Education of a Bodybuilder* (1977), by Arnold Schwarzenegger, whose talent, drive, and exceptionally well-developed muscles transformed him into Mr. Universe (and subsequently into a rich film star, businessman, and international celebrity). Fussell's four-year flesh-and-blood bildungsroman—"a bodybuilder's fundamental task," he writes, "is reinvention" (117)—traces his own transformation from a fearful, gawky, East Coast novice into the 270-pound, aggressive, pumped-up, cut-and-shredded finalist for the California title of Mr. Golden Valley.

The utopian impulse implicit in his bodybuilding finds expression both in the wraparound mirrors that help Fussell measure his progress toward ideal form and in the regular, official competitions, where judges and audience perform the function of mirroring. These competitions do not measure strength. Powerlifters compete to demonstrate strength, whereas bodybuilders create their muscles solely for display. If silicon could be distributed beneath a bodybuilder's skin in the required knots and bulges, it would serve as well as muscle. Visual symmetry—joined with visible and extraordinary muscular development—is the goal. This goal too may reflect dim biological impulses: Deborah Blum in *Sex on the Brain* (1997) mentions symmetry as among the features that seem to affect sexual selection in humans.[15] The bodybuilder's immediate script, however, is cultural. Flesh becomes a living clay on which to impress proportions ("The Apollonian Ideal") borrowed directly from Greek sculpture. Neck, calves, and biceps should be exactly the same circumference (185). The rules of competition demand poses based on works of art that celebrate almost godlike human physiques, including the Farnese *Hercules* and Michelangelo's *David* (133). Fussell in effect obediently redesigns his body to imitate classic statuary and then puts it into motion (while judges watch and the audience roars), flexing and posing to the soundtrack of Isaac Hayes's "Shaft!" The combination of music, motion, sculpture, and body creates a consummate postmodern multimedia artifact—all style and surface—mingling its eclectic, deracinated sources in a kinetic audio-visual performance worthy of the most theatrical rock concerts.

Intense physical training plays a crucial role in the bodybuilder's art, and Fussell says he advanced quicker than his training partners because of an exceptionally punishing regimen. "No one else," he writes, "was willing to suffer this kind of pain" (80). Yet, his self-inflicted pain went beyond the normal four-hour training sessions in which he bench-pressed four hundred pounds or squatted five hundred. Fussell's backside constantly ached from huge knots produced by steroid injections; crash diets eliminated so much body fat that merely standing upright, with no internal padding for his feet, produced excruciating torment. He worried about the premature deaths of bodybuilders and weight lifters who wore out their hearts and livers with muscle-building drugs like his. He refers to other bodybuilders as "diseased" (149) and to the nationwide bodybuilding craze as a malady of "epidemic proportions" (83). Although his references to illness seem at first merely metaphoric, the metaphor brushes dangerously close to literal fact, and he does not hesitate to summarize his immersion in the all-consuming world of bodybuilding as a form of pathology: "I had failed to see the symptoms of my own disease" (249). Elsewhere he specifies some of the costs entailed in attaining a perfect body: "degenerative arthritis, cirrhosis of the liver, hypertension, heart disease, and the host of problems associated with long-time drug use."[16]

What matters in the bodybuilding arena finally is not the pain that bodybuilders endure, not their brush with illness, pathology, and premature death, but rather the role of self-discipline in creating an illusion of health. The competition-honed body, oiled, beefed up with drugs, and bronzed with Dye-O-Derm, conveys an appearance of well-being that is largely fictitious. When Fussell wonders why (despite having achieved an almost godlike physique) he feels so awful, his bodybuilding mentor, Vinnie, bluntly reminds him of the unspoken rules: "Big Man, this is about *looking* good, not feeling good" (193).

The subtext that accompanies Fussell's quest for a utopian body concerns his attempt to escape an interior torment. The utopian body conceals a dystopian spirit. Inseparable from his pursuit of ideal form is a nausea he feels at his own shortcomings. "I hated the flawed, weak, vulnerable nature of being human," he writes, "as I hated the Adam's apple that bobbed beneath my chin. The attempt at physical perfection grew from the seeds of self-disgust" (138). His perfect muscles thus offer more than armor against urban violence. They are an effort to ward off an extreme "self-hatred" (248), just as the extreme discipline required to achieve them serves as an oblique form of self-martyrdom, as a way of "purifying" himself (249). They also provide a weapon with which to retaliate against the father and mother whose divorce so badly wounded him. Bodybuilding, he knows, constitutes a pursuit so anti-intellectual that it is guaranteed to leave both academic parents hurt and stunned. His father for a time disowns him. The gym meanwhile provides an insulation from the inner distress that he refuses to acknowledge: "a place in which I wouldn't have to react or feel" (247).

The relationship between external perfection and internal distress is a theme that Fussell returns to often. We glimpse one source of his torment when Fussell seeks to explain why the only woman he allowed himself to love was (safely) unattainable, engaged to another man. "It guaranteed a kind of distance on my part," he reasons. "The real connection between lovers was something I could never stomach. The rare times I tried the pain was awful" (250). Here again the bodybuilding quest for physical perfection seeks to mask or deny a torment that cannot be located in tissue damage. The utopian ideal hammered into the flesh is thus destined to fail—not just because bodies always rebel, inevitably aching and aging, but because Fussell has attempted to split off body from mind and emotion in ways ultimately impossible and always self-destructive. Pain, as we have seen, always involves our beliefs and emotions as they combine with the biology of neurotransmission to produce complex experiences (albeit some as ordinary as a stubbed toe) that defy neat Cartesian splitting.[17] The long history of psychosomatic illness shows that mental and emotional distress often takes the form of bodily symptoms, and surely we all have known the difficulties of preventing our bodily symptoms (a toothache, a bad cold) from affecting how we think and feel.[18] Although bodily perfection might once have served as an allegory or symbol signifying other forms of perfection, in a postmodern culture that continues to divide minds from bodies there is no higher solace in perfect muscles. Muscles and psyches belong to separate, almost detached, spheres of action. Fussell, as he looks back on his career as a bodybuilder, recalls how "behind that huge frame and those muscular sets, I felt shut up in a kind of claustrophobic panic" (249).

Sam Fussell's attempt to use bodybuilding to resolve problems that reach far beyond the body ultimately turns his flesh into an icon of misjudgment and incipient illness. Photographs of his chiseled and punished body reveal a hollow, haunted look. This is a picture of fitness on the edge of breakdown. Breakdown, in fact, occurs immediately after his almost superhuman regimen of diet and drugs leading up to the Mr. Golden Valley competition, in which he places second. It seems pertinent that Fussell's recovery begins only at the moment when—after his second-place finish—he chooses to forgo his twice-daily ritual at the gym and to abandon the quest for physical perfection. He comes to regard his self-hatred as an unacceptable form of egotism, affirms the value of feeling and caring, and soon reverts to his former size and shape, "like I'd never lifted a weight in my life" (251). Others, however, are not so fortunate as they embark on the postmodern quest for a utopian body.

POSTMODERN BODIES

No topic has received more discussion among postmodern academic analysts than the body.[19] Postmodernism, we might say, has not just rediscovered the body but almost wholly reinvented it. What postmodern analysts see in the body—beginning influentially with the work of Michel Foucault and extending powerfully through feminist studies—is a space for the inscription of social and political power.

The body is seen as "inscribed" (the verb rarely varies) with whatever meanings, shapes, and constraints the dominant social discourses of the day imprint upon its surface. This description may sound abstract, but the process of inscription leaves tangible marks. Some are trivial. We can read them on teeth covered with orthodontic braces in order to produce a socially acceptable smile. Some are disturbing. We can read them on the faces of battered wives, on the scarred backs of torture victims, on the shaved scalps of white-supremacist skinheads. Some are no less horrible for being internal and—until the effects prove unmistakable—unseen. The bodies of black volunteers enrolled in long-term U.S. government research on syphilis bear the imprint of the racist science that secretly denied infected volunteers access to antibiotic medication.[20] Bodies, from a postmodern point of view, are never mere biological entities that constitute (as one medical dictionary puts it) "the material part of a man."[21] They are culturally constructed and hotly contested social spaces where we can observe the complex signs of human fantasy and of human trespass.

The power that cultural discourses hold over individual bodies has been described mainly—again following the work of Foucault—as a form of discipline: like Victorian ladies squeezing their tightly corseted waists to the contours of feminine fashion, we regiment our behavior and even our flesh to conform with the dictates of culture. Medicine is implicated among the cultural forces of discipline by virtue of what Foucault has called a clinical "gaze" that transforms the body into an object of scientific scrutiny. Patients often note how the power implicit in the physician and in the medical setting can reduce us to a state of passive and dependent helplessness, in which we sit for hours in a crowded waiting room until the busy doctor at last finds time to see us. Yet the power implicit in medicine reaches far beyond the clinic, and its impact is often quite positive. We employ the latest biomedical knowledge, for example, to help us regulate our diets, our leisure pursuits, and our sexual relationships. We employ the latest biomedical technology to examine a fetus in the womb, to open a blocked artery, to transplant a life-saving organ. The point here is not to praise or blame the power implicit in medicine but rather to recognize its impact in changing the ways in which we understand and experience our own bodies.

Few developments in postmodern culture have proved more influential in changing our experience of the human body than the rise of sports medicine. Athletics in the modernist era can certainly point to proud achievements, such as the performance of Jesse Owens at the 1936 Olympics. Yet until recently the doctor's role in sport was mainly to treat injuries. The advent of television has transformed both professional and amateur sports into multibillion-dollar businesses and has resulted in added pressure upon athletes for ever higher levels of performance.[22] Doctors now prescribe or supply drugs not just for treating an injury but for enhancing strength and improving endurance. Steroids have invaded the locker room along with exercise physiologists and sports psychologists. While medicine cannot take full responsibility for transforming athletes into ever more finely tuned machines, it certainly has achieved remarkable breakthroughs in surgical techniques and rehabilitation procedures, returning an injured athlete to competition in record time. In this pursuit of individual or team achievement, the postmodern athlete has an indirect but compelling cultural purpose: to persuade us that there are now no natural limits set for the performance of the human body.

The discipline of the body, which is demanded by sport and accepted by athletes, operates more subtly in the related arenas of entertainment and fashion. Most postmodern movie stars, pop singers, and fashion models must project their bodies into a performance as a kind of sexual subtext. Sometimes the subtext is the performance. When *The Ed Sullivan Show*, famous as family television, filmed Elvis Presley from the waist up, viewers were left in no doubt about what portion of the singer's body they were not allowed to see. Sexual subtexts vary greatly, of course, but (to cite only popular singers) the androgyny of David Bowie, the lesbian edge of Melissa Etheridge, or the street-smart sensuality of Tupac Shakur are not just adjuncts to a musical performance. Performance projects an image of the postmodern sexual body in its multiple possibilities. A new breed of designers and supermodels—from Calvin Klein to Cindy Crawford—has helped extend the concept of fashion from a mere display of clothing (in which anonymous and often asexual young women walk down runways) to a highly personal and dramatically sexual choreography of bodies in motion. The annual Oscar presentations in Hollywood, where male as well as female movie stars are quizzed about their designer apparel, no doubt constitutes a crowning moment when fashion, performance, and bodies coalesce under the disciplinary "gaze" of television cameras to constitute a single electronic commodity.

There are few better premonitions of the postmodern ideal of utopian bodies in an environment redesigned by commerce and by popular culture than Richard Hamilton's 1956 collage *Just what is it that makes today's homes so different, so appealing?* (figure 4). The muscle man and his pinup wife—who come, like the work's title, straight from a magazine—strike exhibitionist poses in a room dominated by electronic appliances and modish furnishings: the ensemble a metaphor of consumer capitalism. Outside the window, blotting out the natural world if it could be found, is a movie theater, a privileged source for the culturewide dissemination of images, while the television set offers a domestic image of female beauty and commerce, a woman holding a telephone, no less commodified than the two almost naked householders or the prominent can of ham. The inescapable grip of commerce extends to the heraldic shield identifying the Ford Motor Company; a pop art print hangs on the wall, reproducing the comic book cover of *Young Romance.* Hamilton, who is regarded as a founder of British pop art and who later designed the famous cover of *The White Album* for the Beatles, has written admiringly about the mythic qualities of mass-media culture and about the importance of commercial design in stimulating desire. His collage cannot be reduced to satire, although (as with his favorite artistic predecessor, Marcel Duchamp) ironies abound.[23] Today it looks more like prophecy: the ceiling is an early scientific photo of the lunar surface. Hamilton designed the collage to serve as the poster for an exhibition entitled *This Is Tomorrow,* and contemporary viewers

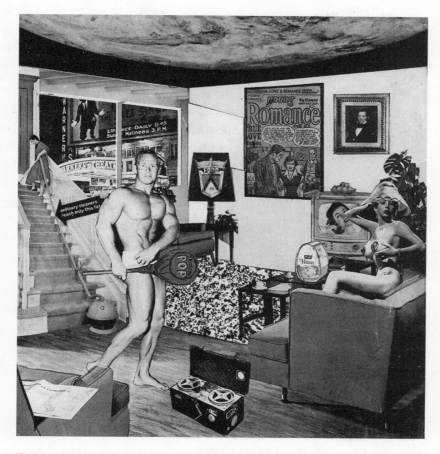

Figure 4. Richard Hamilton, *Just what is it that makes today's homes so different, so appealing?* 1956, collage. Courtesy Kunsthalle Tübingen. Copyright © 1998 Artists Rights Society (ARS), New York / DACS, London.

need add little more than a computer and a CD player (replacing the 1950s vacuum cleaner and tape deck) in order to update his vision of sexualized perfect bodies amid glamorous futuristic commodities. In buying the goods, we consume the myth of postmodern utopia.

The innocence, or at least the triviality, in much popular display of bodies goes without saying. Does it matter if a basketball player dyes his hair green and covers himself with tattoos? In an age of self-promotion, the sexual body can serve as a sandwich board for the diminished or empowered individual ego. Yet, mass advertising has also exposed us to an unprecedented display of bodies culled for their photogenic features—and the consequences are unclear. Even within a single culture women see their own bodies differently because of differing social and economic backgrounds.[24] A cocktail of new drugs and sex hormones unavailable to modernist self-manipulation now lends plasticity to postmodern bodies as people scramble to negotiate the hurdles of advancing age, spreading waistlines, impotence, and infertility.[25] Amid the more frivolous innovations such as an ointment to reverse male pattern baldness, some tendencies should trouble anyone concerned with health and illness. The discipline that cultural discourses and images help to inscribe upon the body does not invariably produce supermodels and rock stars. It is worth giving some thought to the casualties left behind in our fixation on stardom and on images of bodily perfection.

THE ANOREXIC BODY

The superstar status that American pop culture conferred in the late 1950s on crooner Pat Boone—the wholesome, middle-class, God-fearing alternative to Elvis Presley—did not make life easier for his daughter Cherry. It brought perks that any teenager would appreciate: a birthday visit from a TV heartthrob, a backstage meeting with the Beatles. But when Pat Boone revived his flagging career in 1969 with a tour of Japan, his act, now called The Pat Boone Family, pressed into willing service his wife and four young daughters, including fourteen-year-old Cherry. An already fragile perfectionist, who in school expected nothing less than straight A's but was terrified of exams and piled up numerous absences by feigning illness, she was not prepared to handle the normal strains of adolescence compounded by the abnormal strains of a performance—offstage and on—designed to uphold what she calls "our image as the ideal

American family."[26] As she puts it: "Being Pat Boone's daughter was very much like being a celebrity's kid and a preacher's kid all at the same time: maintaining the Boone image was like balancing on a tightrope" (15). At fourteen, on the high wire of semicelebrity, she commenced a deadly ten-year struggle with anorexia nervosa.

Historian Peter N. Stearns, in tracing the links between culture and body weight, argues that it was between 1890 and 1910 when middle-class Americans began their ongoing battle against fat.[27] This modernist struggle provides the basis for innumerable distinctive postmodern tactics, from the rise of nonfat cookies to the Abdominizer. Occasionally, however, our comic self-contradictions—as diet plans vie with cookbooks on the weekly best-seller list—take a tragic turn. Some cynics might contend that membership in the "ideal American family" is a guarantee of illness, yet Cherry's three younger siblings escaped the trauma that awaited their perfectionist sister. It is thus impossible to place all the blame on the father whom Cherry depicts as loving but career-driven, insensitive, authoritarian: the creator and strict enforcer of "seemingly endless rules and regulations" (15). The origins of her struggle with anorexia lay not only in her family and in her role as a performer but almost everywhere, even in the passing comments of a teenage boy. As Cherry says:

> For a performer, physical appearance becomes of primary importance. Self-consciousness is inevitable when you are constantly being stared at on stage or scrutinized in a fan magazine. Suddenly, every imperfection, real or imagined, is a focal point for alteration and improvement. Having developed early and grown more rapidly than the average girl, the excess "baby fat" that I retained looked out of place. I had become self-conscious about my size by age thirteen. And when an eighteen-year-old male friend of our family commented on the value of thinness, I began dieting immediately. (23)

The gaze of the audience or the fan ultimately becomes the gaze of the self upon the objectified body. It is fair to say, in at least two senses, that what Cherry saw in her body made her sick. She began a monomaniacal regime of diet and exercise including a two-hour daily workout that she "followed uncompromisingly to the most minute detail for years" (40). The result: at five feet seven inches tall, she weighed ninety-two pounds.

The ribs protruding from Cherry's emaciated back—exposed by chance when the baggy clothes she wore to disguise her thinness slipped off—so shocked and appalled her mother that a doctor was called in. With medicine adding its discipline to the rigor of a family in which Cherry still received spankings at eighteen, the agonizing ten-year war against the body commenced in earnest, and war is not too strong a metaphor. Despite medical treatment, 5 to 15 percent of known anorexics eventually starve to death.

In *Starving for Attention* (1992), Cherry Boone O'Neill writes about her illness from the perspective of a veteran. The extensive psychotherapy that she credits with saving her life also, however, colors her description. She reproduces in her own story much current medical thought about anorexia, emphasizing, for example, the influence of her troubled family, her desperate need for control, her relentless perfectionism ("Even my pet had to be perfect" [51]). There is no reason why she should suppress such important features, but the assumptions of psychotherapy also shape how she understands and tells her own story. At moments, the constructed language of psychotherapy becomes like a native tongue. ("My body image determined my self-esteem," she observes [73].) Hers is a compelling narrative about a young woman's struggle to control her own fate by starving her body into what she considered a perfect (almost fleshless) form, but in its truth to experience her story leads to insights beyond the conventional wisdom that she openly endorses. The vision of perfection that she pursued and the origins of her illness cannot be located entirely within her family or her psyche. The circle of anorexia nervosa reaches far wider, into the general culture that enfolds and manufactures this peculiarly postmodern illness.

There is no doubt that anorexia nervosa belongs to the same postmodern culture as Andy Warhol and the Boone family tour of Japan.[28] Earlier records exist of women who fast to the point of starvation, especially among Christian mystics of the Middle Ages, but the emergence of anorexia as a diagnosable illness dates specifically to the last decades of the twentieth century.[29] The American Anorexia and Bulimia Association was founded in 1978—the same decade when strange stories about young women who refused to eat first appeared in the popular press. Moreover, the simultaneous emergence of the binge-and-purge disorder called bulimia suggests the rise of a whole new class of illnesses known as eating disorders. Although anorexia affects less than two people per hundred thousand, its impact among young women in high school and college is significant: 1 to 4 percent suffer from either anorexia or bulimia.[30] These alarming percentages have quadrupled since the 1970s.

Anorexia is a disease of women, white women, especially middle- and upper-class white women in Western industrial countries. Among men and black women, for example, it is extremely rare, so gender, race, and economic status are clearly involved. Researchers believe that the rise of anorexia is directly related to the growing affluence that followed World War II (when food was scarce and eating disorders unknown). The causes, however, are complicated and treatment is difficult. Families can exert a strong influence, even to the point of "psychic incest" with the father.[31] The onset of sexual maturity complicates the search for causes, as some anorexics clearly reject their own emerging femaleness—associated with the fatty tissue that accompanies puberty—and seek instead to approximate the male body. Cherry Boone O'Neill's psychological identification and struggle with her famous father is quite clear. ("Pat exercises regularly but Cherry's even outdoing him," her mother remarks [59].) Cherry seems not to grasp the depth of her resentment. "[A]mong my earliest and even fondest memories," she writes with apparent equanimity, "were jokes about not being the son Daddy had wanted so badly" (75). This is the stuff of personal neurosis (and the unhappiness in which each family is unique) that therapists and doctors must sort out, yet her story also points beyond an individual or family crisis. Recent analysis of anorexia has emphasized two contributing causes over which individuals have little control: cultural fantasies of female beauty and a late-capitalist economy that manipulates consumer desire through images of the sexual body.

Cultural fantasies of female beauty might seem far removed from the punished and emaciated body of an anorexic, but the anorexic simply pushes to its logical limit the ideal of thinness that obsesses educated white women in technologically advanced nations. (Beauty among educated black women in the same cultures seems to focus less on weight than on hair.)[32] If it is true that you can never be too rich or too thin, then the anorexic, however self-deceived, is halfway to utopia. Moreover, many anorexics report an experience of exhilaration, power, and almost angelic purification—an elevation of self-esteem almost druglike in its euphoria—that rises in proportion as the pounds melt away. Yet the euphoria is merely another mask of illness. "[F]urious hatred of my fat translated into a furious hatred of myself" (37), O'Neill writes, and when the fat disappears, the self-hatred simply takes new forms. Feminist scholars have made it impossible to overlook the ways in which culture "disciplines" women by equating female beauty with slim, athletic bodies, creating a cultural discourse (involving industries from cosmetics to advertising) through which femininity is constructed as something that, whatever else it does, inevitably reproduces the already unequal power relations between the sexes.[33] Even at its least oppressive and most fanciful, the cultural system of female beauty (as Kathy Davis writes) encourages "the channeling of women's energies in the hopeless race for a perfect body."[34]

It seems clear, in fact, that postmodern ideals of beauty do not circulate in an innocent realm of fantasy but support and promote a consumer economy. Whereas the industrialized modernist economy created tangible goods in order to meet the material needs of a growing nation, the postmodern economy in order to sell its increasingly intangible products (from services to information) must create new and strangely immaterial needs. The best way to create the new needs suited to an age of electronic technologies is to employ images, and the time-tested images for creating new needs are still images of the bodies of women. Not women only. Advertising agencies understand the buying power of female consumers and openly solicit their desire through provocative, semi-naked images of perfect male bodies. The point is that postmodern advertising pursues a distinctive variation of the formula that "sex sells." The most important feature of postmodern sexuality is its promise—through the images of sexual bodies—of an escape into pure or disembodied pleasure.

Postmodern sex has eluded the modernist bourgeois circle of childbirth and family. The oral contraceptive pill introduced in 1960 opened up an era of what historian Donald W. Lowe calls the "sexual lifestyle."[35] Advertisers were quick to recognize opportunities in evoking the desire of consumers to participate in this new erotic lifestyle. Lowe cites a study that Rosalind Coward made of *Cosmopolitan*—a magazine sold primarily to women—describing how advertisers began to employ photographic images of women in ways that effectively remade the female body. This remaking of the female body occurs through the "sexualization" of areas not previously defined as sexual. Coward writes: "It is the sexualization of eyes, lips, ears, wrists, legs, feet, hair, mouths, teeth, smells, skin, etc. It is not a matter of exploiting a pre-existent, naturally sensitive body, but the actual construction of parts of the body as sensitive and sexual, as capable of stimulation and excitation, and therefore demanding care and attention if women are to be sexual and sexually desirable to men."[36] This supersexual, imagistic reconstruction of the female body—with the consequent anxieties and illnesses facing flesh-and-blood women who seek to conform to a fragmented and impossible ideal—is what for Lowe comprises the new cultural context that creates anorexia nervosa. Anorexia nervosa in his view is far less a psychopathology than "a late-capitalist sociopathology."[37]

The view that anorexia nervosa articulates contradictory and ultimately harmful cultural expectations of women—expectations promoted through a utopian imagery that sexualizes almost the entire surface of the female body as reconstructed under late-consumer capitalism—finds considerable support.[38] Yet something is amiss. With millions of women worrying about their weight and cultivating their looks under the pressure of a relentless cultural imagery of perfect bodies to which they cannot possibly conform, why is anorexia nervosa still comparatively rare? Or, to pursue the problem from another direction: how does it happen that intelligent young women who in many cases consciously reject the fashion-model absurdities of their consumer culture nonetheless find it impossible, even under vigilant medical care, to keep from starving themselves to death?

If anorexia nervosa truly fits the model of a postmodern illness, we should expect that its mysteries are biological as well as cultural. There should be an interlocking biology of anorexia nervosa that addresses some of the questions that cultural analysis alone cannot resolve.

THE BIOLOGY OF SELF-STARVATION

Studies with twins suggest that some people inherit a tendency to develop an eating disorder.[39] The genetics of anorexia nervosa, however, is still uncharted territory, and Cherry Boone O'Neill's story of her struggle reminds us that the postmodern body without organs (the virtual body on which culture inscribes its multiple configurations of power and meaning) does not exist independent of an organic body made up of hormones, tissues, and neurotransmitters that greatly complicate the understanding of illness. For example, Cherry Boone O'Neill, while deeply religious with a strong ethical sense, defended her secretive regimen of self-starvation with an unremitting routine of mendacity and outright thefts. When her parents noticed that diet pills and laxatives were missing or asked about locked doors and skipped dinners, she would invent elaborate falsifications. When family members or doctors probed too closely, she lied. Some of the most awful moments in her struggle occurred when she continued to lie to her husband despite his strenuous efforts to help her. (Her husband finally confronts her with inescapable evidence; she breaks down, promises to stop, but is soon back lying and starving herself again.) Anorexia nervosa eroded her character: she became the kind of unethical person she despised, so that the self-hatred that prompted her war against her body now ironically intensified as the war turned her into a habitual liar and thief. The self-starvation that had once imparted a sense of control now signified a life so far out of control that she watches helplessly as her marriage hurtles toward the abyss.

The uncontrollable self-destructiveness that gripped Cherry Boone O'Neill offers two clues concerning the biological substrata of anorexia nervosa. First, the blindly reckless, uncontrollable pursuit of self-starvation despite its known costs closely resembles the pattern of drug addiction. Second, the maniacal exercise routines and uninterrupted focus on diet have similarities with obsessive-compulsive disorder. Significantly, both drug addiction and obsessive-compulsive disorder are known to employ physiological processes that mere willpower is usually impotent to oppose. By analogy, we might expect that anorexia nervosa too would reveal significant biological changes. One study proposes that anorexia nervosa is a form of auto-addiction caused by a reaction to brain opioids produced by the process of starvation. There is reason to believe that eating disorders involve specific disturbances in mesolimbic and hypothalamic neurochemical function. Anorexics have significantly elevated concentrations of several key neuropeptides in their cerebrospinal fluid, as well as low concentrations of gonadal hormones. Amenorrhea is a regular feature, and it has long been known that anorexics, unlike victims of famine, are frequently hyperactive. Both hyperactivity and amenorrhea require accompanying changes in metabolism and in neuroendocrine function, which are well documented in anorexia nervosa. Moreover, researchers have shown the presence of increased serotonin activity as well as pronounced hypercortisolemia. Finally, several studies have shown that anorexics have a high incidence of obsessive-compulsive symptoms.[40] In many cases, the same biochemical processes associated with obsessive-compulsive disorder will undoubtedly coincide with the biology of anorexia nervosa.

My aim is not to trace anorexia nervosa to a specific biological cause but to suggest that once the necessary combination of postmodern psychological and cultural pressures puts a person on the path to self-starvation, biological changes accompany, reinforce, and perpetuate the original impulse to refuse food, making it enormously difficult to change course. Each new refusal is like an addict's fix: the brain chemistry simply overrides any temporary effort the addict makes to stop. Small wonder, with such complex biological and cultural underpinnings, that anorexia nervosa proves so difficult to treat and to dislodge. The young women who fall under the spell of anorexia nervosa, however, are only the most obvious victims of our culturewide obsession with perfect bodies. We need to ask what effect our utopian yearnings have on people who cannot—by any means or under any circumstances—realistically hope to embark on programs to build the perfect body.

AGAINST UTOPIA

Is utopia really what we want? Is the postmodern quest for a pain-free, disease-free, perfect body really in our best interest? When pain is at its most intense, whether in the unusual cases of end-stage cancer unresponsive to opioids or in acts of political torture, it may unravel the rich interior cosmos we create through perception, as Elaine Scarry has argued.[41] Yet in its milder, normal, intermittent, or even chronic forms, pain can also permit us to build up meaning and to appreciate (perhaps for the first time) a beauty all around us. The rare individuals born with a congenital inability to feel pain live short, freakish, unhappy lives, unable to survive in a world where pain protects us, however inefficiently, against a host of common ills. A world wholly free from pain would rob us of a biological endowment indispensable for knowledge and self-preservation, much as a world without death (requiring invulnerable bodies that never wear out) would not only alter our biology but also change our culture beyond recognition. "Another postmodern sunset, rich in romantic imagery," remarks Jack Gladney in *White Noise* as he watches the evening sky.[42] We view our sunsets (as so many aspects of our culture) only in the afterglow of romantic nature-writing that associates beauty with death. What may give the postmodern sunset its unusually vivid color, Gladney also knows, are potentially deadly pollutants suspended in the atmosphere—another by-product of the utopian quest for a world where bodies, like automobiles, are transformed into the image-rich objects of consumer fantasy.

Utopian fantasies of a perfect body ignore not only the evolutionary functions of pain and the biology of aging but also the social consequences of a failure to reach perfection. In a culture dominated by the vision of utopian bodies, illnesses that twist and distort the human figure will register as vaguely disreputable signs of personal defeat, too often met with silence and denial. Western biomedicine, with its objectifying, materializing, clinical gaze, contributes to shaping a culture in which substandard bodies are relegated to institutions or to the marginal social spaces reserved for the elderly, the handicapped, and the infirm.[43] In the United States an almost inescapable cultural teaching about bodies and illness suggests that the acceptable way for consumers to deal with such imperfections is by making a purchase that wipes them out, like underarm odor. It is not just medicine but the correct medical purchase that rescues the body from peril. Yet, the cultural faith in wonder drugs and smart shopping that has been carefully schooled in all of us complicates the dilemma of chronic pain patients by encouraging the habitual overuse of prescription and nonprescription drugs, so that clinics must often begin treatment with a period of detoxification. No one should have to endure reversible pain or illness, but there is much to be said for learning to respect and to embrace the body in all its inevitable imperfections. Meanwhile, people with infirmities ranging from combat wounds to blindness must navigate their damaged and (in some cases) irreparable bodies through a minefield culture in which the perfection of the body has become almost a national quest, a solemn duty if not a sacred rite. It is a secular religion from which the disabled and the disfigured are, of course, rigorously excluded, unless they are willing to play the ossified role assigned to them in reality-based drama as gutsy models of "personal adjustment, striving, and achievement."[44]

Ancient stereotypes link disabilities and deformities with crime, malevolence, and evil. The wicked witch is always gnarled and ugly.

Postmodern stereotypes, visible in any Disney film, are as damaging as the ancient ones. Frank talk by contemporary women who are fat or disabled provides eloquent testimony to the damage inflicted on individuals by our cultural fantasies of bodily perfection.[45]

It is important, of course, to acknowledge the pleasure we receive from the sight of attractive human bodies. It is also important to acknowledge that not everyone who seeks a perfect body finds—or admits to finding—that the quest is contradictory and barren. The cultural significance of bodily imperfections can differ profoundly according to gender and social class. Cindy Jackson, whose nineteen well-publicized cosmetic surgeries in twenty years have transformed her into what some consider a Barbie doll clone, albeit an aging Barbie, irrefutably argues that she has used biomedical technology as a means of achieving a body that better fits contemporary notions of female beauty. In her postmodern self-fashioning, she seems happily unthreatened by neurosis, and she deftly repels feminist charges that she has capitulated to bogus standards of beauty imposed on women by a male-dominated culture. Cindy Jackson likes how she looks. Who has the right to say she should feel manipulated? We cannot automatically assume that cosmetic surgery and bodybuilding are somehow inherently erroneous pursuits, unlike learning a foreign language or practicing the piano. For some individuals, the pursuit of bodily perfection approaches an art.

Cindy Jackson's pursuit of beauty may seem modest compared with the public performances of the contemporary French artist known as Orlan. A sculptor and professor of fine arts, Orlan initiated in May 1990—at the age of forty-three—a series of multiple cosmetic surgeries entitled "The Reincarnation of St. Orlan." Her project, inconceivable before the advent of postmodern self-fashioning and of reconstructive surgical techniques, involved selecting a specific facial feature from various classic artworks that embody Western ideals of female beauty, blending them by means of computer into a composite sketch, and then transferring the composite sketch (via cosmetic surgery) into her own flesh: her chin borrowed from Botticelli's *Venus*, her brow from Da Vinci's *Mona Lisa*, her nose from an anony-

mous sixteenth-century Diana, and so on. After seven operations, she
has nearly finished reconstructing her face to match the ideal form of
her computerized composite sketch. The transformation does not
stop with her face. Orlan transforms the surgeries into performance
art, complete with costumes, make-up, interviews, and camera crew.
(She transmitted the cheek-implant operation live from the operating
theater to the Sandra Gering Gallery in New York City and simulcast
it to art institutions in such far-flung locales as Toronto, Milan, and
Tokyo.) Whatever its value as art, her secular "reincarnation"—a re-
birth of the flesh—epitomizes the postmodern desire to achieve a
utopian body. Her particular desire is so extreme or forward-looking
that it comes very close to erasing the body altogether—at least the
body understood as a biological category with built-in genetic and
material constraints. As she says: "I think that the body is obsolete."[46] For Orlan, the biological body is an archaic site upon which
she and her visionary surgeons erect whatever reborn silicon-based
human artifact they choose.

Orlan and Jackson, while many may disapprove of their quest for
ideal form, have done nothing immoral or illegal, and reconstructive
surgery can perform wonders in rescuing people from the deformities of accidents or birth defects. The important question is not so
much what will specific individuals choose to do with their bodies as
what values will our culture reward. Clearly, as Orlan and Jackson
remind us, we live in a culture where the rewards lie heavily
weighted toward attractive bodies.

The postmodern impulse toward bodily perfection that stands behind a great many individual programs of self-improvement is not
merely a private matter but a cultural fact with real social consequences. Reformers and visionaries probably need utopia—and have
certainly long employed it—as a model for change. It provides a
space not only for idle dreaming but also for visionary thinking with
direct influence on the future. (Orlan, after declaring the body obsolete, continues: "I want to make art for the 21st century.") Yet the
power implicit in utopian visions is not always benevolent. As we
continue to learn more about such distinctive postmodern conditions

as anorexia, chronic pain, and depression, we may come to recognize that the social obsession with perfect bodies can produce and reinforce debilitating illness. It certainly increases the prejudice and difficulties facing people who cannot possibly measure up. What happens when not even a superhuman effort will overcome innate impairments? What happens when the dominant biomedical model of disease—with its emphasis on human norms—strongly implies that "there is something *wrong* with people with disabilities"?[47] There is much to be learned from utopian thinking, but Wallace Stevens identified one of the most important thoughts to ponder when he wrote that "The imperfect is our paradise."[48]

Suppose that the earth—what Dante emerging from hell called the "shining world" (*chiaro mondo*)—is the only paradise we will know. Suppose that paradise is here and now, not in some future or perfect state: the world and its people with all their glaring deficiencies. We might then be called upon to begin working toward an aesthetics and an ethics of imperfection. The aim would be to base our values not in the quest for perfection but in an appreciation of the imperfect. No longer keyed to lifeguards and swimsuit models, bodies and health might find their best representatives in the community of people who continue to function and contribute to society despite serious impairments. It might take as a heroine the mastectomy patient who overcomes fears about lost sexual or personal identity. "With breast cancer," said Barbara Rosenblum, who died of the disease in 1988, "a woman starts owning her own life."[49] It might find a hero in novelist Reynolds Price, paralyzed from the waist down as a result of spinal cancer. "The kindest thing anyone could have done for me . . . ," he writes of his early struggle to deal with life in a wheelchair, "would have been to look me square in the eye and say this clearly, 'Reynolds Price is dead. Who will you be now? Who *can* you be and how can you get there, double-time.'"[50] Such cold-blooded determination to reconstruct a life in the face of radical damage makes the eroticized perfect body seem not just grotesquely self-indulgent as a cultural ideal but worthless and even harmful: the ultimate escapist artifact.

The challenge that faces us is not to eliminate disability, pain, illness, and disfigurement in a quest for bodily perfection but rather to
understand the continuing ethical and social claims that they make
upon us. We cannot keep replacing organs and removing fat cells indefinitely. We can, however, hope to alleviate some of the suffering
all around us. We must therefore be prepared to resist tendencies
within postmodern culture that encourage us—through an unprecedented flow of erotic commercial images—to view the individual
human body as a privileged site of utopian transformations. We must
be prepared to insist that chronic pain, anorexia, depression, disability, and a phalanx of contemporary pathologies named and unnamed
cannot be reduced to emblems of a private dystopia. We might then
come to recognize in our inevitable imperfections—signs of the only
paradise on earth we will ever know—both the evidence of a shared
humanity that makes an ongoing ethical claim upon us and the occasion for seeking to create a culture in which human life could be, as
Karl Popper put it in his postwar critique of utopian thinking, thinking inseparable from Nazi fantasies of eugenics, "a little less terrible
and a little less unjust."[51]

chapter six

Neurobiology and the Obscene

Personally, I loved porno and I bought lots of it all

the time—the real dirty, exciting stuff. All you had

to do was figure out what turned you on, and then

just buy the dirty magazines and movie prints that

are right for you, the way you'd go for the right

pills or the right cans of food.

ANDY WARHOL,
POPism (1980)

In 1992, in the small upstate New York town of Guilderland, a uniformed officer walked into a music store and hand delivered a letter from Police Chief James R. Murley. The letter explained that the store's owner faced possible arrest under New York State law for selling materials considered obscene. It seems that a thirty-seven-year-old hairdresser had complained to police after her teenage daughter purchased two tapes by a California "gangsta" rap group. The usually unexcitable *New York Times* reported that the tapes contained abundant "racial epithets, vulgarities, and descriptions of sexual acts." [1] What made the event most newsworthy was its strange quality of déjà vu, as if Guilderland were reenacting an ancient rite of outrage that more up-to-date communities had abandoned years ago. A few hundred miles away in New York City customers walking into any adult bookstore could buy videotapes that not only describe but vividly depict almost every sexual act performed in the history of the planet—and no doubt a few known only to space aliens. The police officer in Guilderland bearing a letter from Chief Murley resembled a character walking out of a time warp.

The truth remains that the obscene is somehow in our blood. We cannot seem to get free from it. It is, of course, as historical as utopia, which usually turns out to be a space either wholly innocent of the obscene or (as in Rabelais) wholly given over to oral-genital license. Although postmodern America no longer witnesses the epic battles over censorship that engaged modernist writers such as James Joyce and Henry Miller, the obscene still frays tempers and incites debate. Some feminists argue hotly against pornographic material on the grounds that it constitutes violence against women; other feminists question whether pornography is always violent or valueless; still others openly defend the pornographic and the obscene as a legitimate realm of erotic expression.[2] In any case, both pornography and obscenity (often impossible to tell apart) seem fixtures in the late-night, low-rent postmodern marketplace. Euphemistic labels (even come-ons) such as *adult, explicit, X-rated,* and *hard-core* hold a secure place in consumer culture, drawing big profits for the porn industry and cable TV, while the Internet has turned into a superhighway for sexual information and sleazy services that makes Sodom and Gomorrah look like small towns. Meanwhile, civil libertarians vigilantly guard our right to free speech and the inevitable smut it produces. Even the Guilderland police force speaks a judicious, conciliatory, public-relations jargon. "We're certainly not looking to violate the First Amendment," Chief Murley assures reporters.[3]

The obscene, like the repressed, always seems to return, and law alone is powerless to defeat it. Supreme Court Justice Brennan in 1957 enunciated the basic principle that obscenity falls outside the area of constitutionally protected free speech.[4] The dilemma, reflected in later reports from Guilderland, is that many individuals and communities no longer know what counts as obscene, so prosecutions flounder. Chief Murley, for example, later retracted his warning to the music store, saying, "Maybe they should get rid of the word 'obscene.' What's obscene? I don't know. Apparently no one knows. If the law doesn't apply to anything, then why have it here?"[5]

It is easy to sympathize with a hard-working policeman honestly confused by the shifting and slipping terrain of postmodern community standards. A culture where people no longer understand what constitutes the obscene—a culture unlike, say, that of the early Puritan inhabitants of New England—has not so much severed its ties with the past as slipped into a state of quandary. Suppose, however, that the obscene cannot be pigeonholed as merely a question for lawyers, feminists, and religious fundamentalists to argue. Suppose that the obscene, despite its power to change across cultures and times, constitutes an enduring category of human experience. A biocultural perspective would suggest that the obscene achieves its apparently ineradicable place by weaving together powerful elements of our biology, psychology, and social life. Evidence for such a view—which has significant implications for cultural activities ranging from the practice of law to sodomy—comes from a little-known condition named after the nineteenth-century French neurologist Gilles de la Tourette.

TOURETTE SYNDROME: TICS AND ATTACKS

An oblique but fascinating glimpse into the obscene is provided by the condition known as Tourette syndrome.[6] This disorder—whose exact prevalence is unknown—was once considered rare but is currently estimated to afflict from one to ten persons per thousand. It takes its name from Gilles de la Tourette, who, in 1885, identified a set of tic-like signs and symptoms separate from other movement disorders. Now, as then, the etiology is not known, and there is no specific diagnostic test.[7] Most specialists today think that Tourette syndrome, with its cluster of recognizable and often bizarre symptoms, has a genetic basis.

The disorder originates in early childhood, with the mean age of onset being about seven years, and it occurs some three times more often in males than in females. Tourette divided the symptoms into separate developmental stages. First came motor symptoms such as eye blinking and erratic movement of the upper limbs. Second came somewhat indistinct vocalizations that sounded like barks, grunts, or muffled cries. The third symptom was so unusual that it forced Tourette to invent a new word: *coprolalia*—from the Greek *kopros* (dung) and *lalia* (talk)—which thenceforth entered the medical lexicon as the technical term for an involuntary utterance of vulgar or obscene language.

Tourette was wrong in identifying coprolalia as a distinctive symptom of the disorder that now bears his name. Obscene utterance occurs today in about 30 to 60 percent of Tourette syndrome cases, but it also appears in other neurological disorders such as dementia, nonfluent aphasia, and the violent writhing movements known as hemiballism.[8] The obscenity is not always completely audible—often being slurred or truncated—and it is sometimes unexpressed, resulting in a condition known as mental coprolalia. Yet, if not an invariable accompaniment of Tourette syndrome, coprolalia is surely among its most troublesome symptoms, and the distress radiates in many directions. Adults may live like recluses. Children, one group of researchers reports, are "punished by parents, disciplined by teachers, ostracized by classmates, and shunned by strangers." Parents will often confess with guilt that they washed the child's mouth out with soap.[9] It is hard to imagine a punishment that construes with more direct literalness our everyday metaphor concerning "dirty" words.

Coprolalia, then, is an eruption of obscenity, a normally blocked or inhibited speech surging out of control, and it persists in patients with Tourette syndrome over an entire lifetime—only on occasion showing instances of remission. The question of control is complicated. In a recent study of 135 patients with Tourette syndrome, 92 percent claimed that their tics were not automatic or involuntary but conscious and voluntary responses to an intense premonitory urge.[10] Patients often report that they can briefly defer the tic, and under special conditions the tic may temporarily disappear. Oliver Sacks describes a brilliant surgeon whose distracting verbal and motor tics vanished completely while he was performing surgery, only to reappear afterward.[11] Even if the tic is not wholly uncontrollable, however, most people afflicted with coprolalia act as if in the grip of an uncontrolled impulse.

Today, with the biological revolution in full swing, there is little support for the psychoanalytic explanations, common between 1920 and 1970, that traced coprolalia to unresolved sexual conflicts or trauma. Psychological damage, however, can certainly emerge as a *consequence* of coping with such strange and distressing symptoms as involuntary barking or swearing. Further, patients with Tourette syndrome (especially children) may suffer from other conditions such as attention deficit hyperactivity disorder and obsessive-compulsive disorder.[12] Thus, accompanying mental or emotional dysfunction is not uncommon. Coprolalia—like other symptoms of Tourette syndrome—can be induced by a blow to the head, and thus it is at least plausible that severe psychological trauma equivalent to the impact of a physical blow might trigger Tourette syndrome in someone genetically predisposed.

Most researchers are convinced that the underlying mechanism responsible for coprolalia among Tourette syndrome patients is strictly biological. Thus the likelihood that biological processes may underlie coprolalia offers evidence for thinking that the obscene—or the specific neurological patterns responsible for it—is somehow hardwired in the body. We can reject the unlikely notion of a single and unvarying neurological circuit. Our aptitude for the obscene is far more likely to resemble the "biologically prepared learning" and "gene-culture coevolution" proposed as underlying such specieswide (although not universal) human traits as fear of snakes and spiders.[13] Coprolalia, after all, occurs in Tourette syndrome patients from cultures as diverse as Denmark, Spain, and Japan.[14] Although no one, so far as I know, has attempted to describe a neurobiology of the obscene, such an inquiry is consistent not only with biological hypotheses about Tourette syndrome but also with what linguists and neurologists are learning about how the brain processes language.

It is now well known, for example, that textbook models of language that restrict normal linguistic activity to serial processing in the left perisylvian cortex (at least in right-handed individuals) need major revision. Evidence from patients with brain lesions suggests that neural processing from speech production and speech perception is not narrowly localized but broadly distributed in the perisylvian area. Lesions of the right hemisphere may damage or destroy the ability to make inferences about the relation between sentences, which is essential for understanding narrative. In addition, researchers recently have emphasized the importance to speech of various subcortical structures, including the thalamus, cerebellum, and limbic system. Separate areas of the brain, moreover, seem to handle distinct classes of words, as indicated by lesions that disturb only the naming of specific categories such as fruits and animals. (Other category-specific deficits include abstract words, verbs, geographic names, colors, and body parts.)[15] Coprolalia, of course, draws upon the highly idiosyncratic class of words called expletives, utterances that fall outside the normal categories of grammar. Still, no matter how idiosyncratic expletives may be and no matter how sketchy our knowledge, the coprolalic speech of Tourette syndrome necessarily taps into regions and processes of the brain engaged in the understanding and production of language.

Coprolalia, however, is also puzzling and distinctive, behaving in ways measurably different from normal language. Most researchers presume that coprolalia obeys an involuntary mechanism (like the irregular motor tics typical of Tourette syndrome, which are not preceded by the electrical brain impulse that precedes voluntary acts).[16] Yet, a curious subprocess of linguistic selection is at work in coprolalia. In one well-known case, a nine-year-old boy lost his coprolalia when informed that the words he employed were not obscene, and a bilingual young man regularly switched his obscene outbursts from Spanish to English depending on the language spoken around him.[17] Further, religious profanities rarely show up.[18] Coprolalia, it appears, centers almost exclusively on the body and on its lower-order associations with dirt and sex. A list of common coprolalic terms reads like an honor roll of foul-mouthed smut. Coprolalic utterance also seems to possess a distinctive grammar and style. The words—often slurred, mispronounced, or shortened—are delivered in a tone or pitch louder than usual and are curiously lacking the musical prosody of normal speech. Not only do they interrupt the flow of sentences but they also fill the syntactic pauses like punctuation, leaving the sentence rhythm undisturbed.[19] Maybe the most impressive evidence that coprolalia functions differently from ordinary language is simply this: like other symptoms of Tourette syndrome but unlike ordinary speech, coprolalia disappears or greatly diminishes under the influence of haloperidol and other drugs that block the action of the brain's (mostly subcortical) dopamine receptors.

Tourette syndrome, in short, presents a neurological disorder in which the brain misfires in such a way that a person may be galvanized into bursts of foul speech. Even if patients temporarily defer the overwhelming urge they describe, sooner or later, in the privacy of a bathroom or closet, the obscenities pour out. The inference seems unavoidable that there must be neurological processes for coprolalia both engaged with and at least partially separate from the modes of normal speech. Obscene words must be coded in a distinctive way, like the names of fruits or animals, and they must also establish connections with subcortical structures that permit them to tumble out unbidden, like a shout or cry. I have not found specific studies on the neurological processing of obscene words, although the technology, if not the funding, is available for such research. (The few general brain-imaging studies of Tourette syndrome patients are quite inconclusive.)[20] Thus, until researchers produce better maps of the brain, there is no alternative to constructing what are still necessarily abstract and hypothetical models of obscene speech.

IN SEARCH OF THE OBSCENE

Culture clearly tells us something important about illness. Can illness, as a biocultural perspective implies, also tell us something important about culture? In coprolalia, we confront not just a neurological disorder such as uncontrolled twitching but a mobilization of the complex cultural resource called obscenity. There are formidable problems in seeking to understand the obscene, as opposed to merely banning it. One basic problem, leaving aside disputes about definitions, is how to speak of the obscene at all: obscenity is that which should be unspoken and out of sight. (The state of Kansas passed a legal stricture forbidding the use of obscenity by faculty members on university land.)[21] A paradox reposes here, of course, because obscenities rank among the most common features of human speech. Yet, in order to discuss the obscene, we must self-consciously enter into its domain, and this is an act that scholars have mostly avoided. Consequently, we know little about the obscene, and what we do know often lies scattered in odd corners of specialized or vaguely disreputable journals.[22] I confess reluctance to using words here that I prefer not to use in public. But such reluctance is exactly the point. Despite all that postmodern culture has done to repackage obscenity as art, free speech, or adult entertainment, it is the nature of the obscene to generate anxieties. My gesture toward an eventual definition of obscenity would be to propose that if something is not capable of generating anxiety, it cannot be obscene.

Consider an innocuous but telling example. A New York writer, in 1993, was watching the network television drama *NYPD Blue* when a hard-boiled police detective, using the dialect of his trade, called one of the suspects an asshole. Simple realism. Here is how the *TV Guide* writer reports his own reaction: "I couldn't believe what I'd heard. I found it disturbing. And unsettling."[23] He was disturbed enough to replace the word *asshole* (in his commentary) with a fatuous circumlocution. The incident reminds us that, no matter how accustomed we grow to foul language, the obscene always retains a power—at least in certain circumstances—to get our attention. "Hey, Asshole!" Most people would feel more than unsettled if a stranger were to address them in public with an orotund obscenity.

What unsettles us about the obscene also—in the name of decorum—maintains our ignorance. Paul Cameron, writing in 1969, noted that the famous Thorndike and Lorge word-frequency list (1944), which scholars had been citing for almost three decades, was based entirely on written English and contained almost no profanities.[24] He also observed that another well-known study of English usage based on New York City telephone conversations had excluded from its sample, in the unspoken name of decency, fully 25 percent of the words uttered, which were of course obscene. In a search for facts, Cameron dispatched his students to compile secret frequency lists of words employed in three different social settings. Among the fifty most often repeated words in each setting, he found such predictable staples as articles, pronouns, and prepositions, but four other words made every list of the top fifty: *damn, hell, fuck,* and *shit.*

Here is an idea worth pondering: Americans seem unable to express themselves, at least a good percentage of the time, without recourse to the obscene. Why? Informal social codes governing obscene usage are so byzantine that it is a wonder anyone ever learns to swear. Yet people learn, effortlessly, perhaps because obscene speech at first evokes the enticements of forbidden knowledge. It gives us an early taste of the pleasure of transgression. It connotes daring and freedom. An ease with obscene speech is also a crucial way of showing that you belong to a specific group; unskilled foreigners trying to swear in English, for example, almost invariably sound absurd. In this sense, a working knowledge of the obscene imparts power. It provides a useful tool for entering a new environment, for finding your way around, for dealing with trouble, for feeling at home.

The challenge, then, is not how to justify thinking about the obscene but how to face up to its demands. An emphasis on language makes sense not only because obscene speech is so pervasive but also because obscenity so often lies in the word rather than in what it represents. As sociologist Murray S. Davis observes, it is lower-class words (prick, cunt, fuck, suck) that today are censored as obscene, while educated, upper-class, Latinate terms referring to identical activities or organs (penis, vagina, intercourse, fellatio) are acceptable.[25] It is less obscene acts than the public circulation of obscene words and images that causes most of the trouble, as in Guilderland. Even if obscenity sometimes seems about to vanish forever in a last flash of postmodern smoke and mirrors, the disturbing power of the obscene stakes a claim rooted in the human nervous system and reaffirmed at the deepest levels of human social life. No single feature—including upright posture and the opposable thumb—is more important in the development of human society than the emergence of language. Obscene words are somehow an inseparable part of the biocultural speech system that links us together. How, then, should we think about the nature of obscene speech?

A biocultural model of obscene speech must account for two crucial features: the emotional quality of obscenities and the neurological process of inhibition. Obscene words are learned along with the highly emotional knowledge that they are powerful, dangerous forces that can get people punished or attacked. Psychological research confirms that we process obscene words differently from ordinary language, with measurable differences in recall and recognition, as well as variations dependent on gender and social situation.[26] We learn obscenities, further, at an impressionable age, which helps assure they are coded within the brain bearing the unusual caution—no doubt expressed through neurological processes of inhibition—against uttering them except under special circumstances.[27] I know a psychiatrist who docks his child's weekly allowance in punishment for each obscenity uttered. Comedian Lenny Bruce built a tragic and brilliant career out of saying what you were not allowed to say in public.

Although, as we have seen, speech is for the most part controlled by the left hemisphere of the brain, the right hemisphere appears to hold dominant responsibilities for modulating the emotional components of language. Moreover, certain kinds of emotional speech belong not to the highly evolved centers of the neocortex but rather to the older, deeper structures of the midbrain and limbic system. Stimulation of specific areas of the human thalamus, for example, produces monosyllabic yells and exclamations, which researcher Georges Schaltenbrand takes to be utterances of surprise, fright, or pain. "The function of the thalamus in speech," he argues, "cannot be defined as building up sentences and propositioning abstract concepts. Its function must be of a more technical type, namely the releasing and silencing of preformed patterns."[28] Obscenities easily fit the definition of a technical type of speech that we utter mainly in preformed patterns, like the colorful descriptors that stream out fully formed the instant another driver cuts us off in traffic: a special class of emotionally charged words not fully bound by the brain's normal left-hemispheric rules for speech.

Arguments for the importance of midbrain and limbic structures in the control of obscene words also find support in research strongly suggesting that human speech, however it developed during the long history of evolution, did *not* develop from the cries and vocalizations of nonhuman primates.[29] Human speech differs fundamentally from animal cries in the sense that it proceeds from an entirely different region of the brain. Typical cries of rhesus and squirrel monkeys, for example, proceed not from the neocortex but from centers of emotion in the midbrain and limbic area. Thus, when researchers remove large areas of a monkey's neocortex, the cries continue unimpeded. Human speech, by contrast, entirely disappears when lesions destroy appropriate cortical regions of the left hemisphere. There is, however, one fascinating and well-known exception. Aphasias that cripple or destroy normal speech, leaving patients unable to talk or write, sometimes preserve untouched the ability to swear like a sailor.[30] Obscene speech comes like a voice issuing from somewhere beyond the space of normal language.

A full model of obscene speech, then, would seem to require an extensively distributed network of paths—perhaps, as Ronald Melzack has proposed for pain, a neuromatrix—connecting the ancient midbrain to higher levels of cortical processing in the left and right hemispheres. An obscenity, after all, is more like a cry than a word. Or, rather, it belongs to a special class of words that serve as the direct expression of emotion. The linguist's favorite example of meaningful language—"the cat is on the mat"—is an archetype of words drained of emotion, unless perhaps you love cats (or mats). Obscenities, however, are fighting words, gross words, dirty words, words charged with power; they are hurled like insults, heaped up to contaminate and defile, to incite or inflame, or just to let off steam. They leap out before we can stop them. They draw attention, they get us in trouble.

The emotion and the obscenity proceed together, as if fused, overriding cortical inhibitions in a quick, involuntary burst.

An impressionistic sketch might represent the obscene as an ancient subcortical creature ordinarily kept under lock and key by higher cortical inhibitions, but able to escape in moments of crisis through hidden tunnels and secret passageways. Interestingly, several biomedical researchers have characterized Tourette syndrome as a disorder of the brain's inhibitory mechanisms.[31] Others have posited neural pathways linking the disruptive motor and vocal symptoms directly to the midbrain and limbic system.[32] Linguist Colin Martindale, in a study of coprolalic verbal tics, proposes that word-selection activity in the posterior cortical speech area somehow triggers an interruptive burst of activity in a subcortical system involving the thalamus and corpus striatum. M. R. Trimble and M. M. Robertson speculate about a possible role for the cingulate gyrus, one of the largest structures within the limbic system, which, when stimulated, leads to vocalizations both in animals and in humans.[33] Such proposals do not amount to an explanation, but they clearly point out the general direction in which research is looking. A neurobiological explanation of coprolalia that links obscene speech to the midbrain and limbic system, however, holds implications that reach far beyond Tourette syndrome. Tourette syndrome, in fact, offers strong evidence that the obscene is not something wholly outside the self, that it is not simply an annoying or emancipated cultural behavior like smoking cigars in a restaurant, which can, in theory, be legislated out of existence, but rather something permanently, intractably, and uncomfortably located in the biocultural space where outside and inside converge.

POSTMODERNISM AND THE OBSCENE

Henry Miller is a useful guide to a biocultural version of the obscene as created at the crossroads of culture and human neurobiology. In 1961 Grove Press reprinted his long-suppressed book *Tropic of Cancer*, first published in 1934, thus creating an occasion for the reappearance of a classic modernist text in a postmodern context. The ensuing legal battles showed that even in the early 1960s obscene narratives still held an important place in the bourgeois politics and poetics of transgression.[34] Certainly the federal, state, and local bureaucrats who sought to ban *Tropic of Cancer* indicated something quite specific about American relations to the obscene circa 1960. They described the obscene as a kind of hellish opponent of everything lofty and ideal. It had to be banned or expunged in order that the ideal could survive.

Chief Justice Charles Desmond offers a typical American response to the obscene in writing about *Tropic of Cancer* for the New York Court of Appeals: "From first page to last it is a filthy, cynical, disgusting narrative of sordid amours. Not only is there in it no word or suggestion of the romantic, sentimental, poetic or spiritual aspects of the sex relation, but it is not even bawdy sex or comic sex or sex described with vulgar good humor. No glory, no beauty, no stars—just mud."[35] Mud, of course, is an apt metaphor for the obscene as dirt, filth, pollution, and defilement (topics to which we will return). Mud suggests the existence of a lowdown, viscous, indeterminate substrate of human life that threatens to swallow up and defile everything decent and noble and civilized. In 1961 a narrative of sex that failed to acknowledge reigning cultural pieties about beauty and romance was simply too dangerous for official sanction. It had to be roped off and banned as obscene.

American law still defines obscenity as material that deals with sex in a manner appealing to "prurient interest." Various lower courts and public servants agreed with Justice Desmond that *Tropic of Cancer* appealed to prurient interest, and their decisions entangled Miller and Grove Press in a cross-country marathon of legal action stretching from Brooklyn to Los Angeles. The Supreme Court nonetheless finally upheld publication on a split vote, in a judgment remarkable for containing no arguments and no opinions. Nobody, it appears, wanted to go on record. Yet two significant results drifted out of this judicial silence. First, the obscene had begun to slip through legal barricades that had previously suppressed or forced it underground. Obscenity would thenceforth be a visible player in the public culture. Second, the litigation, censorship, and public disapproval surrounding Henry Miller were not without benefit because they drove him to air several particularly shrewd discussions of the obscene. Turning from courtrooms to the shadowy world within the self, he depicts the obscene as a mirror that exposes some unpleasant but liberating truths we prefer to keep hidden.

Miller's mirror theory finds clearest expression in a long essay titled *Obscenity and the Law of Reflection*, first published in Paris in 1945 and then reprinted in 1964 during the controversy that surrounded the reprinting of *Tropic of Cancer*. The essay is recognizably modernist in its claim that the artist always engages in a struggle with the vast bourgeois masses, whom Miller calls "the unthinking public." In this struggle, Miller views the obscene as an instrument with almost religious power to transform human consciousness. "Its purpose," he explains, "is to awaken, to usher in a sense of reality. In a sense, its use by the artist may be compared to the use of the miraculous by the Masters." [36] Sex for Miller—at least in his more reflective moments— becomes almost a spiritual practice designed to break through the deadness of bourgeois daily life, with its secular agenda and sterilized eroticism. The truth that obscenity retrieves for Miller is far more than a coarse realism captured in the depiction of forbidden sexual acts. It is the illumination of a primal mystery suppressed or repressed within us. In ways less preposterous than the idea appears when plucked from the heart of Miller's argument, sex thus becomes a vehicle for achieving a kind of intuition of the divine within the human sphere. The eroticized spirituality of the world's great religious mystics, he believes, implied no less, and Miller feels at home in their company, although they doubtless would have been a bit puzzled by their earthy guest.

Miller's quasi-mystical psychology of the obscene, with its implicit debt to the Freudian concept of repression, is so clearly a document of high modernism that it carries little persuasion in the postmodern era of blinking neon sex shops and AIDS. Postmodern erotic life has been cycled through innumerable how-to manuals as bland and explicit as a cookbook. What better author to domesticate a power formerly deemed obscene than a physician with the improbable last name of Comfort, who creates books entitled *The Joy of Sex* and *More Joy of Sex*, as if an erotic life were no more exciting or hazardous or uplifting than a good dinner. What makes Miller still important in the age of safe sex is that he never really removed sexuality from the dangerous arena of the obscene. He never sought to domesticate it. Instead, he relied on its shock value, valued its unsettling power to enlighten us, and insisted on the unification of obscenity with the divine. In this sense, he recognized the sameness of mud and stars, where Chief Justice Charles Desmond saw only irreconcilable opposition. The value in returning to Miller's point of view is that it suggests why the obscene should have aroused such anxiety and why we should defend against it with such potent processes of inhibition, including the stratagems of domestication. The deep fear aroused by obscenity, he suggests, is a fear of the half-formed and repressed life moving blindly within us.

A version of the obscene as a projection of something dreaded and suppressed within the self is useful in suggesting why it should be obscene words, with their childhood aura of the forbidden and unclean, that pour forth spontaneously in various neurological disorders. The obscene for Miller is not an innate or archetypal category but something we have put within ourselves and in effect forbidden to come out. His psychology of the obscene is firmly based in the processes of human culture, and it thus offers a useful complement to current theories that emphasize a purely biological account of coprolalia. In the recent history of Tourette syndrome, for example, the effectiveness of new drugs such as haloperidol has led to a near total rejection of psychological accounts. One example of the flight from psychology is the account of coprolalia by neurophysiologist Marc R. Nuwer, who shows that computer-generated strings of high probability English letters and phonemes will produce, within a very short time, common four-letter obscene words.[37] This statistical principle, he argues, not a psychiatric disturbance, is what accounts for the presence of coprolalia in Tourette syndrome. Nuwer fails to note, however, that computer-generated strings also produce such common four-letter words as *hope* and *love*, which of course are not among the common verbal tics of Tourette syndrome. Why is it, Henry Miller forces us to ask, that only some of these four-letter strings get us so dreadfully upset?

From a biocultural perspective, neurological and psychological accounts of coprolalia need not be in conflict.[38] Indeed, they require each other to generate an explanatory power sufficient for understanding a complex neurolinguistic disorder such as Tourette syndrome. Henry Miller helps us understand why it is not just statistically or linguistically basic words but rather basic forbidden words—primal obscenities—that Touretters cannot prevent from streaming forth.

The mysteriously primal qualities of the obscene are what for Miller supply its potential for crisis and regeneration. "If any one had the least feeling of mystery about the phenomena which are labeled 'obscene,'" he writes in *Tropic of Cancer*, "this world would crack asunder."[39] For the modern artist, he insists, obscenity contains the same magical force accruing to ancient forms of language such as spells, incantations, and curses, in which words hold the power to cure or to kill. "Voodoo death," for example, is an extreme variant of the nocebo effect—nocebos cause symptoms in the same scientifically inexplicable fashion that placebos relieve them—and occurs when culturally potent language seems to induce chaos in the autonomic nervous system of the victim.[40] "It is my honest conviction," Miller writes, "that the fear and dread which the obscene inspires, particularly in modern times, spring from the language employed rather than the thought. It is very much as if we were dealing here with primitive taboos."[41] Just so. The trials of Henry Miller, in this context, are connected not only with the biology of Tourette syndrome but also with the experience of early humans struggling to survive in an environment where certain forms of language—prototypes of our obscenities and taboos—might prove the difference between life and death.

CULTURE, ENVIRONMENT, AND OBSCENITY

Anthropologist Weston La Barre made the basic point that our ideas of the obscene are an artifact of culture. As he writes: "We perform with indifference a great number of acts (such as drinking milk, blowing the nose, eating a beefsteak, or holding food in the left hand) which various oriental peoples view with inexpressible horror." The obscene, far from constituting a specific Western obsession, appears in so many places in so many guises as to constitute an enduring presence in human life. "A Haida Indian woman," La Barre continues, "is embarrassed to be caught by a strange man without her labret or lower lip plug. Among many Negro groups in Africa, propriety requires the buttocks to be covered, not the genitals. Philippine Islanders and Samoans think it indecent for the navel to be exposed, though every other part may go uncovered. In China, it is an obscenity for a woman to expose her artificially deformed feet to a strange man."[42] While Guilderland struggles with its postmodern confusions, the fundamentalist Parliament of Iran approves legislation requiring the death penalty for producers and distributors of pornographic videotapes.[43] The role of culture in the construction of obscenity is unmistakable.

A postmodern perspective makes it both unnecessary and unwise to ask whether obscenity is absolutely universal, given the wide range of human cultures and their power to modify genetic predispositions. Instead, research in the new field of evolutionary, or environmental, psychology encourages us to ask a somewhat different question. Has obscenity proven so pervasive across cultures and across time because—like sex, with which it is deeply entangled—humans could not have survived without it? Or, less sweepingly, did the biologically coded ability to recognize certain categories of experience as obscene confer advantages that favored human survival? Perhaps the process of human evolution has left us predisposed to recognize and respond to obscenity in such a way that (no matter what legislation the courts uphold to forbid it) we cannot easily give up our need for obscene speech?

The persistence of the obscene, I want to argue, depends in part on what obscenity contributed (and still contributes) to the development of human culture. Stephen Kaplan and Rachel Kaplan—whose work traces human preferences for certain qualities in landscape—observe that the "pattern of survival has been, throughout human evolution, a social one."[44] They point out that humans from the earliest times have hunted together, defended themselves together, and together challenged other human groups, although with a cohesiveness that is rarely secure. As any nightly newscast will confirm, humans can also prove extremely dangerous, especially when they feel competitive, frustrated, angry, confused, or betrayed. Cultures thus must develop ways to counteract these potentially disruptive threats from within, or else the entire social structure—and with it the possibility of individual survival—will collapse.

Evolutionary psychology and its various cognate fields would ask us to consider how evolution has endowed humans with a biological structure keyed to interaction with the surrounding environment (including other humans and their cultures). This human biological structure evolved to favor behavior and needs that promote survival, so that at a relatively late point in development of *Homo sapiens* the physiology of our remote ancestors changed to favor the possibility of speech.[45] Certainly the advent about 100,000 years ago of spoken language, with its dependence upon the growth of the neocortex and the upward migration of the larynx, permitted new forms of communal labor and new modes of social organization that had a major impact on human survival. It seems unthinkable that we would possess some six thousand spoken languages today (some in areas nearly inaccessible to outsiders) unless the possession of language conferred survival advantages, unlike, say, the possession of six toes. So far the claims seem quite probable. Yet some reputable scholars have recently pushed the underlying argument much further.

Ellen Dissanayake in *Homo Aestheticus* (1992) argues—against postmodern skepticism about universal features—that the universality of making and enjoying art is best explained within what she calls "the long view of human biological evolution."[46] This Darwinian view sees art as a form of behavior drawing upon neural structures of perception, thought, and feeling that originated from and played a critical role in human biological adaptation. Aesthetic acts like singing, dancing, and hitting a baseball illustrate for Dissanayake our species-centered capacity to distinguish a realm of the "extraordinary" and ultimately depend upon a biological substrate established because it contributed to survival. The playlike behavior of numerous mammal and primate species suggests that a disposition to play is connected with survival, and many important cultural activities are, at base, variations on play. Moreover, Walter Burkert in *Creation of the Sacred* (1996) has offered a similar account to explain the extraordinary persistence of religious behavior across cultures and times. Religion, he argues, extends to a supernatural realm the biologically hardwired need for hierarchy that we also observe in numerous mammal and primate species.[47] Supreme deities (whether Apollo, Lord, or Terror of the Universe) not only serve as the highest authorities on behavior and values basic to social survival but also are believed to command the rites and ceremonies that constitute the glue of human culture and group identity.

The arguments advanced in evolutionary psychology—arguments that are far more complex than I have conveyed here—cannot be dismissed as merely speculative; the physiological evidence on which they are based is compelling and demands an explanation.[48] The human recourse to obscene speech is as fundamental as play or prayer, with which, as we have seen, it seems closely connected, and one way to ask what advantages obscenity might provide in the development of human social life is to examine the place of obscenity in non-Western, indigenous, preliterate cultures. Such anthropological evidence links the obscene directly to issues of peril and survival.

A full anthropological study of the obscene does not exist, but one good starting point is Mary Douglas's fascinating study of ritual pollution. The remote peoples whom she examines in her book *Purity and Danger* (1966) help reveal how the organization of human thought and social life depends on the identification of specific areas as forbidden, unclean, and defiling: in short, as taboo. The word *taboo*—an import from the nonindustrial world, Polynesia to be exact—refers to prohibitions that, if not observed, are believed to result in immediate or inescapable harm.[49] The rules against incest offer one example of a taboo, as do the famous prohibitions in Leviticus against eating animals deemed "unclean." Although the concepts of taboo and obscenity are not identical, they are related in ways helpful in illuminating Chief Justice Desmond's anxiety about certain forms of artistic expression as mud or dirt or filth. The premodern response to experience deemed unclean (including language rooted in excremental functions and in the problematics of human sexual life) is to fence off the danger zones with prohibitions and taboos.

It is easy to imagine an evolutionary and adaptive value in traditional taboos against incest, which prevent weakened offspring and cement patriarchal social ties through the circulation of women. No doubt religious laws designating certain foods as "unclean" also protected against disease and thus strengthened the social group. There are good reasons why early peoples whose prohibitions kept dwellings and settlements free from human waste—as is the case with current nomadic tribes—would experience better health than people without such taboos. Jeffrey A. Gray in *The Neuropsychology of Anxiety* (1982) speculates that natural selection may have favored fear of dirt as much as it favored fear of snakes or of enclosed spaces.[50] Yet Mary Douglas would caution against assuming too quickly that the only purpose of pollution rituals is to protect against disease or debility. The concept of taboo incorporates a belief, stretching back to human prehistory and to the earliest religious cults, that nature is crisscrossed with malign, threatening, uncontrollable forces, not just ferocious animals and destructive storms but hostile demons ready to attack at the slightest provocation. The important point, Douglas insists, is that dirt, filth, and pollution stand as the image of matter-out-of-place, the image of disorder, anomaly, ambiguity, and danger, with their threats to human survival. The danger lies less in the filth, as a material fact, than in the disorder it represents. Filth, however, is not only a direct image of disorder but also an indirect sign of social cohesion. "Where there is dirt," Douglas writes, "there is system. Dirt is the by-product of a systematic ordering and classification of matter."[51]

The taboo, with its links to dirt and pollution, thus constitutes for Douglas far more than merely a mechanism for hygiene or eugenics. Rituals of pollution, like other rites and ceremonies, represent a strategy of control over a universe that seems in their absence uncontrollable and deeply threatening. The sense of control that all rites provide in their formal repetitions may be ultimately less important for group survival than the belief in coherence that such rites affirm and that accompanies any culturewide system of order. As Douglas sees it, pollution rituals and taboos are an essential means of imposing order on a world that at any moment threatens to collapse into a chaos of black magic and destruction. They are not miscellaneous superstitions but rather the indispensable underpinnings for an entire system of belief. The coherent belief systems provided by a culture—far more than a few scattered taboos—are what offered real protection against a hostile environment and against the dangers that human beings pose to other human beings. Remove the principle of dirt and you risk damaging the sense of coherence provided by a systematic order. Our need for a sense of coherence, as the new evolutionary psychologists see it, is not a random or adventitious cultural taste, like our occasional desire for rocky-road ice cream, but a hardwired biological drive. A scene of complete randomness in which for a prolonged period humans experience nothing except unrelieved confusion provides all the ingredients necessary for breakdown. Dirt, understood through the lenses of evolutionary psychology, is a social expression of our underlying biological need to find an order in experience.

While dirty words and traditional Western obscenities do not occupy Douglas in her study of taboos, other anthropologists show clearly that language often proves central to the social experience of defilement and purification. In the Ethiopian province of Gurage, for example, the words for certain animals—serpent, leopard, antelope—are taboo and a woman is forbidden to utter the name of her husband.[52] In other cultures, the name of a dead relative must not be spoken. Such words and names hold a dangerous power. So strong is the sense that certain forms of language hold power to pollute and contaminate that, even today, bilingual speakers of English will often refuse to utter words from their own native tongues that sound, even vaguely, like obscenities in English.[53] Mothers and police chiefs and TV critics are not the only people who find obscene language upsetting. At the heart of the obscene lies the power to evoke dirt, ambiguity, anomaly, disorder, outrage, and danger. If we want to imagine how obscene language could create a special category of brain function, we need only imagine a point in human prehistory when language itself was attributed magical power. Or consider patients who suffer from the degenerative brain condition known as Huntington's disease: while they vary in the inability to identify and interpret various emotions, they usually cannot even recognize the emotion of disgust. To German neuropsychologist Reiner Sprengelmeyer this pattern strongly suggests that disgust is an emotion that arose so early in our evolutionary history—perhaps as a nonverbal warning of spoiled food—that a specific part of the brain was dedicated to its recognition.[54] The parallels with obscenity are hard to miss. We need not make the strongest claim, which I believe to be true, that the obscene or its prototypes once held a direct relationship to human survival; it is sufficient for my argument simply to observe that obscenity remains, at very least, a by-product of other social and linguistic features that are indeed adaptive.[55] Its roots, in any case, reach deeper than any historian can delve.

The power of the obscene to create fear and confusion must be regarded as dynamic rather than static. As we have seen, the particular acts and words regarded as obscene change across cultures and across time. *Tropic of Cancer*, once so scandalous, is now ignored, and instead rap groups, adult videos, and skin magazines draw the wrath of anti-obscenity forces. An understanding of the cultural forces that periodically reconstruct the obscene would require a sociology of swearing and a history of blasphemous speech.[56] (*Vulgarity*, for example, another name for obscene speech, refers to language once identified solely with the common people in aristocratic societies.)

Geopolitical forces as real as the English Channel and the Atlantic Ocean subdivide and historicize obscene language. By the fifteenth century the English were known throughout France as *Goddams*, referring to an expression apparently indispensable to English soldiers.[57] The rise of Puritanism in England, H. L. Mencken has suggested, in effect transferred swearing from England to America, where it has certainly thrived.[58] *Fucking*, I learned one summer, is an adjective that can be applied indifferently to hammers, boards, nails, or almost any inanimate object that a carpenter might order his lowly assistant to fetch. The social context changes, but the obscene remains an instrument of power.

A biocultural approach requires an awareness of how changing historical and social forces help give obscenity its particular shape. Although the obscene relies on neurological processes encoded in the tangles of evolution, it is reshaped even by the changing means taken to disseminate and to combat it. Walter M. Kendrick in *The Secret Museum* (1987) notes that methods emerged toward the end of the eighteenth century for restricting access to obscene materials so as to exclude women and the lower classes. It was in 1818 that Dr. Thomas Bowdler published his famous edition of Shakespeare, removing all words and expressions "which cannot with propriety be read aloud in a family." The first recorded use of *pornography*—from the Greek *porne* (prostitute)—appeared a little later, in the 1857 edition of Robley Dunglison's *Medical Lexicon*, referring to "a description of prostitutes or of prostitution, as a matter of public hygiene." Thus, while pornographic writing and pictures far predate ancient Rome, our term for describing and implicitly condemning such material had to await Victorian medicine and its moralized attention to public health.[59] Today the pornographic and the obscene come reshaped not only by Victorian morality and modernist resistance to Victorianism but also by postmodern commerce, so that, as Andy Warhol puts it, you now choose the dirty magazines that are right for you with the same freedom and well-honed consumer skills with which you buy pills or groceries.

This historical reshaping of the obscene raises a possibility that the coprolalia of Tourette syndrome may at times take an altered form. In postmodern America, religious profanities evoke measurably less negative response than do sexual obscenities.[60] In a culture that attributes immense importance to religious language, the vocal tics of Tourette syndrome might take the form of profanities instead of sexual obscenities, helping to account for cases of blasphemous speech that previous eras explained as diabolic possession. Again, the important point is to view the obscene not as universal and timeless but rather as biological and cultural. The pervasiveness of obscenity across so many societies, despite its shifting historical shapes, lends credence to a view that taboo language and the obscene are far more than local customs. A biocultural perspective would view them rather as enduring forms of cultural behavior rooted in human anatomy.

Taboo language offers one final clue to the prehistory of the obscene. Quite possibly, words stigmatized as dirty or polluting not only proved indispensable to the development of cultural systems but also conferred immediate practical advantages on early humans. Consider the value of words so saturated in dirt and anxiety that they, like the name of Yahweh at the opposite pole of linguistic usage, are held unspeakable. To utter these emotionally charged words was to risk unleashing terrible forces, which explains the need to recruit strong neurological inhibitions to prevent their inadvertent use. The advantage of possessing such dangerous, unspeakable words is that their use automatically guarantees maximum attention. They reach us—at least they did before cable television and First Amendment rights made them as common as daisies—with the force of a slap in the face.

Any device for guaranteeing maximum attention is useful and sometimes life saving, like an air raid siren. Obscene words also serve especially well for acts of aggression, and not just on the highway. Australian aborigines use obscenities for the explicit purpose of arousing anger, and arguments between two aboriginal women quickly fill the air with abusive epithets referring to filth and excrement.[61] Then, too, taboo words prove useful for purposes of eroticism and sexual display; they often pour out spontaneously during orgasm, the moment when coprolalia ceases for Tourette syndrome patients.[62] Consider the words of an eighth-grade American boy explaining why the sexual harassment of girls occurs most often when boys cluster in groups: "Then everybody's competing for attention. And one way to get it is to do something obscene."[63] There is even clear psychological benefit derived from obscenities employed for letting off steam. Finally, best of all, these solid advantages may be bought quite cheaply. The wonderful thing about taboos, Douglas reports, is that most acts of pollution have a simple remedy for undoing their ill effects. "There are rites of reversing, untying, burying, washing, erasing, fumigating, and so on," she points out concerning taboos, "which at a small cost of time and effort can satisfactorily expunge them."[64]

The problem of obscenity today may not be the inevitable (if misguided) attempts to police it, since by definition the obscene is that which disturbs, but rather the loss of a ritual context that allows cultures to acknowledge the obscene while erasing the danger that it releases into the community. ("Excuse me"—spoken after a coarse remark—is a rudimentary purifying rite.) Henry Miller believed that the world is healthier when people confront rather than repress the obscene within them. Acceptance of the obscene, he argues, brings significant changes: it changes the person, and it changes how the person views the world. Obscenity itself alters. As Miller writes of the obscene in the last sentence of *Obscenity and the Law of Reflection*: "When it is recognized and accepted, whether as a figment of the imagination or as an integral part of human reality, it inspires no more dread or revulsion than could be ascribed to the flowering lotus which sends it roots down into the mud of the stream on which it is borne."[65] What Miller envisions here is not really the end of the obscene but a radical transformation. Traditional obscenities would still exist in Miller's world, but no longer would they cluster around sex. Sex, free from dread, would be free from the stigma of obscenity.

What remains truly obscene, Miller says, what deserves every resource of our fear and loathing, is the spectacle of men in closed rooms laboring over weapons of mass destruction.

The disgust, revulsion, and dread associated with obscenity have potent uses in a world still full of dangers, so perhaps we should not be so quick to domesticate and defuse the obscene as merely an annoying issue of free speech. Humans continue to encounter situations requiring a language of anxiety, anger, outrage, and alarm. The archaic category of matter-out-of-place may still retain crucial uses in underwriting our fragmented and diffuse postmodern systems of social order. Sexuality moreover is a powerful force in childhood development, seldom untouched by anxiety, while dirt and excrement have long held a powerful grip on the human imagination, as satirists know. It seems unlikely that such potent forces will all gradually lose their capacity to disturb us. Miller, however, makes a fascinating point. It is possible, as he suggests, that a wise society can learn how to narrow or expand or redirect the range of the obscene. Think of the obscene as an ancient survival mechanism, the product of a biocultural process embedded in human evolution, as impossible to legislate away as the tics of Tourette syndrome. We might then begin to appreciate the uses of obscenity and apply our ancient language of filth and outrage somewhat more selectively to whatever it is within the vastly altered postmodern world order that truly threatens our survival.

chapter seven

The Plot of Suffering

About suffering, they were never wrong,

The Old Masters: how well they understood

Its human position . . .

W. H. AUDEN,
"Musée des Beaux Arts" (1938)

"Our continued existence as gay men upon the face of this earth is at stake," wrote playwright and novelist Larry Kramer in 1983. "Unless we fight for our lives, we shall all die."[1] His impassioned, angry, alarmist outcry about AIDS occurred at a time when the number of known victims killed by the mysterious new disease had recently climbed over one thousand. In the two years prior to 1983, widely scattered news reports and medical bulletins had referred to a shadowy fatal ailment called GRID, gay-related immune deficiency, so-called because most of its victims were male homosexuals. Why were they dying? Nobody knew, although wild theories, paranoia, and outright antigay bigotry began to circulate almost at once. (With graveyard humor, New York City hospital staff invented their own acronym for the disease: WOGS, or wrath of God syndrome.) Only in mid-1984 did scientists isolate the cause of AIDS in a retrovirus—labeled HTLV-III by Americans, LAV by the French, and ultimately HIV. Two years later, the U.S. Public Health Service estimated that between 1 and 1.5 million Americans were infected with HIV. Early in the next decade, the World Health Organization concluded that by the year 2000 the number of HIV-positive people will stand at some forty million worldwide. According to United Nations figures, sixteen thousand people are now infected each day. What the popular media first described as a "gay plague" has grown into a global pandemic that threatens even newborn infants. The gay community in the United States has been hit especially hard. "Because fate had placed me on the front line of this epidemic from the very beginning," as Kramer explained the role (part jeremiah, part foot soldier) that he felt thrust upon him, "I was a witness to much history that other writers were not." [2]

There is no doubt that AIDS has reshaped the postmodern era. The fear and suspicion that it introduced into human sexual relations have, as philosopher Jacques Derrida observes, "irreversibly affected our experience of desire." [3] Fortunately, the prognosis of imminent holocaust is not so grim as when Kramer issued his 1983 alarm to the gay community. Advances in pharmacology are beginning to transform AIDS—at least in the West—into a manageable chronic illness. Throughout central and East Africa, however, and elsewhere across the developing world, death from wasting symptoms of the so-called thin disease is swift and sure. Even where treatment is affordable, AIDS continues to destroy lives, families, and communities. A new literature has emerged that chronicles how AIDS has turned parent against child, straight against gay, employer against employee, lover against lover.[4] AIDS also still carries the stigma attached to high-risk groups such as homosexuals, intravenous drug users, and prostitutes. As a sexually transmitted fatal disease, it evokes the emotional charge always latent in the volatile bond between death and eroticism, so that real effort is required to see AIDS patients as merely people who are ill. Patients are too often viewed as helpless victims. The science-based public television series Nova employed the horror-film scenario of victims in the grasp of a hideous creature to provide the structure for a widely shown documentary on AIDS, with doctors and scientists cast as heroic dragon slayers.[5] The person who falls ill with AIDS today falls unavoidably into this net of tacit meanings and subliminal narratives.

No contemporary affliction illustrates better than AIDS how the biology of human illness intersects with cultural practices that increasingly reshape it.[6] In effect, while the human immunodeficiency virus was silently digging into the genetic material of the billions of cells it attacked across the globe, activists with the passion of Larry Kramer (including his critics within the gay community) were generating an unprecedented discourse of protest, analysis, argument, fear, elegy, and denunciation. Talk about AIDS filled the air and encircled the virus in meaning, with widely varying results. Such talk helped some patients and activists to work out a new sense of their own identity, but for others the babble of conflicting voices threatened to undermine a stable sense of self. Public health posters and (to a lesser degree) televised ads reinforced the discourse with images of healthy, beautiful, erotic bodies threatened or poisoned by AIDS.[7] As Paula A. Treichler has shown, people who suffer from AIDS in the developed world suffer within a cultural context in which their illness has been saturated with multiple meanings and ambiguous information.[8] The role of culture in helping to construct this distinctively postmodern affliction raises an issue that connects AIDS with other forms of traumatic illnesses. How far is human suffering a state which we experience in ways given or taught to us, however indirectly, by our cultures?

SUFFERING, VOICE, AND NARRATIVE

Biomedicine, with a few distinguished exceptions, has left the issue of suffering nearly untouched, delegating (or relegating) it to pastoral care.[9] Most major religions, in fact, take suffering quite seriously as a central question to be addressed, often inseparable from the problem of evil. Within biomedicine, by contrast, there is not even an agreed upon vocabulary with which to define suffering or to frame the questions it raises. It is at least clear that suffering and pain are conceptually distinct, in that you can be in pain without suffering or suffer without being in pain, so that suffering cannot be defined merely as a heightened degree of pain. Moreover, patients with various painful illnesses such as cancer or AIDS frequently experience simultaneous suffering that goes well beyond the expected consequences of tissue damage. Such suffering can ultimately prolong and aggravate difficult problems of pain until pain and suffering become, for practical purposes, inseparable. How, then, do you tell them apart? Does each require its own mode of medical treatment? It should not seem a surprise that biomedicine has mostly ignored suffering in favor of problems—not always equally pressing—where the boundaries are less vague and the complications more responsive to innovations in technique and in pharmacology.

The biomedical model faces particular difficulties because suffering seems to resist the methods of science. Suffering cannot easily be studied in a lab, and the variables are numberless. What do you measure when you measure suffering? Yet, indirectly, experimental science has already offered powerful insights into suffering. Jay M. Weiss in 1972 described experiments in which two rats were given electrical shocks equal in duration and intensity. One rat was permitted to learn how to predict and to control the shocks. The second rat had no means of prediction or control—learning only that it was helpless in the face of unpredictable, uncontrollable pain. Weiss called the state experienced by the second rat "learned helplessness," and he demonstrated that (compared with the rats receiving shocks absolutely identical in duration and intensity) rats in a state of learned helplessness showed significantly greater weight loss, gastric ulceration, and neuroendocrine changes.[10] It seems axiomatic that human suffering involves learned helplessness, since almost no one would choose to suffer if help were available. Weiss's study makes it logical to expect that human suffering involves significant biological change, as indeed occurs in chronic pain. Pain specialists C. Richard

Chapman and Jonathan Gavrin explored this idea in devising a model of suffering based partly on the stress response and its relation to the hypothalamo-pituitary-adrenocortical (HPA) axis.[11] The profession of nursing, with its strong tradition of clinical observation and hands-on care, has raised other questions about suffering and helped to remind biomedicine about the problem it prefers to ignore.[12] Still, while we know little about the biology of human suffering, we have not even begun to ask more difficult questions about what a full biocultural perspective might look like. As a start, it is certain that a postmodern perspective on suffering would need to introduce a serious discussion of narrative.

Narrative over thousands of years has constituted a special resource (often used to great advantage by philosophers and theologians) given over to the knowledge of suffering. What narrative can tell us about suffering, however, and ultimately about the suffering of people with AIDS, is a question that from a postmodern perspective at first opens up onto a bottomless chaos. Contemporary theory has forced us to ask hard questions about the nature of interpretation and about the relations between text and world. A loose alliance of new academic disciplines has shown how earlier canonical works of Western literary tradition relegate minority figures—women, blacks, Asians, gays—to, at best, marginal status. What narrative turns out to tell us about suffering, in short, depends on basic decisions about what counts as narrative, how we interpret it, and whose suffering matters.

Difficulties mount because postmodern theory makes it often hard to say what narrative has to tell us about *anything*. Some theorists hold that all texts are inherently undecidable—or else receive temporarily stable meaning only through their receptions by historically changing interpretative communities. A move from theory to practice does not promise firmer ground. The individual texts to consider are numberless. "It is probably no exaggeration to say that the single most common subject of art," writes Walter Slatoff, "is some form of human suffering."[13] Practical critics in the analysis of specific texts often simply replicate contested theoretical assumptions. We can expect that Marxist critics will show how suffering is bound up with social class and with the means of production; psychoanalytic critics, how it taps into mechanisms of desire; feminist critics, how it follows the fault lines of gender. Although recent debates have left us in no danger of oversimplifying a discussion of suffering, they may also appear as merely endless conflict among partisans of wholly irreconcilable ways of reading.[14]

A final difficulty—the presumed need to define suffering and to distinguish it from related or overlapping states such as grief and pain—would seem to constitute an impassable barricade. Yet, some barriers can be safely sidestepped. There is much to be learned through invoking an exploratory spirit and a provisional vocabulary as a means of respecting both the vast diversity of suffering and the urgent need for dialogue among disparate disciplines, which always tend to see things a bit differently. One useful way to continue the explorations that a few scholars have already begun into suffering and its relation to narrative is to consider the concept of voice.[15]

Voice matters both to suffering and to narrative. T. S. Eliot in "The Three Voices of Poetry" (1953) argued that poetry demands an encounter with intricately layered nuances of human speech expressing tone, attitude, and character.[16] Voice for a modernist writer such as Eliot means something different than it does for a postmodern writer. As the postmodern self becomes increasingly fragmented and indeterminate, the voice of the text becomes correspondingly attenuated and many sided, the echoes from a linguistic no-man's-land where apparently free-floating speakers address free-floating listeners, where phrases and words often seem detached from individual speakers.[17] Nonetheless, even granting significant differences between modern and postmodern texts, what every concept of voice holds in common is the relationship to its opposite: silence. Silence stands in opposition to every voice, weak or strong, ordinary or unique, prosaic or poetic, modern or postmodern. This absolutely basic opposition between voice and silence matters here because suffering, like pain, with which it so often intermingles, exists in part beyond language.

The silence of suffering has, paradoxically, turned into something of a cliché—despite the contrary evidence of an almost interminable discourse of contemporary complaint, lament, litigation, symptom mongering, and public confession. The paradox may simply acknowledge our power to tune out unwelcome news—suffering appears silent because we do not want to hear it—but clichés also often express complex and basic facts.[18] Suffering is truly voiceless in the sense that silence becomes a sign of something unknowable. It implies an experience not just disturbing or repugnant (not just something we do not want to hear about) but inaccessible to understanding. We might say that suffering encompasses an irreducible nonverbal dimension that we cannot know—not at least in any normal mode of knowing—because it happens in a realm beyond language. The quality of such suffering remains as resistant to thought as the void opened up by a scream.

The scream might serve as a potent image for the metaphorical silence at the heart of suffering. A scream is not speech but the most intense possible negation of language: sound and terror approaching the limits of absolute muteness. Like the ceremonial wailing of grief, it seems to come from a region where words fail. Even a typical Hollywood scream, while it shatters a preceding silence or calm, also deepens the silence it shatters, as if it gestured toward something radically inexpressible. One function of narrative is to bring this deeper silence to awareness, to make such silences "speak" by extending our recognition of an irreducible, nonverbal dimension of suffering. The impossible project of giving "speech" to silence is important because it exposes how we simplify and betray suffering, as in many standard psychological tests, when we ignore its power to elude every linguistic and conceptual tool that humans employ to understand it.

Silences convey a wide range of significance, from a pregnant pause to a stunned wonder. The silence of suffering, in addition to gesturing toward an inexpressible dimension, also points to very practical breakdowns of speech. Such silence expresses experience that is not ultimately ungraspable but merely resistant to description. Suffering tends to make people inarticulate, and the voicelessness of people who suffer often resembles the silence of chronic pain patients who discover that months of complaint finally just exhaust caregivers and even family. Such patients, who have learned their own helplessness, withdraw into an uncommunicative isolation constructed in response to an environment where effective aid has all but vanished. Here the challenge for narrative analysis is to distinguish the inexpressible from what is merely hard to describe or a sign of learned helplessness.

What narrative can teach us about silence is especially important in showing that silence is not simply an experience of the solitary individual but a social consequence almost built in to the interpersonal structure within which suffering occurs. That is, even when words prove at least partly adequate, even when speech occurs, communication fails. Thus W. H. Auden observes in his famous poem "Musée des Beaux Arts" (1938)—based upon the painting *The Fall of Icarus* (1555) by Pieter Brueghel the Elder (figure 5)—that suffering is embedded in a social world where nonsufferers always find their own lives infinitely more immediate and absorbing.[19] The problem, as Auden poses it, is not that witnesses deliberately turn away from disaster, unable to bear it or refusing to assist, although in fact people often do turn away. Auden does not represent an aversion to suffering as moral failure, a lapse, say, of charity or courage. Instead, he depicts aversion or detachment as the outcome of a structural position we cannot help but occupy. In his poem, the ploughman never looks up at the white legs of a boy (who has fallen out of the sky) almost disappearing into the sea in the lower corner of Brueghel's painting. The expensive ship sails on. Should suffering fall unavoidably within our field of vision, Auden insists that we cannot escape our built-in detachment, so suffering might as well occur in silence. Not even the Old Masters could somehow place us in direct relation to another's suffering, he suggests. Their triumph—straining the limits of art—lies in forcing us to recognize and to contemplate our fated detachment as each person, like Icarus, inevitably suffers alone.

The significance of Auden's poem, from a postmodern perspective, lies in the artfulness with which it presents the modernist myth that suffering is a quintessentially private act. Auden employs

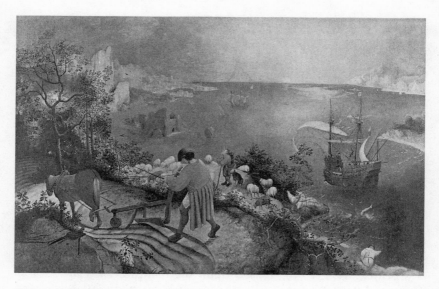

Figure 5. Pieter Brueghel the Elder, *The Fall of Icarus*, 1555, oil on canvas. Courtesy Musées royaux des Beaux-Arts de Belgique, Brussels. Photo: Giraudon / Art Resource, New York.

Brueghel and the Old Masters in order to elevate into the position of universal truth what is merely a historically and culturally specific modernist interpretation of suffering as exclusively private and internal. As heirs of modernism, we may readily affirm in Auden's poem a sense that the normal "human position" in regard to suffering mandates a glasslike separation and detachment. This modernist narrative about the solitude and privacy of suffering is not, however, an inevitable interpretation of Brueghel's painting. It is not at all certain that Brueghel takes suffering as his subject. The fall of Icarus can as easily depict violent death or the folly of overreaching. (In reaching beyond the human, Icarus ignores the beautiful humanly cultivated world that, in return, ignores him.) Nonetheless, Auden has succeeded so powerfully in describing Brueghel's work that most readers seem to believe Brueghel not only confirms the poem's view of suffering but also (as one of the "Old Masters") confers a kind of universality upon it.

The postmodern experience of suffering is somewhat different. After a debilitating stroke, an eighty-seven-year-old woman was kept alive for five days in the intensive care unit by means of a respirator and a feeding tube. Her daughter, Elisabeth Hansot, describes what she calls a "harrowing" ordeal that unfolded as she desperately sought to convince doctors in the ICU to respect her mother's explicit legal directive not to have her life prolonged by artificial means. The cadre of cardiologists, neurologists, and pulmonologists had their own views. Voice, it appears, is not just a matter of speaking but of being heard. The suffering of the elderly Mrs. Hansot—a "distress" her daughter calls "palpable"—soon became hard to bear. "During her ordeal," Elisabeth Hansot writes, "my mother became increasingly frantic. She continually leaned against her restraints, trying to get her hand close enough to her feeding tube to tear it out again. My sense of being trapped in a nightmare intensified."[20] In one sense, this double nightmare occurs in private. Yet, like Elisabeth Hansot's letter to a prominent medical journal describing it, the event also becomes a semipublic drama in which suffering manages to find a narrative voice.

The modernist narrative of suffering as a quintessentially private state is not the last word or the only word on suffering. A postmodern perspective exposes the dissent and dialogue that leave open other possibilities for a richer narrative of recovered voices. It hears the differences even within modernist accounts of suffering. Samuel Beckett, for example, spent a lifetime creating minimalist texts in which voice seems caught, like the Cheshire cat, in the process of imminent disappearance.[21] Either the human state in its seriocomic bleakness leaves almost nothing to say, as in *Waiting for Godot*, or stable identity crumbles toward anonymous incoherence, as in *Not I*, where a spotlight shines on a single mouth-sized hole in the curtain through which a nameless voice utters its nonstop woe. Yet, on the edge of linguistic breakdown—where suffering is not a trial of faith or noble burden but an almost meaningless charade in the cosmic theater of the absurd—Beckett manages to portray speech as a kind of existential imperative amid postwar confusion and emptiness: to speak is, in a minimal but ineradicable assertion, to be. Beckett's art is to represent this diminished, almost nullified state of suffering with such droll precision that it seems almost tolerable: "I can't go on. I'll go on."

A postmodern perspective finds in narrative a compendium of diverse voices with a potential to readjust the "human position" of suffering. The voices are far from always wise or composed. The voluminous writing in response to the experience of World War I contains, like the Book of Job, halting and troubled voices, voices that are angry and confused, voices that are hurt, exhausted, foolish, or blasphemous.[22] The content of the utterance, while crucial to its writer or speaker, matters less from a postmodern perspective than the evidence that affliction has broken through into language. We are brought into the presence of words that cross over, imperfectly, from the other side of torment. Indeed, narrative voices convey such an enormous diversity that—taken together—they approximate an encyclopedia of suffering. What matters from a postmodern point of view is the sheer plurality of voices. No single utterance is complete or sufficient. Women's voices convey a different experience of suffering than men's voices; black voices speak differently from white voices; the voices of Protestant martyrs differ from the voices of Catholic martyrs; medieval voices, speaking of sin and damnation, differ from secular modern voices.[23] Narrative employment of voice offers an opportunity to open up the interior or private life of a character, revealing an aspect of affliction that we rarely see. It can also infuse suffering with an unusual power to capture attention, to move emotion, and to compel a response. Such narrative voices create the occasion for an answering empathy inaccessible to Auden's eye-to-the-ground ploughman. They hold a power to address or even reverse the pressure within affliction toward isolation and silence.

"The use of language," as Joyce Carol Oates said in accepting the National Book Award in 1970, "is all we have to pit against death and silence."[24] As a native postmodernist, Oates never guarantees that the opposite of silence is truth, yet she also insists that narrative, in giving voice to affliction, is a significant force in the struggle to alter and improve our difficult relation to suffering. Certainly as Western medicine grows dependent on high-tech machines and complex pharmacokinetics, the uses of an instrument as basic as the human voice seem greatly underestimated. Support groups—the postmodern social equivalent of one-on-one modernist psychoanalysis—provide evidence that shared narratives of suffering, under the right conditions, can hold healing powers. There is evidence now for a therapeutic benefit in prayer, which is a shared and ritualized as well as personal language.[25] Reynolds Price, who lamented the inability to find helpful voices in print when he faced his personal struggle against spinal cancer, soon after publishing his 1994 book about the ordeal was receiving dozens of letters each week from people seeking his assistance. Voice ranks among the most precious human endowments suffering deprives us of, removing far more than a hope that others will understand or assist us. Silence and the loss of voice may eventually constitute for some a complete shattering of the self. Even as it threatens to immure the sufferer in a speechless, destructive silence, suffering also intensifies our need to hear and deploy the human voice, as we can recognize in letters, diaries, and journals written in situations of great duress by people now famous or obscure, from John Keats to unknown slaves or soldiers. The modernist myth of private suffering, in short, is a cultural narrative that the postmodern voices of Larry Kramer and AIDS activists—who work under the slogan Silence = Death—can teach us much about resisting.

GENRE AND THE SHAPES OF SUFFERING

Narrative and voice are important in understanding the suffering that so often accompanies illness, but there is a problem with much postmodern analysis that employs them without an attention to genre. Narratives or stories always require form—they are never simply formless utterances, much as voices are never simply an expression of individual speech. Drawing upon the work of philosophers and sociolinguists, recent theorists have argued that speakers are always engaged in dialogue with other speakers in the encompassing social network of language. Each voice speaks with a distinctive, maybe unique, timbre. No one can communicate in language, however, without employing the innumerable speech acts—asking, telling, promising, begging, urging, and the rest—that typify the intricate, shared, cultural and linguistic codes that underlie every utterance. These ordinarily unnoticed codes reflect the widely shared social patterns that Russian theorist Mikhail Bakhtin calls "speech genres."[26] Genre, of course, refers to the traditional forms of literary composition—such as pastorals, epics, and sonnets—including the innumerable varieties of mixed forms (from tragicomedy to novels) as well as relative newcomers like Westerns and sci-fi thrillers. The concept of speech genres is valuable because it calls attention to the various formal codes that underlie every utterance or communication: conversational asides, legal briefs, football cheers, jokes, government documents, postcards, papal bulls, telephone calls, letters of recommendation, whatever. Voices are comprehensible less because we understand language (the simple prerequisite for understanding) than because we come to recognize the social and formal patterns that shape and underlie any act of speech.

Every utterance constitutes a miniature text, and Jacques Derrida makes the crucial point when he writes that "there is no genreless text." "A text," he insists, "cannot belong to no genre, it cannot be without or less a genre."[27] Like written texts, voices communicate by means of genres that not only impose loose or strict demands on speakers but also depend on the existence of specific discourse communities. A football cheer is meaningless in a culture without sport. An Islamic call to prayer makes no sense in a world devoid of Muslims. Yet, speech genres do more than assure that there is never simply a voice speaking. They help to shape the substance of what is said. Ralph Cohen shows how a single oral narrative (about the unfortunate apprentice George Barnwell) undergoes crucial changes as it is retold in the differing eighteenth-century literary genres of ballad, domestic tragedy, chapbook, and novel.[28] *Romeo and Juliet* takes on more than new characters when it passes through Broadway and a (romanticized) urban gang culture to emerge as *West Side Story*. In its conventions and social forms, the Broadway musical reshapes a Renaissance story about star-crossed lovers and feuding families into a portrait of immigrant experience in the postmodern land of opportunity.

Why does it matter for people suffering with AIDS that every voice is shaped and constrained by speech genres? It matters because how we talk about suffering and how we talk when we suffer are always constrained by the speech genres of specific discourse communities. Even the groaning or silence of a woman in childbirth reflects the values a specific culture places on expressions of pain. (In Micronesia, I was told, only by placing a hand on a woman's abdomen can a Western doctor know if she is in labor.) Discourse about suffering in a scholarly journal, for example, will take the form of academic essays. There will be footnotes to contemporary thinkers, correct grammar, titles with colons. Obscenities will be expunged. Authors will place an invisible premium on intelligence, employ specialized terms, reject the ideas of previous writers, and strive to appear boldly original. Methodist hymns, by contrast, treat human suffering within a speech genre where none of the social patterns governing scholarly essays applies—or even makes sense.

Subtly or overtly, then, genre molds facts, events, and speech to fit its contours, and a narrative of suffering will undergo significant changes depending on whether it takes the form of, say, a documentary film, a TV miniseries, an experimental novel, an obituary, a comic book, or even such deeply personal utterances as the testimony of Holocaust survivors. Narratives will often betray traces of generic patterning no doubt invisible to the speakers, since we employ the resources of genre almost automatically, just as interviewers may not recognize how they subtly steer a speaker toward narratives they consider palatable.[29] Arthur W. Frank in *The Wounded Storyteller* (1995) identifies four main patterns that distinguish postmodern stories of illness: he calls them testimony, restitution, quest, and chaos narratives. The tendency among some anthropologists and historians to treat all narrative as homogeneous—mere undifferentiated discourse—ignores how, as in Frank's four examples, genre always shapes the representation (and, inescapably, the experience) of suffering. Suffering, no matter how isolating and horrific, occurs only within a context of social life. In effect, there are never simply narratives of or about suffering: suffering at the point that it coincides with language can take only the generic forms we are prepared to recognize. Anything else, until we learn how to read it, will prove as incomprehensible as an unknown tongue.

The shaping force of genre extends beyond form and content to meaning. We depend on generic patterns to provide a framework for interpretation. Such frames, for example, let us know whether we are watching a tragedy or a dark comedy, whether we are reading sacred scripture or a blasphemous parody: the language at times may be almost identical. In fact, the same utterance that would seem incoherent within a tragedy may make perfect (non)sense in a farce. Understanding the meaning of any utterance, E. D. Hirsch Jr. says of genre (invoking a crucial metaphor from philosopher Ludwig Wittgenstein), is "like learning the rules of a game."[30] The rules may change and new games may appear. It is important to remember that genres are historical creations and, like tragedy or romance, change over time. Thus medieval tragedies and postmodern romances have their own distinctive qualities that set them apart from ancient Greek tragedies and romances. It is genre, however, in every age, that tells us what language game we are playing.

There is something uncomfortable in thinking about the genres of suffering in terms of game and play, but, following Wittgenstein, postmodern theorists have employed games as a dominant metaphor to describe the rule-bound, arbitrary, socially constructed arenas of language and culture. It is culture that governs how we employ the biological resources of sadness and laughter; it is culture at work teaching us that behavior perfectly appropriate at an Irish wake would be an outrage among orthodox Jews sitting shivah. As in traditions of courtroom testimony, culture and genre not only shape what we say but, equally important, what we are *permitted* to say. Moreover, specific genres often carry explicit or unspoken cultural values.[31] Suffering, as we will see, is thus infused with values specific to the genre in which it is expressed. Indeed, genre even influences the shape of human knowledge. Hayden White has argued that historians write history—and hence that we know our own past—only within the conventions of literary genre: we get not unvarnished facts but rather facts set within and shaped by a specific kind of story, such as epic, romance, tragedy, comedy, farce.[32] It is thus highly relevant to the situation of people with AIDS that two powerful literary genres—tragedy and the novel—have dominated Western discourse on suffering. The unavoidable question is this: what values, constraints, or conditions do tragedy and the novel impose on our knowledge and experience of suffering?

TRAGEDY AND NOVEL ON SUFFERING

Serious illness, especially when it seems to cut short a life rich with promise, is often described as tragic. Tragedy is so basic to Western ideas of suffering that newspapers still call almost any large misfortune tragic. Behind this casual usage lies a tradition that stretches back to Aristotle, who begins from a point so basic that we may overlook its significance. Suffering (Greek *pathos*) is for Aristotle indispensable to tragedy. Drama without *pathos*, he writes, cannot be tragic. Illness, of course, has all the ingredients of drama, as every soap opera writer knows, and when (in the West) the arc of illness includes suffering, we may find it hard to disentangle our experience from its heritage of Aristotelian thought. So it becomes a matter of some importance to know what exactly Aristotle said about tragic suffering.

Aristotelian tragedy, in its implicit cultural assumptions, involves a view that not all suffering (and not everyone who suffers) is equal. Unknown before the fifth century B.C., the term *pathos* indicated not just misery or misfortune but what classicist Thomas Gould calls "catastrophic suffering, undergone by some great figure, man or god, far in excess of the sufferer's deserts."[33] In effect reproducing ancient Greek assumptions about social worth, it holds at its core the values of an aristocratic, slave-owning culture in which ordinary suffering and ordinary people lie beyond its scope: excluded, marginalized, or personified in a passive, hapless chorus. Aristotle's cultural assumptions are also reproduced in his insistence that tragic poets write in an elevated style appropriate to powerful individuals and great acts. The catastrophe befalling a prince or general involves the fate of whole families or armies or cities, so that Aristotle helps confirm our normal assumption that suffering is invariably serious. Yet, a belief that suffering is invariably serious—tragic—belongs to the history of Western thought since Aristotle. Other cultures do not invariably share it.[34]

The novel—the other major genre that shapes our knowledge and experience of suffering—complicates the emphasis in tragedy on high seriousness. Complication arises in part from the mixture of styles and voices that Bakhtin calls "heteroglossia."[35] It is heteroglossia—the clash of social dialects and discourses—that for Bakhtin distinguishes the novel from more homogeneous, elevated genres such as tragedy. In addition, novels in his view extend heteroglossia to an underlying principle: novels put all beliefs and knowledge into dialogue, such that no single voice emerges from the text as delivering the authorized version. The contrast with Aristotle is instructive. Whereas tragedy for Aristotle is implicitly aristocratic, the novel for Bakhtin is implicitly democratic in its mix of voices and in its subversion of hierarchies. Where Aristotelian tragedy focuses on characters of high birth, the novel for Bakhtin focuses on widely differing social classes. Where Aristotle sees tragedy as always serious, Bakhtin views the novel as inherently comic, a prose carnival, where laughter and a license to speak freely call into question every solemn or single-minded view, including the view of suffering implicit in tragedy. The novels of Samuel Beckett, for example, tend to undermine tragic seriousness and to dramatize a view that suffering is finally absurd—absolutely devoid of meaning—in which case a tragic insistence on the high seriousness of human suffering appears almost comic.

Tragedy and the novel, then, embody quite different outlooks, and it makes a big difference which genre shapes our knowledge of suffering. Yet, it is not necessary to choose between them; most people absorb both perspectives, and in one respect each genre reinforces an implicitly unified view of suffering: they both rely on the fascinations of plot. Plot is one of our most important cognitive resources with which to understand suffering. Plot, not suffering, is for Aristotle the soul of tragedy: it is what elevates suffering to tragic status. Thus, while he insists that tragedies must include *pathos,* suffering alone does not create tragedy. It is action or plot that creates the structure within which tragic *pathos* makes sense. Moreover, with some quirky exceptions such as *Tristram Shandy,* plot is so central to the novel that some popular novelists and screenwriters seem little more than machines for mass-producing plots. Novelistic suffering, even when extended deep into the consciousness of a particular character, fundamentally demands the construction of plot. Plot, we might say, is crucial to the generic framework within which both novels and tragedies place human suffering.

What does plot have to tell us about suffering? Through their emphasis on plot, tragedy and the novel implicitly represent suffering not as a mere state of being—persisting like a viral infection almost independent of human agency—but as an event embedded within a matrix of related actions. Plots illuminate the connections among individual events. One reason why Aristotle values plot so highly is because plot allows the cognitive clarifications that make tragedy, in his phrase, more philosophical than history.[36] History in Aristotle's view provides a mere record of actual happenings, which often include ridiculously improbable coincidences. Tragedy, by contrast, employs its artful plot not to dramatize what did happen (the possible) but to show us what, in any series of important actions, ought to happen (the probable). It demonstrates, almost like a theorem in geometry, that suffering is an unavoidable outcome given a sequence of specific, connected actions. Novels, too, although less consistently than Aristotle might like, place suffering within a framework of plot that reveals the connections among events. Both genres show us suffering as more than a persistent theme in the human condition. Their emphasis on plot usually transforms suffering from a static condition—

a changeless and thus inherently undramatic state of being—into an event, an event enfolded within the context of a larger, surrounding action.

Suffering in tragedy and the novel—despite regular invocations of fate—loses its ancient aura of fatalism because it is never merely the experience of a debilitating passivity. In these genres, it is an action. It is represented as the outcome of a series of preceding acts. This plot-centered view holds the promise of cognitive clarifications that may lead to personal or social change. Although the hero of a tragedy or novel may be trapped within a surrounding action too intricate or complex to reverse, audiences occupy a position in which the modernist detachment that Auden depicted in "Musée des Beaux Arts" is not inevitable. For example, a plot-centered view of suffering holds important consequences for Gustavo Gutiérrez, the Peruvian priest who founded liberation theology, another postmodern invention. Gutiérrez does not view the suffering of the impoverished masses in the slums of Lima as a changeless state rooted in original sin or in the human condition, as is implied by theological narratives that explain suffering as God's will. For Gutiérrez, the poverty, illness, and suffering that daily face millions of Latin American poor are embedded in an extended and continuous historical plot. This plot—a sequence of connected actions, not an outright conspiracy—takes the form of political and economic oppression sponsored by an elite class (including leaders of his own church) that has secured power through an appalling series of injustices.[37] Gutiérrez insists that suffering in the slums of Lima will be reversed not by medicines or compassion or improved services, welcome though they might be, but only by material social change—connected action—that signifies the creation of a new and just historical plot.

AIDS: THE PLOTS OF SUFFERING

Plot has at least as much impact on the lives of people with AIDS as does the biology of the human immunodeficiency virus. Scholars seem agreed that AIDS is a socially constructed disease, and an extensive literature traces how social attitudes and public policies have shaped its course. Yet the social construction of AIDS is not somehow isolated from biology—HIV, like other microbes, can change in response to human activities—and it is at the crossroads of biology and culture where the AIDS epidemic has been created.[38] Historian Charles E. Rosenberg comes closest to articulating a biocultural view when he describes AIDS, in the readjustments it requires in traditional thinking about illness, as a postmodern epidemic. "After a generation of epistemological—and political—questioning of the legitimacy of many disease categories," he writes, "AIDS has exposed the inadequacy of any one-dimensional approach to disease, either the social constructionist or the more conventional mechanistically oriented perspective."[39] Rosenberg adds the offbeat perception that all epidemics tend to follow the pattern of a drama in four acts, from the initial slow revelation of danger to a "flat and ambiguous" last act. The two middle stages of the drama (which he calls "managing randomness" and "negotiating public response") are where we stand today. Within this biocultural drama played out as the AIDS epidemic unfolds there are numerous subplots, although they are distinct enough that (for convenience) we can call them separate plots. Three such subplots merit special attention not only for their impact on people suffering from AIDS but also for their place within the larger cultural struggle to control the AIDS narrative: the plot of origins, the victim plot, and the plot of resistance.

Suffering must come from somewhere. The plot of origins allows the community to assign both a cause and a trajectory to its misfortune. In the case of AIDS, one consistent public response was to conflate the epidemic with earlier notions of plague, with consequences reaching far beyond the metaphorical language common both in everyday speech and in scientific writing. Metaphors are often poetic accounts of origin, and AIDS quickly achieved what Susan Sontag calls a "dual metaphoric genealogy": it was understood as both an invasion and a pollution.[40] Microbiology soon made it clear how the invasion occurred, often with recourse to the military metaphors that remain a regular feature of contemporary thinking about disease. Yet, the AIDS virus did not operate exactly like other related pathogens, such as the agent responsible for syphilis, which causes symptoms after an incubation of twelve to thirty days. Syphilis was like a visible army whose advance could be mapped and therefore opposed. The exact moment of infection could be determined, in retrospect, and therefore responsibility could be determined. HIV, because it remains dormant within the body often for many years, operates more like a terrorist, penetrating at unknown points, lurking unseen, striking in ways impossible to neutralize with a counterstrike. AIDS is unlike a traditional disease that targets a specific organ: it is the cause of multiple illnesses that finally wear down the body's defense. The invasion plot in the case of AIDS can leave us feeling as if defense is ultimately a losing, futile strategy.

The plot of origins that focuses on pollution is even less satisfactory. AIDS in the West emerged with an unmistakable link to the recently and imperfectly liberated world of gay sex. It was thus linked with a group for many years openly oppressed and despised, a group whose sexual practices were reviled by various religious leaders and politicians as unnatural, ungodly, and unspeakable. Even prominent members of the gay community such as Larry Kramer and Randy Shilts argued that sexual practices associated with the gay bathhouse in its heyday—anonymous coupling, multiple partners, prolific activity, and group sex—were in the context of the AIDS epidemic at the very least unhealthy. With the public alarmed at learning that AIDS is an infectious disease, fears of contagion simply intensified homophobic antagonisms and revulsion: gays who contracted AIDS found their suffering enveloped by a poisonous air of stigma.[41] With the risk of infection unknown, many dentists suddenly appeared before their patients wearing masks and rubber gloves. A rule appeared almost overnight to protect professional basketball players from the blood of injured competitors. The heterosexual traffic in one-night stands reportedly dropped off as people in bars grew worried about disease. Everywhere the so-called gay plague carried with it the fearful subplot that the straight world too might soon be dragged down into a murky pool of viral pollution and death. Gays with AIDS suffered within the social context of a mythology as virulent as any fundamentalist rhetoric about divine censure.

Plots of origin associated with past epidemics usually share a single pattern: the plague always comes from elsewhere. One scenario popular in the mid-1980s had AIDS originating with green monkeys in central Africa, transmitted via infected Africans to Haitians visiting Zaire, then passed to American homosexuals vacationing in Haiti, who brought it back to New York City and passed it on to intravenous drug users.[42] The only story line missing is a loop in which New York IV drug users conspire to infect an international convention of hemophiliacs. The green monkey theory has been fully discredited. Physician Paul E. Farmer has shown how the high incidence of AIDS in Haiti functions to provide the developed world with a scapegoat satisfying the need to affix blame.[43] Despite such demythologizing, there is no end to plots of origin, especially plots that seize on the exotic, the unfamiliar, and the remote, on some distant site of deviance and otherness. Thus, while Americans usually locate the origin of AIDS in Africa, a majority of people sampled in Rwanda believed that AIDS came from the United States.[44] No matter where you are, plague always comes from somewhere else. What makes this plot of revolving origins less than comic is its implicit melodrama of villains and victims. The moral condemnation widely and early affixed to the gay community—as if every case of AIDS originated in some forbidden sexual act—reveals how our dominant culture composes and rewrites the plots of suffering in ways that ultimately justify and perpetuate its dominance.

The victim plot is nested within the plot of origins, in the sense that dominance requires submission and submission often requires or generates a victim. AIDS has certainly produced original twists on the plot of victimization. Gays, of course, find themselves often cast by the dominant culture in the role of self-victimized victim. Viewed as responsible for their own suffering, they are thus inherently denied the sympathy extended to people infected through medical accidents, transfusions of tainted blood, or the follies of a spouse. Americans seem disposed to grant women and children the special status of innocent victim, but AIDS complicates even this questionable tendency. Fearing infection, neighbors band together to exclude children with AIDS from local schools. AIDS activist Mary Fisher reports meeting a beautiful young woman in Harlem, perhaps twenty, who told her: "I wish I had cancer instead of AIDS. I could stand the treatments and the pain and my hair falling out. And I'm going to die anyway. But then, at least, my family wouldn't reject me. I could go home."[45] Women face special hardships. During the years when AIDS was considered a gay disease, women who suffered from the disease were mostly erased from policy decisions and media accounts. Later, as media and medical professionals began to acknowledge that women contracted AIDS, women's other familiar roles emerged to taint or call into question the role of innocent victim: woman as prostitute, nymphomaniac, evil parent, and African "other."[46] Here too culturally scripted plots determined the context in which people with AIDS would not simply suffer but suffer in their appointed role as victims.

There has been much comment, but little research, on the postmodern lure of victimhood. Almost everyone today with a grievance or injury seems eager to establish a claim as victim. The sources of this trend are complex, and they include zealous attorneys, social service programs, paranoia, and a growing awareness of the institutionalized racism, sexism, and disenfranchisement that prove genuinely, if often subtly, oppressive. What matters is both the force that such victim plots add to the experience of illness and the social context that they create for understanding the AIDS activists who boldly began to rewrite their own suffering as a narrative of resistance.

A radically new plot demands a new language. "We condemn attempts to label us as 'victims,' which implies defeat," declares one activist manifesto, "and we are only occasionally 'patients,' which implies passivity, helplessness, and dependence upon the care of others. We are 'people with AIDS.'"[47] AIDSpeak is what this new dialect of resistance came to be called, and it had immediate political consequences in changing the way in which officials discussed public health issues.[48] More important, however, is the decision that AIDS activists and individual AIDS patients made to reject the plot of the suffering victim. As Max Navarre wrote from firsthand experience: "The point is to see AIDS, when it happens to you, less as a defeat and more as an opportunity for creative life management. That might seem glib, but, given the choice between what the *New York Times* recently called 'a shattered life' and seeing AIDS as a chance to live fully on a daily basis, it doesn't take much to realize which view is the more helpful. Taking the bull by the horns is a means of escaping the sentimental soap opera that the media has created around the experience of having AIDS."[49] Navarre accurately recognizes that televised soap opera constitutes one of the major cultural genres that shape the postmodern experience of suffering. A helpful alternative to the script of shattered lives (what Arthur W. Frank calls chaos narratives) is not necessarily ready-made.[50] As traditional plots fail, AIDS activists in many cases transform or revalue existing genres into postmodern vehicles of resistance. Larry Kramer turns the open letter into a personal art form. Others see a new prominence and purpose in obituaries and memorial services. The NAMES Project transforms a traditional non-narrative American folk art, the quilt, into an immense language-rich memorial that tells its own tale about the innumerable lives stitched into its fabric.[51] Maybe the most important implicit narrative conveyed by the AIDS Memorial Quilt is the plot of a scattered community that (as if for the first time) constitutes and recognizes itself in the experience of shared grief. The community thus constituted by the artwork—the implicit audience imagined by the text—is not restricted to gays or to the families of people with AIDS. The Quilt, in its communal spirit, enfolds everyone who feels moved in its presence. It creates a spontaneous bond among strangers who experience its power and recognize its assertion that suffering must be understood and respected as something other than a narrative of victimhood.

The Quilt, like much AIDS discourse, rewrites the narrative of suffering in a fundamentally elegiac mode.[52] Despite the bright color and joyousness of specific panels describing individual lives, we cannot escape an overwhelming sense of loss as we move through the assembled artifact, even if loss is now contained within a formal structure of lament and implicit consolation. Elegy, however, is not the only genre that AIDS activists have changed in rewriting the narrative of suffering. One especially controversial contribution of Larry Kramer is his role in founding ACT UP (the acronym for AIDS Coalition to Unleash Power). ACT UP even in its name serves as a metaphor or mininarrative, suggesting irrepressible, high-spirited, and deliberate departures from the norm of good behavior. It is bad children who "act up," disrupting the decorum of the classroom, challenging the top-down distribution of power, and the activists who banded together in ACT UP saw their founding purpose as disruption and challenge. In creating its disruptive counternarrative, ACT UP borrowed many of its tactics from the antiwar and civil rights movements of the 1960s, which brought with them a rediscovery of guerrilla theater. In claiming this activist heritage of social protest, ACT UP saw its role as being not just unruly but, in yet another meaning of *act*, deliberately and publicly theatrical: guerrilla texts authored by members of the ACT UP collective included such performances as chaining themselves to government buildings, throwing vials full of bloodlike liquid, and chalking outlines of the dead on city streets. In January 1991, taking street theater directly into the television networks, they staged an on-air invasion of the studio in which the CBS Evening News broadcast was in progress.[53]

Maybe the most notorious ACT UP performance occurred during services in December 1989 at Saint Patrick's Cathedral in New York City. Joined by the Women's Health Action Mobilization and other groups, ACT UP demonstrated against Cardinal John O'Connor by shouting, passing out information, and lying on the floor as O'Connor attempted to keep on speaking.[54] The demonstration, beyond mere disruptive tactics, constituted a postmodern speech genre now as recognizable in its general features as a church sermon. The purpose of the demonstration, in fact, might be described as an effort to insert a secular, censored, unruly text about suffering into a sacred text (the church service) that had seemed to turn its back on AIDS sufferers. Certainly, Cardinal O'Connor had become a symbol of the Catholic church's intransigent stance on the subjects of homosexuality and AIDS education, and the activists dragged out of the cathedral used their bodies to produce a vivid countertext, a protest not only against O'Connor and the church but also, more important, against what John M. Clum has called "the victim mentality of many AIDS narratives."[55] Here was a narrative of refusal: a defiant rejection of elegiac sadness and the posture of victim.

Narrative is an entirely appropriate term to describe what was an improvisational audio-visual artifact. In fact, the ACT UP demonstration at Saint Patrick's Cathedral received intense media coverage and even prompted a documentary film, *Stop the Church* (1991), directed by Robert Hilferty. O'Connor's parishioners were outraged and dismayed, of course, as intended, but this was not just another outrageous nonviolent protest designed to attract the media and to challenge public policy. Sociologist Stanley Aronowitz sees in ACT UP a conscious shift away from the politics of modernism with its belief in the electoral legitimacy of the liberal state. ACT UP, he argues, challenges the *ethical* legitimacy of liberal institutions, institutions such as medicine, health care agencies, pharmaceutical companies, and even the church. It is this direct challenge to the ethical legitimacy of the liberal state that makes ACT UP, in his view, "the quintessential social movement for the era of postmodern politics."[56]

Suffering, as the work of ACT UP affirms, is from a postmodern perspective never strictly an internal, private affair. It is better understood as inevitably social—better reconceived as social suffering.[57] This rethinking opposes the modernist refrain that suffering is radically individual and unknowable. The qualities of individual suffering extend beyond language, as we have seen, and we can never entirely penetrate the experience of another person. The disruptive texts of ACT UP, however, show how culture offers important insights into what is also public and sharable in suffering. An understanding that suffering is always social allows us to recognize the implicit narratives and speech genres that shape our individual experience. It allows us to create new genres and new plots to replace narratives that prove harmful or inadequate. Narrative served this creative function in the past by extending the boundaries of a moral community to encompass the suffering of people previously dismissed as outcasts: for example, slaves, chimney sweeps, the mentally ill.[58] Harriet Beecher Stowe provides an especially clear example of this power to reinvent suffering in *Uncle Tom's Cabin; or Life Among the Lowly* (1852), the first American novel to sell over a million copies, which so strongly engaged popular feeling that she has been cited among the causes of the Civil War. Her narrative moved contemporary readers not only to weep at the ordeals of a fictional slave but also, implicit in such emotion and far more important than tears alone, to recognize slave experience *as* suffering and thus, sooner or later, to disrupt and rearrange the existing social order that had denied it.

Suffering, in short, is not a raw datum—not a natural phenomenon we can classify and measure, despite its links with biological processes—but a fluid social state: a status that we extend or withhold. We extend or withhold it depending largely on whether the sufferer falls within our narratives of moral community. When an Iraqi truck driver in the Persian Gulf War died in a firestorm of laser-guided missiles, the incident played on American TV as one more proof of U.S. pinpoint technology. (Iraqi soldiers seemed to find Kuwaiti civilians equally disposable.) We do not acknowledge the agony of people outside our moral community as suffering, but instead detach ourselves from their pain as if it were an incomprehensible behavior encountered on some Swiftian island. Inside a moral community, we employ names like *martyr* and *hero* to inscribe the suffering of our own party within narratives of hallowed sacrifice and epic achievement. The perspective opened by these examples might be called the postmodern view of suffering. It sees our relation to suffering not as fixed—in Auden's universalized "human position"—but as mobile and contingent, set in motion or frozen in place by the specific cultural narratives we construct. The challenge, which AIDS has dramatized so clearly, is to find genres appropriate for our era that validate, illuminate, and authenticate suffering—especially the easily ignored suffering of minority groups—while seeking to alleviate and oppose it. We need narratives of resistance, such as ACT UP provides, but we also need a knowledge of narrative, knowledge sufficient to help us resist whatever cultural forces directly or indirectly transform human suffering into an occasion for the perpetuation of victimhood.

chapter eight

Illness in the Time of Disney

When asked at one of Disney's pricey

management seminars whether anyone ever

died at Disney World, the group leader, on cue

from a supervisor sitting in the back of the room,

said simply, "No."

PROJECT ON DISNEY,
Inside the Mouse (1995)

An odd reversal has altered postmodern intellectual relations between Europe and the United States. American writers important in the invention of modernism—Henry James, Ezra Pound, and T. S. Eliot, for example—embarked on a compulsory pilgrimage to Europe, as if journeying to the origin of art, culture, and civilization. (Eliot even took out British citizenship.) Although there was always a trickle of return traffic from Europe to America, as in the famous nineteenth-century lecture tours by Dickens and Oscar Wilde, today numerous European writers and intellectuals find a journey to America not only advantageous but also—given the role of America in the formation of international postmodern culture—impossible to resist. One somewhat surprising feature of recent journeys by the distinguished European academics Jean Baudrillard, Louis Marin, and

Umberto Eco is that each visitor (celebrated for the depth and originality of his thought) makes an excursion to the world of Walt Disney.[1]

Disneyland (1955) and Walt Disney World (1971) are significant postmodern inventions that Americans tend to see as a national tradition, like the presidents sculpted on Mount Rushmore. Even when reproduced in Europe or Japan, the Disney cosmos is an American export, embodying the basic myth and marketing strategies that transformed a struggling film company into a diversified, transnational powerhouse.[2] The Disney-backed myth of childhood as a brief period of imagination and pleasure in life's dusty trek through the real world means that for the price of admission anyone can reenter this oasis of fantasy. (Most adults exorcise their guilt by bringing children along.) The carefully engineered experience envelops the visitor in a hermetic space where architecture and landscape conspire to keep us wholly within its boundaries. As the Japanese scholar Mitsuhiro Yoshimoto observes: "To create a space of fantasy, any elements which remind visitors of their daily life and the outside world are carefully excluded."[3] Americans respond on cue by viewing the twin theme parks, like childhood, as a space somehow insulated from everyday life. A trip to Disneyland is the archetypal family vacation, a rite of passage, a commodity without which children can consider themselves officially deprived. This almost automatic perspective makes it significant that Baudrillard, Marin, and Eco all view Disneyland and Disney World not as set apart from the rest of the United States but rather as an extension and magnification of its basic character.

There is surely something right in this European view of the Disney parks as an extension of daily life, as metaphors summarizing America, as centers of postmodern experience. A bit sourly but incisively, Marin finds Disneyland a "degenerate utopia": the "representation of the makeup of contemporary American ideology." More upbeat but not unironic, Eco sees Disneyland as America's Sistine Chapel, an embodiment of the postmodern faith that technology gives us more reality than nature can, as a place where spectators

openly admire "the perfection of the fake." Baudrillard views Disneyland as a "microcosm" of the Western hemisphere: a "parody of
the world of the imagination" where reality has achieved a state indistinguishable from images and simulations.[4] Some Americans will
find these interpretations too solemn and overintellectual as accounts
of what is merely good family entertainment. In viewing the Disney
parks as an extension of everyday life, however, the European visitors implicitly invite us to recognize how far postmodern culture has
become an extension of the entertainment industry. This is not to
judge entertainment as trivial but, on the contrary, to notice its significance.

"Entertainment," writes film critic Michael Wood, "is not, as we
often think, a full-scale flight from our problems, not a means of for-
getting them completely, but rather a rearrangement of our problems
into shapes which tame them, which disperse them to the margins of
our attention."[5] The value in noticing how the Disney cosmos tames
and disperses our problems lies in the possibility that such a recognition provides for noticing what specific problems *cannot* be tamed
and dispersed—but only excluded. We need to ask, that is, what, in
addition to the interminable lines of waiting customers, the engineers
of fantasy do *not* want us to see. Violence, crime, deformity, and even
death, it turns out, despite or through the best efforts of the supervi-
sors, are visible throughout the Disney parks, albeit suitably tamed,
dispersed, and controlled (as, for example, in popular attractions like
the Pirates of the Caribbean). One dilemma, however, automatically
gets excluded from the Disney cosmos and its fantasized extension of
everyday life: chronic illness and the process of dying.

No one would fault Disney for excluding chronic illness and dying
from the Magic Kingdom: they have nothing to do with contemporary myths of childhood or with consumer fantasies. Most contemporary readers fault the brothers Grimm precisely for *including* in childhood too much that is upsetting. The Disneyland exclusions,
however, tell us something useful about a culture that, as the Eco-
Marin-Baudrillard wing contends, constitutes a seamless extension of
the Disney enterprise. Chronic illness has almost no place in popular

self-representations of the postmodern world. It is nearly absent from network television, which prefers to focus on acute illness that is curable, curable especially by handsome, heroic, young doctors using drugs, technology, and the resources of biomedicine.[6] The denial of death is old news, and oversold, given the cameras rolling and clicking at every local disaster. What we are really determined to deny is not so much death as the extended process of dying. Cameras do not like the nursing home or sickbed.[7] While death is photogenic and uncanny, even an entertaining spectacle in well-crafted horror films, serious illness and dying represent a wasteland devoid of redeeming images and utterly without entertainment value. The effort to reclaim chronic illness and dying from biomedical reductiveness and corporate Disneyfication is a major unfinished project of postmodern culture.

UNNATURAL KILLERS: THE BIG THREE

The three most common causes of death among adults in postmodern America are, in ascending order of magnitude, stroke, cancer, and heart disease. Each has been described for many years through a biomedical language of organic dysfunction that gives patients little recourse but to see themselves as victims of their own bodily processes. Treatment has been typically aggressive, as doctors and surgeons rally their forces: radiation and chemotherapy to burn out the cancerous cells, bypass surgery and angioplasty to improve the flow of blood, clot-busting drugs to dissolve obstructions. These procedures sometimes save lives—or at least buy time. Yet in addition to the development of technical procedures that successfully extend the mechanistic philosophy of biomedicine, the last few years have seen new attention to the ways in which stroke, cancer, and heart disease seem responsive to influences from the surrounding culture. The data are not unambiguous; the evidence is not all in. It is clear, however, that the biomedical model can provide neither a full explanation of cross-cultural patterns in illness nor an effective program of prevention, so there is good reason for thinking that the three main killers of adults in postmodern America are best understood as biocultural illnesses.

Stroke, according to the World Health Organization, is the third most common cause of death in the developed nations. In the United States a stroke occurs almost every minute, leaving at present some two million stroke survivors in varying degrees of physical, emotional, or financial disability. A stroke is defined as an impairment in neurologic function following a decrease in arterial blood flow to the brain, and strokes assail the elderly in especially high numbers. The effects range from immediate death to brain damage, paralysis, imbalance, slurred speech, visual deficits, and a series of minor quirks, some so small as to pass unnoticed. The accumulation of small strokes accounts for the plight of nearly 10 percent of the elderly patients diagnosed with dementia.[8] It might seem evident that the biomedical model offers a perfect description of a condition that depends on something so mechanical as the flow of blood to the brain. A plumber could describe the process. Yet, while stroke has everything to do with the failure of oxygenated blood to reach brain cells, we have begun within the last fifty years to appreciate the less vivid but nonetheless crucial contribution made by the flow of knowledge, images, and cultural practices.

Although blood flow is something all humans share, one study offers the surprising conclusion that immigrants to the United States have a markedly lower rate of mortality from strokes than does the American-born resident population.[9] Why? The study does not say. The higher risk faced by U.S. natives is not shared equally. African Americans have what is known as "excess stroke mortality": they die from stroke at higher rates than white Americans do. What causes this difference? Lower socioeconomic status plays a role in excess stroke mortality among black males, but not among black females. A substantial portion of the overall excess in African American stroke mortality is due to other causes, including "social resources," lifestyle, genetics, and cerebrovascular risk factors unrelated to socioeconomic status.[10] A role for biology seems likely in accounting for overall excess stroke mortality among African Americans, even if the

processes remain obscure, but it is also clear—especially in euphemisms like social resources—that excess stroke mortality among
African American males has much to do with culture and with the
consequences of a history of racism.

The cumulative evidence is pretty strong, although individual
studies must be interpreted with caution. As research has shown, one
major source of risk for stroke is a diet high in cholesterol and saturated fats. Diet, of course, varies with particular cultures and ethnic
groups. In contrast to the diet of natives raised on double cheese-
burgers with fries, a low-fat, low-cholesterol diet among immigrants
to the United States might help account for their lower stroke mortality. Exercise is another cultural influence that might help account for
the lower stroke mortality rates of immigrants, who tend to work at
vigorous manual jobs and may not have a gallery of labor-saving appliances. (As a compensation for the sedentary effects of affluence,
the postmodern unisex health club owes some of its popularity to the
well-advertised role of exercise in reducing hypertension and thus reducing the risk of stroke.) In addition to a role in affecting mortality
from stroke, culture also plays a significant role in later stages of the
illness. One study showed that elderly stroke patients with fewer
limitations in physical function also had larger social networks. (It
also turns out that among 276 healthy volunteer subjects, people with
more diverse social ties proved less susceptible to common colds.) In
other research, stroke patients who received high levels of emotional
support showed dramatic improvement. In particular, elderly male
stroke patients who perceived an absence of social support, especially from a spouse caregiver, were significantly at risk for depressive disorder, whereas men who received active social support had
less depression.[11] Culture, in short, seems to influence not only mortality from stroke but also recovery.

Cancer shows a similar pattern. One-third of the people in the
Western world will develop some form of cancer. There are over 100
individual types of cancer, and a full discussion would need to treat
each type separately—lung cancer, breast cancer, prostate cancer,
leukemia, melanoma, and the rest. Yet, some basic similarities are

clear. Up to one-half of all cancers in the United States are of unknown origin, while a very small percentage can be traced directly to
the action of bacteria, viruses, and genes. The remainder, even when
we assume that unknown genetic features may predispose individuals to risk, have a demonstrable link to lifestyle, diet, occupation, and
environment: in short, to culture.

Surprisingly, in the United States about 20 to 25 percent of cancers,
excluding skin cancer, are related to diet.[12] Nutrition can both promote certain cancers (for example, through a diet loaded with carcinogens and high-fat foods) and promote the resistance to certain
cancers (for example, through dietary fiber that protects against cancer of the colon). Diet, however, is only one cultural influence closely
related to cancer. Approximately thirty substances are known to
cause cancer in humans, and human cancers have occurred following
low-level exposure: asbestos brought home on the clothes of workers
has caused fatal cancers in family members.[13] Utah, with its predominantly Mormon community committed to the avoidance of alcohol
and smoking, has a low cancer mortality compared with rates almost
250 percent higher in New York and the District of Columbia. In addition to cigarette smoking and asbestos, other risk factors firmly related to cancer include air pollution, radiation, and ultraviolet light.
Even survival after diagnosis (with certain cancers) has a demonstrable link to culture. Women receiving mammograms had a one-third
reduction in mortality from breast cancer compared to a control
group who followed their normal patterns of medical care.[14] Such
early detection of breast cancer is more than a biomedical practice
that enhances survival. It is also an event with profound cultural implications. African American women have higher mortality rates
from breast cancer and cervical cancer than do white women, in part
because of cultural limitations on their access to medical care.

Cancer is a complex disease—or set of closely related diseases—
that in many cases has multiple causes, so that culture often plays
merely a contributing role. From a biocultural point of view, however, both biology and culture play contributing roles, and culture
may offer the most effective opportunities for prevention. For exam-

ple, African American males have the highest known rate of prostate cancer, almost double the rate of white American males, which may be related to 15 percent higher average levels of testosterone in young black men but certainly has something to do with cultural access to medical care.[15] We must not simplify cancer by overemphasizing its cultural components, but a single-minded focus on genetics and cell biology also produces simplification. The good news is that cultural change—in reducing air pollution, cigarette smoking, and environmental carcinogens, as well as in increasing social access to medical care and altering exposure to sunlight—could go far toward reducing the general levels of cancer. As with stroke, culture can help not only reduce general levels of disease but also improve recovery. Social support is beneficial to cancer patients as well as to stroke patients in helping them adjust to the stress of a traumatic disease that still carries a heavy burden of stigma, anxiety, and mental-emotional turmoil.[16]

Heart disease outstrips stroke and cancer as the most common cause of death among adults in the postmodern era. Here again the importance of biology is not in dispute. Although some doctors are skeptical about what role psychosocial factors might play in coronary heart disease, a recent review of the scientific literature concludes that life stress can increase rates of mortality, while emotional support can both reduce mortality and promote recovery.[17] As with stroke and cancer, the biology of heart disease has a great deal to do with cultural processes. Once again, we encounter an ancient illness that the best current medical research is teaching us to see as biocultural.

The influence of culture on heart disease extends beyond well-known dangers such as cigarette smoking, alcohol consumption, obesity, and lack of exercise to include complicated variables that appear to reduce risk, such as the quantity of fish in one's daily diet.[18] Race, gender, and social class also seem to affect heart disease. Women, although they develop cardiac problems some ten years later than men do, die of heart disease at higher rates, so heart disease is more threatening to women than to men. This striking gender inequality doubtless has less to do with biology than with unequal access to medical care, with differences in risk factors, with the fact that women live longer, and with a history of medical inattention to women's health. At least through 1993, published clinical trials in the prevention of heart disease all used male subjects, so the role of gender is still undecided. Recently documented risk factors for women include low social class, limited education, the double load of work and family responsibilities, lack of social support, and chronic troubling emotions (a phrase that may betray the same gender bias it addresses).[19] Race remains of uncertain influence, but the facts are clear enough: the highest rate of death from heart disease—among six ethnic groups studied in California between 1985 and 1990—occurred for all ages in African American men and women.[20] Among black men in America, mortality rates from coronary heart disease are newly accelerating.[21] Why? A biocultural perspective suggests that significant statistical changes in the biology of health and illness will correspond to significant changes in the body politic.

Fifteen hundred Americans die each day from coronary heart disease. Coronary heart disease is the medically registered cause of about 25 percent of all deaths in the United Kingdom.[22] This is a lot of dying to remain more or less invisible, despite the occasional dramatic clutching at the chest in television versions of a heart attack triggered by grief or fright. A worker at Disney World reports: "We had a guy last summer who went to EPCOT, stood in front of the golf ball, took a gun, and blew his head off. But he didn't die. He stood right there in front of all those tourists and went 'click' and brains blew everywhere. But he didn't die there. The medic told me that they are not allowed to let them die there. Keep them alive by artificial means until they're off Disney property, like there's an imaginary line in the road and they go, 'He's alive, he's alive, he's dead.'"[23] Even if apocryphal, this story exposes a tacit imperative concealed in the American way of dying: absolute denial until the patient crosses over into death. The arsenal of biomedicine always contains another drug or procedure, until the final technologies fail and the ineffectual specialists at last slip away, outgunned. Today, as medical attitudes and medical economics begin to change, it is often families who insist that doctors keep hopelessly ill patients alive on life-support machines, as if racing away from Disney World toward some invisible line in the road.

The postmodern world is beginning to reject this behind-the-scenes, cure-driven, technocratic charade of death. Public clamor for physician-assisted suicide is an understandable effort to reassert the claims of human dignity. We are also seeing, however, the emergence of a more hopeful approach to dying that does not transform physicians into compassionate executioners. Before we examine this approach, it will be helpful to look at two illnesses that bear a close relation to death and that tell us much about the changing arena of postmodern medicine: depression and Alzheimer's disease.

DEPRESSION AS DEATH-IN-LIFE

Even the statistics are alarming. In the United States alone, severe depression is estimated to affect over fifteen million people at a cost of some twenty-seven billion dollars annually. It is a major health hazard that helps shape the postmodern condition. As we have seen, major depression in the United States occurs among 2 to 4 percent of the community, among 10 to 14 percent of medical inpatients, and women are twice as likely to suffer depression as men are.[24] (The less prevalent bipolar disorder, formerly called manic-depressive illness, affects men and women equally.) Over a lifetime, one in four women will suffer a serious clinical depression, a figure which radiates with multiple implications for families. It turns out that caretakers for young children—caretakers who are doubtless mostly women— show a significant incidence of depression, and the depression of parents has a demonstrable impact upon children.[25] The family, of course, is a social institution open to historical change, as in the advent of the famous "nuclear" household, so that the biology of depression today often unfolds within the changing social structure of the postmodern family, with inevitable feedback loops: depression affects the family, the family affects depression. Some changes in the recent profile of depression as our risk increases and as the age of on-set decreases no doubt derive in part from improved diagnosis, from more effective treatments, from the role of insurance, and from a greater willingness to seek medical help, but clearly something else is going on: we cannot speak about the postmodern condition without also addressing depression.

The most encouraging news about depression concerns the recent discovery of effective drug treatments. Some 80 percent of patients with serious depression now improve significantly with treatment. The effectiveness of drug treatments created a rapid consensus among doctors—rapidly transformed into public conviction—that depression is a biochemical disorder of the brain's neurotransmitter systems. For patients, this shift meant that depression no longer bore the stigma formerly attached to the shadowy realm of mental illness. "Depression is a real disease," *Parade* magazine in 1988 trumpeted in Sunday newspapers across the United States (implicitly demeaning the status of other mental illnesses unresponsive to medication).[26] Depression was thus reconceived as a chemical imbalance in the brain requiring the same type of corrective drug therapies employed to treat, say, a hyperactive thyroid gland. No need for long, expen-sive, ineffectual sessions of psychotherapy. One welcome by-product of this drug-centered demythologizing, which doubtless serves to pump up the statistics that surround depression, is that people now feel less threatened in seeking medical help. Real assistance—in pill form—is available for a real disease. In effect, depression has been detoxified and slipped quietly back inside the biomedical model.

The so-called biological revolution in psychiatry, however, is not a complete victory for patients. Because pills are easier and cheaper to dispense, needed psychotherapy (perhaps addressing a trauma that triggered or followed the depression) may be ignored. While drug treatment of a neurochemical imbalance certainly corrects a biologi-cal disorder, it does not explain why or how the imbalance occurred. Moreover, leaving aside serious concerns about the implications of long-term, nationwide reliance on drugs and about the chemical production of normalcy, we need to ask questions that a successful course of treatment with Prozac leaves completely unaddressed. How far is the biological revolution supported by pressure from insurers to medicalize depression? Would everyone hospitalized for depression need to be on medication to qualify for coverage? Outpatient review considering insurance coverage for psychotherapy would doubtless press for medication as a prerequisite for continued financial support. Such pressure is not just medical in origin but cultural. Are there additional reasons to think that depression is not wholly a biological illness but rather, as a postmodern perspective would lead us to suspect, biocultural?

The truth is that we lack a full understanding of depression. Depression does not have reliable and valid biological markers, although there are probable genetic correlations, along with demonstrable contributions from neurotransmitters and hormones. We still do not fully understand what depression is, though, or how and why it occurs, and we are thus thrown back on competing accounts: psychoanalytic, biological, cognitive, and descriptive.[27] One approach that has begun to ask difficult questions about depression goes under the name of "cross-cultural psychiatry." Psychiatrist and anthropologist Arthur Kleinman in collaboration with anthropologist Byron Good published in 1985 a groundbreaking collection entitled *Culture and Depression: Studies in the Anthropology and Cross-Cultural Psychiatry of Affect and Disorder*. Kleinman and Good do not pretend that the collection of cross-cultural studies solves all the conceptual problems surrounding depression, but they strongly challenge what they call the "growing consensus in the psychiatric community that the current criteria of depression are valid and represent criteria of a universal, biologically grounded disease."[28]

Postmodern skepticism about claims to universality seems especially pertinent when it comes to claims that depression is no more than a problem in biochemistry. In fact, the symptoms of depression differ widely across cultures. A study comparing patients with depression in Greece and Australia found that—while *levels* of depression, anxiety, and somatic symptoms were almost identical—Greek patients scored significantly higher on complaints of dizziness, tingling in the extremities, and (the oddness is pertinent in illustrating cross-cultural differences) spasms while chewing. Australian patients scored significantly higher on complaints of drowsiness, hypersomnia, and nonrefreshing sleep. The clinical assessment of a disorder that shifts its symptoms across cultures is obviously a difficult matter.[29] Even more difficult—from a biomedical point of view—is the question of why a strictly chemical and genetic illness should appear as a sleep disorder in Australia, while in Greece it involves an experience of disorienting sensations.

The research collected by Kleinman and Good offers fascinating illustrations of cultural influences on the experience of depression. The dysphoria basic to depressive illness—"sadness, hopelessness, unhappiness, lack of pleasure with things of the world and with social relationships"—has quite different meanings and values across cultures. Buddhists in Sri Lanka, for example, view dysphoria as the first step toward salvation and a turning away from worldly things, while the Balinese and Thai-Lao seek to "smooth out" emotional highs and lows in order to preserve a pure, refined, and untroubled inner self.[30] Such contrasts are reflected in the experience of middle-aged Asian immigrants to Britain when compared with the experience both of middle-aged native Britons and of young Asian immigrants. The middle-aged Asian immigrants differed not only in their beliefs about depression but also (despite the existence of measurable psychiatric morbidity) in not reporting depression in themselves or in others. In effect, they preserved the attitudes and practices of their own culture toward dysphoria, while young Asian immigrants assimilated the cultural attitudes and practices of the native British.[31] The main difference was not between age and youth but between assimilation and nonassimilation to quite different cultural understandings of illness.

It is important not to overstate the significance of culture or to overlook pertinent distinctions. Psychosocial influences seem relatively insignificant in altering the course of severe and recurrent depressions, although they are significant in the *onset* of severe depressions and in the outcome of milder depressions.[32] Still, while depression runs in families and clearly has a genetic component, individual psychological makeup plays a role in vulnerability to depression, especially among people with low self-esteem and consistently pessimistic outlooks. The National Institute of Mental Health reports that depressive episodes can be triggered by such clearly psychological and social events as a serious loss, a difficult relationship, financial problems, or an unwelcome change in life patterns.[33] The considerable evidence suggesting an interaction between culture and biology in depression, while easily ignored within a biomedical model of disease and a strictly biological model of psychiatry, seems in fact very hard to refute.

We get a rare patient-centered look inside this distinctive postmodern illness when novelist William Styron in *Darkness Visible: A Memoir of Madness* (1990) provides an extended account of his nine-month struggle with depression. In Paris to receive a prestigious literary prize, he felt, inexplicably, as if cast down into the lowest depths. The dominant sense he conveys is that depression defeats ordinary comprehension. "Depression," he writes, "is a disorder of mood, so mysteriously painful and elusive in the way it becomes known to the self—to the mediating intellect—as to verge close to being beyond description."[34] There are ominous twitches and pains—"Nothing felt quite right with my corporeal self" (43)—but soon these puzzling ailments pass into something far less familiar. "I was feeling in my mind a sensation close to, but indescribably different from, actual pain" (16). Styron's words suggest that his dilemma is not just linguistic but perceptual. How can we make sense of a torment wholly alien to normal life? "For myself," he offers, "the pain is most closely connected to drowning or suffocation—but even those images are off the mark" (17).

An illness that immerses the sufferer in an experience close to drowning or suffocation has certainly intermingled life with death. Pain is notoriously resistant to description, but the pain of depression, Styron insists, is strangely abnormal, hard to localize in a specific limb or organ, as if endless and unrelenting. "If there is mild relief," he writes, "one knows that it is only temporary; more pain will follow. It is hopelessness even more than pain that crushes the soul" (62). Styron's language here too, like his title evoking Milton's description of hell, carries on a running parallel with the theological state of damnation—perhaps the ultimate degree of despair and near-death hopelessness—which extends beyond conventional analogies linking depression with chronic pain. The kinship between depression and chronic pain has, in fact, been a major theme in the medical literature of the past twenty years.[35] Patients with chronic low back pain, for example, experience three to four times higher rates of depression than does the general population. While the exact relationship between chronic pain and depression remains obscure, the two conditions are not identical. The inexact picture emerging from studies in comorbidity portrays a nightmare of loss: pleasure, energy, libido, sleep, appetite, self-esteem, and normal life vanish beyond hope of recovery. The sufferer moves in a dysphoria so static and so frightening that the familiar world has been thoroughly shattered, even though outwardly little appears to have changed. Not even pain is the same. This is more like what we might imagine as the pain of dying.

Styron's account proves helpful in exposing a typical postmodern confusion. He is confused not so much about what he feels—he offers a chilling description of torpor and despair—as about how to understand it. He continues to insist on a qualitative difference between what he calls physical (or actual) pain and the pain of depression. In effect, he is reproducing confusions implicit in the myth of two pains. His account grows especially revealing when the ready-made distinction between mental pain and physical pain begins to break down even as he professes to uphold it: "What I had begun to discover is that, mysteriously and in ways that are totally remote from normal experience, the gray drizzle of horror induced by depression takes on the quality of physical pain. But it is not an immediately identifiable pain, like that of a broken limb. It may be more accurate to say that despair, owing to some evil trick played upon the sick brain by the inhabiting psyche, comes to resemble the diabolical discomfort of being imprisoned in a fiercely overheated room" (50). The torpid, immobile, joyless, defeated, hellishly overheated body of the depressive patient lies at an opposite pole from the postmodern utopia of glowing health. The patient suffers not just an illness but an exclusion, like exile or damnation, which is of course an experience defined and constituted by culture. While pain in Milton's *Paradise Lost* at least served a traditional purpose as divine punishment, Styron's punishing illness seems to him wholly meaningless. The meaninglessness extends to his entire world, which appears to be a place of multiple losses (56). He tells us he has lost his mother to death, lost his self-esteem to a powerful sense of "self-hatred" (5), lost even the comfort he once received from the heavy daily use of alcohol. From the depths of this suffocating postmodern hell he imagines that the only available release is suicide.

Suicide is twenty-four times more common among patients with a history of major depression than in the general population.[36] Styron's multiple and unresolved losses, added to despair and unrelenting pain, finally push him to the brink of self-destruction, which in effect makes literal the metaphor of depression as death-in-life. He escapes only by means of a self-imposed hospital stay, which (as he pursues the imagery of death-in-life) he compares to a season in purgatory (69). Happily, while Styron's allusions to Milton intensify the aura of hellish disaster, they also hold out the promise of upward movement. *Darkness Visible* ends with a vision of recovery: the prospect of a return to health and something like the familiar world transfigured. Styron's final sentence explicitly compares his own escape from depression to Dante's ascent from the inferno: "trudging upward and upward out of hell's black depths and at last emerging into what he saw as 'the shining world' [*chiaro mondo*]" (84).

Despite the availability of effective drugs, not everyone who suffers from depression can tell such a heartening story. Patients with Alzheimer's disease lose even the powers, biological and cultural, that permit them to give their lives the form of a coherent narrative. Their fate too lingers somewhere in limbo between living and dying.

ALZHEIMER'S DISEASE AND MYTHS OF OLD AGE

Alois Alzheimer (1864–1915), a German neurologist, has given his name to what many feel is an illness more frightening than death: it is the death of the self while the body lives on. Recognized in 1907, Alzheimer's disease (AD) emerged in its current conception during the 1970s, and research since the 1980s has led to what one specialist calls "an almost dizzying accumulation of knowledge"—including knowledge of neurobiological perspectives, of neurotransmitter lesions, and of substances that typically accumulate in the brain.[37] AD refers to a condition in elderly persons in which progressive degeneration of nerve cells in the brain disrupts memory, learning, and higher cognitive functions that ultimately have much to do with the constitution of selfhood. Increasing impairment of these mental powers leads not only to senile dementia but also to an apparent emptying out of the self. In its later stages, patients afflicted with AD cannot recognize family members, cannot remember their own lives, and have lost a grip on their own identities:

LEO: Who am I?

MAY: What do you mean, you know who you are. You're Leo. You were a boxer. You're my brother.

LEO: Boxer? Was I?

MAY: Yes you were.

LEO: Where am I?

MAY: In Cleveland, where you've been living for years.

LEO: Mobile?

MAY: No, you were born in Mobile, but now you're in Cleveland.

LEO: Who am I?[38]

In this terrible situation the trauma may be worse for their loved ones than for patients. Alzheimer's patients come as close as we are likely to see to a literal embodiment of the undead. They have lost most of the qualities that we associate with humanness.

No one knows what causes AD, and no one knows how to cure it. It currently affects more than 11 percent of the American population above age sixty-five, and as the population ages the number of Alzheimer's patients will create an immense public health dilemma. (In America, AIDS, by comparison, may come to look quite manageable.) Research confirms an association between AD and a genotype called apolipoprotein E, so a genetic and hereditary predisposition is likely.[39] (Other contributing factors from head injury to occupation have been explored with inconclusive results.) The biology of this neural degeneration is clearly visible under a microscope: a telltale residue of tangled hairlike fibrils remains after the cortical cell has disintegrated. Thus, although cause and cure remain a mystery, there is no doubt that AD belongs to the neurodegenerative afflictions for which a biological explanation will eventually be found. The stories of people reduced to blank infantile humanoids by this terrible disease are too numerous and familiar to rehearse here. Everyone knows, or will soon know, a patient or family undone by AD. The question from a postmodern perspective is what contribution to our understanding, if any, is left to the role of culture.

Culture, we might say, is the silent partner in AD that constructs our vision of old age. "The aging body," as sociologists Mike Featherstone and Andrew Wernick put it, "is never just a body subjected to the imperatives of cellular and organic decline, for as it moves through life it is continuously being inscribed and reinscribed with cultural meanings."[40] Your age is not just what your biological clock reveals: it is also socially constructed, even as in industrial nations the postmodern demographics of a rapidly aging population is an artifact of culture (including systems of health care). In traditional societies, old age inspires familiar images of wise, almost magical elders. For minorities in American culture, by contrast, old age often means suffering the triple jeopardy of ill health, poverty, and racial prejudice.[41] In a vicious circle, the degeneration of elderly people who suffer from undiagnosed AD has no doubt contributed to the cruel stereotypes of old age that continue to frighten and demoralize the elderly. To complicate matters, a postmodern revision of aging that began in the 1970s has begun to promote a positive vision of the elderly as "healthy, sexually active, engaged, productive, and self-reliant."[42] There is now a rich market of elderly consumers, whom advertisers court with commercials that show vigorous white-haired couples at play in their retirement years. "Postmodern timelessness" is what sociologist Stephen Katz calls this erasure of the boundaries that once divided the human life cycle into distinct stages controlled by the imperatives of biology and cellular function. Elderhood, Katz writes, has been reconstructed in the postmodern era as a "marketable lifestyle that connects the commodified values of youth with bodycare techniques for masking the appearance of age."[43] The danger is that within such a context AD is not so much an illness as a scandal.

The biology of aging and of age-related illness, in short, coexists with cultural images that help shape how we view the elderly and how the elderly view themselves. The fate of the elderly depends to a large degree on what dominant narratives a culture constructs about the last years of life. In the industrial West, aging has been deeply influenced by the omnivorous cultural narrative of medicalization, especially in the field of gerontology, as people increasingly view their lives from birth to death as a sequence of medical events.[44] But old age as a time of ever increasing dependence upon medicine is not the only narrative available. Religion offers very different end-of-life narratives—still powerful in many parts of the world—and among elderly African American women church-related activities are a significant predictor of satisfaction with their lives.[45] It is unclear, however, whether religion can offer more than a minority voice in many postmodern cultures, and difficult questions remain unanswered.

How will our newly commodified images of vigorous and lusty elderhood play back against the realities of an aging population where a significant percentage of all people above retirement age suffer from AD? How will the changing politics of old age affect postmodern culture as the elderly at first demonstrate their united power and ultimately prove as heterogeneous as feminists, academics, or army recruits? A biocultural model does not guarantee answers, but it offers a helpful perspective on difficult problems and prevents us from oversimplifying the questions. The elderly patient adrift in self-forgetfulness has lost more than normal biological function. The disorder is terrible—even if the patient remains sedated or pleasantly deluded—precisely to the degree that it strips away from us everything in our culture, from families to personal identities, that gives our lives meaning.

POSTMODERN DYING

Patients may survive with AD up to a decade or more following diagnosis. It is a hard practical and philosophical matter to say when dying begins. There is little gain in restating the paradox that dying begins the day we are born. The ending to a chess game, technically, begins with the initial move, but endgames differ profoundly from opening gambits. Zygmunt Bauman offers a convincing argument that modernism (as part of its assault upon all constraints) in effect undertook "to deconstruct mortality" by transforming death from an unmanageable and overwhelming (almost unthinkable) threat into a series of small, manageable, biomedical problems: heartbeat, respiration, tumor, blood pressure, virus.[46] It is as if modernist medicine believed that simply by applying enough raw science to the specific causes of illness it could ultimately defeat death. The consequences of this continuing modernist deconstruction of mortality have brought us to the current postmodern impasse in which dying patients are trapped between two evils: a runaway medical technology of ventilators, surgeries, and organ transplants that can keep bodies alive indefinitely and—as if this prospect were not frightening enough—an understandable but reckless public clamor for physician-assisted suicide as the only alternative to such ignominious physician-assisted suffering.

The impasse shows no sign of resolution. Nothing will stop the advance of biomedical technology, which brings great good along with its unforeseen dilemmas. Suicide (with or without assistance) is both a practical option described openly in how-to books and, in some places, a protected legal right. Under U.S. law, patients who are mentally competent can legally refuse or discontinue life-sustaining treatment, which constitutes suicide in all but name. Meanwhile, business as usual in the ICU and hospital wards leaves one-third of the families of dying patients bankrupt. Things get worse. One major study, as we have seen, showed that half of all patients who died in the hospital spent at least half their time (according to family members) in moderate to severe pain.[47] Clearly there is room for improvement in our treatment of the dying patient. It is thus a hopeful sign that, amid the controversies and horror stories, physician Ira Byock is directing an ambitious community-wide effort (the Missoula Demonstration Project) designed to rethink the contemporary way of dying.

The basic shift in vision required for such rethinking, in Byock's view, comes when we abandon the traditional biomedical model focused on cure. "Modern clinical training, procedures, record-keeping, and economics," he writes in his own critique of the deconstruction of mortality, "constrain doctors and force them to approach dying as if it were strictly a set of medical problems to be solved."[48] Doctors wedded to the biomedical model of scientific problem solving may even deliberately avoid the word *dying*—which is scientifically imprecise—in favor of something more seemingly objective like *multiple organ failure.* Such biomedical euphemisms do the patient and family a serious disservice in preventing a recognition that the process of dying (as distinct from accelerated medical treatment) is under way. The new model of dying that Byock proposes, based on the experience of hospice care, stresses what from a modernist point of view is an unimaginable end-of-life goal: personal growth and development.

The Missoula Demonstration Project offers an experiment in creating a new community-based biocultural model of dying. Biology has a fundamental role. Byock's approach demands as close as possible to absolute control over pain and other symptoms, and dying patients thus receive the full benefit of drug therapies and other bio-

medical advances. With the biology of pain and symptom management securely under control, however, the other fundamental role of
caregivers is to facilitate what are basically nonmedical processes of
individual learning and social interaction. Storytelling, music, and
opportunities for reviewing life histories may prove as therapeutic as
medication. The dying patient is the focus, of course, but the patient
and family *together* (including extended and nontraditional families)
constitute the basic unit of care: personhood extends beyond the skin.
In effect, the complex cultural web of human relationships gets as
much attention as biological processes. Indeed, biology and culture
provide intersecting and mutually reinforcing principles of care in
this bold new model of postmodern dying.

Dying, Byock believes, while by definition irreconcilable with
cure, is highly compatible with healing. It is a time when patients,
families, friends, caregivers, and even the wider community can experience meaningful connections and beneficial changes despite
fears, conflict, and progressive illness. An important underlying
metaphor that Byock applies to the process of dying comes, paradoxically, not from gerontology but from pediatrics: stages of growth and
development. "Someone who is dying," he writes, "like the developing child, goes through stages of discovery, insight, and adjustment
to constantly changing circumstances. . . . Mastering the taskwork
may involve personal struggle, and even suffering, yet it can lead to
growth and dying well."[49]

Hospice is the one organization today devoted to a philosophy of
dying well, not just dying quickly or dying painlessly, and it has
made a crucial contribution to whatever is positive and hopeful in
postmodern illness. The first American hospice opened in 1974 in
New Haven, Connecticut, inspired by and modeled on St. Christopher's Hospice outside of London, which founder Dame Cicely
Saunders opened for inpatients in 1967.[50] Since then, thousands of
patients have lived their last weeks or months mostly at home, pain
free, with dignity and with a chance for meaningful reconciliation,
growth, insight, and healing. In the best-seller *Megatrends* (1982),
John Naisbitt discussed the hospice movement as one of ten "new di-

rections transforming our lives" and noted its significance as part of the larger social trend away from institutional care and toward "self-help."[51] The benefit of hospice—and every U.S. citizen may be entitled to a hospice benefit—unfortunately reaches too few patients. Almost 20 percent of hospice patients are referred only in the last week of life, far too late to derive maximum assistance. As heirs to the modernist deconstruction of mortality, we cling to the cure-centered vision of biomedicine, even when cure is impossible. Hospice, however, offers something better than the vain hope of a last-minute medical miracle while the patient suffers. It offers the radical idea (with its recovery of wisdom implicit in ancient tribal rituals) that dying is not only a biological event but also an occasion, despite its sadness, suffused with positive cultural values and meaning. Even the implacable biology of an approaching death, in this postmodern view, can be reshaped by culture into an occasion for individual growth, family healing, community sharing, and a final leave-taking that comes amid such social and personal achievements as peace, loving care, and human dignity.

THE COUNTRY OF THE ILL REVISITED

The postmodern revision of death both suggests the need and establishes a precedent for rethinking what we mean by health. It is odd that we know so little about health, considering the vast number of state, federal, and worldwide agencies devoted to its analysis and pursuit. The budgets, mission statements, and bureaucratic good works have left us, finally, much better at opposing illness than at understanding health. This is not entirely our fault. Health, as philosopher Hans-Georg Gadamer puts it, "is not something that is revealed through investigation but rather something that manifests itself precisely by virtue of escaping our attention." Health, as he says, is an "enigma."[52] Most often, it seems to describe a time rather than a condition: it indicates a period that *precedes* illness, so that we recognize *when* we have lost it, even if we cannot say exactly *what* it is we have lost. Significantly, most definitions start by staking out negative ground, identifying health with something it is not. "Health does seem to require the absence of disease or illness as a necessary condition," writes ethicist Arthur L. Caplan, "but it is not clear that this absence is by itself sufficient to define the nature of health."[53] As the formula runs: health is not just the absence of illness, it is x or y or z. The World Health Organization in its constitution (1946) no doubt provided the basis for most such formulaic definitions. "Health," writes the organization in what remains its credo, "is a state of complete physical, mental and social well-being, and not merely the absence of disease or infirmity."[54]

Today the mysterious x, y, and z of health frequently center on physical, emotional, and psychological fulfillment attained through programs of nutrition, exercise, stress control, and lifestyle engineering all associated with the new philosophy of *wellness*.[55] Wellness, as a program, aims not just at preventing illness but at maintaining the highest possible health and quality of life. It is hard to criticize such a worthwhile aim, except for its reinforcement of almost irresistible tendencies in postmodern culture toward bourgeois self-absorption. Yet the widely shared assumption that underlies both the philosophy of wellness and the World Health Organization's definition of health seems seriously flawed. Complete physical, mental, and social well-being is a fantasy borrowed from modernist utopian fiction. From a postmodern perspective, health (in all its variations) is something that happens not so much in the absence of illness as in its presence.

The paradox of postmodern understandings of health—as a state not only consistent with illness but interpenetrated by it—rests on a rejection of the binary thinking that supports most modernist biomedical conceptions of health and illness. It is simply not true, from a postmodern perspective, that the absence of illness is a "necessary condition" for health. Postmodern health, it stands to reason, must be as biocultural as postmodern illness. A biocultural vision implies far more than the recognition that different cultures define health differently, in ways that undermine a single, universal, or even worldwide criterion of well-being.[56] A biocultural vision implies that health is not a biological state at all—meaning not solely or strictly biological—but rather a condition in which biology and culture necessarily converge. Moreover, it insists that we go wrong precisely by thinking that health and illness are opposite, incompatible, antagonistic states—one more dualism—as if they embodied an eternal contest between good (health) and evil (illness). A biocultural, postmodern understanding of health escapes from the dualism in which we are either sick or well.

This concept of health as inevitably contaminated by illness sounds so counterintuitive that skeptics, if they cannot be persuaded to consult their personal experience, may be surprised by a few facts and figures. First an informal survey. How many people reading this book are currently experiencing not just the absence of disease or infirmity but complete mental, physical, and social well-being? How many are in pain, under the weather, down in the dumps, recovering, injured, or just plain indisposed? The following list, compiled from reliable sources, offers a view of illness and medical disabilities in the United States for the hypothetical year 1994.[57] The year must be hypothetical because even the most reliable sources often list figures for different years and because all numbers are conservative and rounded off, sometimes violently. Still, the results are rather appalling:

Illness and Disability in America, 1994 (in millions)

AIDS	0.5	Hemorrhoids	9
Alcoholism	14	Hepatitis C	4
Arthritis	33	Hernia	4
Asthma	14	HIV infection	1
Cancer	7	Hypertension	28
Cardiovascular disease	60	Lung disease (chronic)	28
Cataracts	7	Migraine	11
Deformities or orthopedic		Osteoporosis	10
impairments	31	Sexually transmitted	
Depression	11	disease (not AIDS)	1
Dermatitis		Sinusitis (chronic)	34
(including eczema)	9	Stroke	0.5
Diabetes	7	Tinnitus	7
Hay fever	26	Ulcer	4
Hearing impairments	22	Visual impairments	8

Total = 391 million

The total population of the United States in 1994 was around 260 million.[58] Thus by a conservative count—leaving out drug addiction, hospital infections, epilepsy, and a host of common ailments—the country boasting the most advanced medical technologies in the world theoretically had far more people suffering from significant illnesses and disabilities in 1994 than it had people. This is what postmodern life is really like inside the Magic Kingdom.

Statistics lend themselves to various interpretations, of course. Some people unfortunately suffer from multiple conditions—diabetes, for example, exposes people to numerous comorbidities—so any final figure must be fictitious. Fictions, good or bad, are all we have. The point is that nobody knows the absolutely correct number to describe the extent of significant illness and disability in the United States. The estimate here is useful because it suggests something important and normally overlooked about the unknown actual state of affairs. Health, statistically and conceptually, makes no sense when understood as a state that belongs only to the few people lucky enough to escape illness, injury, or disability. Such a state is as fleeting and untenable as youth—and subject to the same nostalgic, idealizing misrepresentations. Health, we might add soberly from a postmodern perspective, is far too important to be wasted on people who are perfectly well.

A postmodern prospect on health opens when we imagine that—except at the extremes of terrible illness and perfect comfort—most people live within a trajectory exposing them to intermittent trauma and even chronic damage. Arthritis, diabetes, multiple sclerosis, lupus: many people suffer from difficult and debilitating conditions that make daily living uncomfortable and often difficult. Yet, many chronic conditions may be managed. Although the most dire consequences of diabetes (including blindness or loss of limbs) are clearly traumatic, even people who suffer from diabetes to the point of serious impairment can still live full, productive lives. Despite diminished function, they exercise, eat well, hold jobs, serve the community, raise families, provide loving homes, and pursue spiritual satisfactions. Is there something more that would constitute a good life? No doubt they would be happy not to deal with illness. Dealing with illness, however, does not take away the opportunity to enjoy a healthy life. Postmodern culture offers us the vision of a future in which health can be redefined—in opposition to modernist fantasies—as the manner in which we live well despite our inescapable illnesses, disabilities, and trauma.[59]

SEARCHING FOR WALT DISNEY

We do not think of Disneyland and Disney World as representations, but they are: triumphs of simulation. Far more than mere ordinary theme parks, they are three-dimensional narrative structures—fragments of film come to life—in which famous cartoon characters emerge from their stories to walk among the audience, shaking hands like politicians. The audience no longer consists of passive spectators but of active participants who move through a carefully constructed flow of attractions from entrance to exit, from morning to night. Some attractions constitute an actual, if miniature, narrative— a jungle cruise, say, with a recognizable beginning, middle, and end—resembling the course of a carefully varied novel rather than the arbitrary and identical repetitions of a carnival ride. They confront us with an experience carved out in advance to preclude interference from anything that is not a well-scripted and often well-recognized representation. The nature of our experience in Disneyland and in its copies scattered around the world cannot be disengaged from the postmodern context in which life has become the perpetual engulfment in a world built out of simulations.

The qualities that make Disneyland a distinctively postmodern enterprise are recognizable by comparison. The power-driven Ferris wheel (invented by American engineer G. W. G. Ferris in 1896) might stand as an example of modernist entertainment. An employee pulls a lever and the machinery clanks into motion as the giant wheel slowly turns. Postmodern Disneyland, by contrast, keeps the machinery out of sight: computers rather than engines are the driving force.

Each visitor, rather than rotating in the same upright circle, is wrapped within an exfoliating myth that connects childhood fantasies (given a Disney spin) with adult dreams of pleasure and success. Every American who achieves an Olympic medal or a championship ring knows the mantra: "I'm going to Disneyland." Their trip is not merely a public-relations event. Disneyland has become an unofficial conclusion to the postmodern cultural narrative of making it. Even the ordinary visitor with no recent victories to celebrate implicitly constructs a personal story to tell the folks back home, often with the aid of snapshots or video camera. ("We made it to Disneyland!") In contrast to the Ferris wheel, Disneyland is a high-tech consumer paradise in which pleasure flows from our immersion within an image-rich, shared, multimillion-dollar structure of representations. We like it because it is the opposite of affliction, but its radiance is not entirely innocent. The self-serving fantasies promoted by a huge international corporation have—as Baudrillard, Marin, and Eco implicitly affirm—something to do with a culture in which illness appears increasingly as an anomaly or scandal that must be excluded from the consumer paradise of pleasure and health. It is thus worth briefly distinguishing the flesh-and-blood Walt Disney, man and artist, from the corporate functions now carried on in his name.

Disney's work in film was never completely removed from issues of public health. Enlisted by the U. S. government, Disney Studios during the war years of the 1940s produced for Latin American audiences fifteen Spanish-language films on health care. The films used animation to promote a well-meaning biomedical imperialism that traced illness to contagion and personal hygiene—wholly ignoring the ways in which states and corporations collude in policies that sustain poverty and even increase disease.[60] Yet something else was going on in Disney's career at the same time. "*Bambi*," wrote the admiring Russian filmmaker Sergei Eisenstein as he considered the arc of Disney's career, "is already a shift towards ecstasy—serious, eternal: the theme of *Bambi* is the circle of life—*the repeating circles of lives*."[61] What Eisenstein sees in Bambi is not a humanized animal (the staple of animated cartoons) but rather what he calls "a 'redeerized' human." *Bambi* (1942), he suggests, returns spectators to a primal condition: we are no longer sophisticates amused by cartoon creatures but rather we experience a profound change, akin to totemism, in which animal and human have become one. This unity of human and animal in the mythic circle of life plays out in our responses to the terrifying forest fire in which Bambi's mother burns to death. Such a scene is utterly foreign to contemporary corporate fantasies of childhood, where death is usually just another special effect, but it has a certain relevance to the life of Walt Disney. Typhoid fever put him seriously at risk as a boy. In his teens, he falsified his birth certificate to drive an ambulance in World War I. Biographers can easily show that he was not the lovable Uncle Walt he sometimes portrayed. He was ultimately something better. What is healthy in his films has little to do with bluebirds and singing rabbits. It lies in a vision that includes facing threats as serious and sometimes as irremediable in their losses as illness and death.

The hopeful thing about postmodern illness is that, by giving us a knowledge of the relationship between biology and culture, it gives us an opportunity for identifying unhealthy conditions in our surrounding environment that are as insidious as ponds full of mosquito larvae. Postmodern illness occurs in a world in which representations and simulations have as much power as microbes and mosquitoes. Some representations help us, some hurt us, some put a little harmless pleasure into our lives: the point is to learn the difference. We cannot ban or legislate out of consciousness every potentially harmful image. We can, however, enlist the power of representation in promoting what is healthy, in refusing to glamorize what is harmful, and in helping us to understand and to confront the world we inhabit and construct—a world that includes not only well-scripted simulations but also people suffering from serious illnesses and disabilities in part shaped and constrained by the surrounding world of images. Illness, if we learn how to see it in a biocultural vision, can be far healthier than we know. It is a thought that might have pleased Walt Disney: a chain-smoker, he died of lung cancer at sixty-five.

Conclusion

NARRATIVE BIOETHICS

You don't have anything

if you don't have the stories.

LESLIE MARMON SILKO,
Ceremony (1977)[1]

Postmodern writing has a special difficulty with conclusions. "I think my work has always been informed by mystery," Don DeLillo said to an interviewer: "the final answer, if there is one at all, is outside the book. My books are open-ended."[2] Many postmodern writers share DeLillo's sense that an open-endedness in contemporary life defeats the traditional purpose of a conclusion. We have endings all around us, but few summings-up. DeLillo sees in the 1963 shooting of John Kennedy—which forms the occasion for his novel *Libra* (1988)—a pivotal moment in the making of postmodern America. "We seem much more aware of elements like randomness and ambiguity and chaos since then," he says.[3] Consumer culture offers another source and reflection of postmodern resistance to closure. Television soap operas have learned how to cultivate the ambiguity and potential for chaos in human relationships by means of a narrative structure that, in principle, defies finalization. Postmodernism may even develop in audiences a taste for incompleteness, along with a nostalgia for times when marriage and other social institutions seemed stable, or at least less shifting. Each blockbuster movie generates a sequel, every hemline and strip of chrome holds place for a season. As in weekly episodes in a sitcom, any apparent closure is temporary, illusory, and arbitrary. We know that the ending is not a finale but merely the resolution of today's entanglement. Besides, we can catch it all again in reruns.

The study of postmodern illness, for a combination of reasons, cannot properly conclude but only arrive at a temporary closure, in which final answers lie outside the text. Such an inconclusive finish, while necessarily open-ended, does not preclude a backward and forward glance.

The vision of postmodern illness as biocultural has offered a way to understand, if not necessarily to resolve, some of the confusions we are living through. It provides a corrective to the modernist belief that a knowledge of disease at the molecular level will inevitably produce effective treatments. Molecules alone, as we have seen, cannot wholly account for the human experience of illness. Culture as it intersects with biology twists and turns molecular structures. What happens under laboratory conditions, where variables are carefully controlled, does not always correspond to what happens elsewhere: pain on the battlefield differs significantly from pain induced by attaching electrodes to the tail of a mouse. Meanwhile, the microbes responsible for many illnesses keep changing, often in response to changes introduced by humans into the surrounding culture. Two humans sharing roughly identical molecular structures (but coming from different cultures) can respond quite differently to roughly identical microbes and medications. Culture, in short, captures illness within a shaping field as powerful and sometimes as invisible as the force of gravity.

The importance of articulating this new biocultural vision lies not merely in the possibilities it offers for improved treatment. A slightly improved medical treatment for lung cancer is less valuable, in the long run, than successful efforts to modify the cultural practice of smoking. A biocultural perspective proves valuable especially in the opportunities it opens for interdisciplinary collaborations, for bringing biomedical knowledge into contact with the insights of anthropologists, sociologists, philosophers, historians, and others who make cultural knowledge their field of study. Unfortunately, medical schools still show little inclination for contact with disciplines and activities outside their traditional curricula. A routine psychosocial workup is simply no substitute for a vigorous engagement with the complications of culture as it affects human illness. No one expects doctors and nurses, in addition to their other weighty responsibilities, to be anthropologists or philosophers. The point is simply that a biocultural perspective invites unusual forms of collaboration that ultimately will provide more effective tools in helping people deal successfully with their afflictions.

The one nonscientific discipline that has found a relatively secure place within contemporary medicine is bioethics. In the clinic or office, doctors regularly confront situations that impinge on the rights of the patient. They must deal not only with patients but also with insurance companies, lawyers, and family members, whose conflicting interests at times create knotty moral dilemmas. Large questions loom behind every casual encounter. Do physicians have a moral or professional duty to provide a drug-addicted patient with pain-killing narcotics? What are the ethical implications of a world where the United Kingdom—for every 100,000 people—prescribes some 4,000 milligrams of morphine, while Mexico prescribes almost none?[4] Is there now a de facto racial or ethnic geography of pain? The questions seem to proliferate with every scientific discovery and technical breakthrough. Is it unethical to clone humans? Do employers have a right to learn about the genetic defects of an employee that might cost stockholders millions of dollars in medical expenses? Bioethics is the discipline developed to deal with such vexing questions. Although it offers one example of the fruitful collaborations possible at the crossroads of biology and culture, bioethics nonetheless tends to operate within a rather narrow domain sketched out for it by medicine, which normally pays the bills. Its more radical implications emerge when we ask what might happen if bioethics paid serious attention to something so apparently trivial and nonmedical as the human activity of telling stories? The outrage is already under way, with a few doctors and bioethicists in the vanguard.

THE NARRATIVE TURN

One infallible sign that you have entered the gravitational field of postmodernism is a swerve toward narrative. *Narrative* in the modernist era was mostly a deluxe word for *story*. Story, even in literary criticism, was the preferred term. "We shall all agree," wrote E. M. Forster in 1927, "that the fundamental aspect of the novel is its story-telling aspect."[5] Narrative in the postmodern era has turned into a far more comprehensive concept that embraces the storylike qualities that novels share with other genres and modes, including ballads, sitcoms, films, myths, dreams, and the unconscious. Stories do not exhaust the possibilities of "telling"—Latin *narrans*—implicit in narrative. Thus postmodernism reinvented the nonfiction novel. It reshaped narrative subgenres from news reports to garden manuals. It incorporated into magazine prose such fragments of narrative as dialogue, character, landscape, talk, letters, anecdotes, and innumerable materials also found in novels. As postmodern thinkers increasingly doubted that reason could provide access to noncontingent, absolute, universal truths, they found increasing use for narrative as a term to describe the various explanatory structures that intellectual disciplines offer. The result has been described as a wholesale "narrativist turn" in the human sciences.[6]

Meanwhile, new and unforeseen dilemmas continue to arise. In modernist medicine, no one needed to ask what constituted death. Nobody had to ask how to choose a sperm donor, or who was eligible for a liver transplant. Such questions were not just unasked but (in any practical sense) unthinkable. The acceleration of medical sci-

ence and technology during the 1950s and 1960s in effect called forth
a new ethical knowledge that might help guide physicians and manage the dilemmas generated by rapid change.[7] The term *bioethics* first
appeared in the 1970s, and today most medical schools provide training in ethics, most hospitals maintain an ethics committee, and most
television networks keep a bioethicist on call to comment on the latest controversial research. What has gone without saying—an assumption lodged in medical thought too deep for recognition—is
that bioethics and narrative must surely belong to separate worlds.

Medicine in its aspirations to scientific status not only avoids narrative but treats it with a disdainful mixture of hostility and con-
tempt. "The hospital," says physician and ethnographer Barry Saunders, "can be a profoundly anti-narrative institution."[8] Lab reports, X
rays, statistics, these non-narrative staples of clinical decision making
reflect the powerful tendency within medicine to distance itself from
the undisciplined, verbose, contingent realm of narrative. Like law,
medicine prefers to cleanse its discipline of narrative. Attorneys sure
of their ground will sometimes lob clients a softball invitation to narrative—"Tell me, Mr. Morris, what happened on the night of . . . "—
but rambling replies are cut short, and the only authorized legal narratives appear in the summarizing arguments of the attorneys. As
Arthur W. Frank contends, in modernist biomedicine the sole authorized narrative of illness is the physician's account. In recent years,
however, Kathryn Montgomery Hunter and others have begun to
show how medicine—despite its official disdain for storytelling—is
shot through with narrative, from the medical tales swapped around
the water cooler to a professional education based on case histories.
Physicians Oliver Sacks and Arthur Kleinman have argued that medicine needs to embrace the extended narratives of illness (Sacks calls
them "clinical tales") that permit a fuller account of the patient's experience. Interest in narrative is now starting to grow within medicine, at least in a few selected specialties. Professional storyteller
Richard Stone often works in hospices with dying patients. "When
people have a chance to tell their stories," he says, "they're able to see
the meaning of life, to see the path they've taken, and approach the

whole event of their death very differently."[9] There are good and timely reasons why postmodern illness should lead us at last to the curiously hybrid concept of a "narrative bioethics."

THE CHICKEN AND THE SNOW SHOVEL

Narrative, like illness, is a biocultural phenomenon. This controversial statement opposes the normal view of narrative as wholly a product of culture. Certainly, different cultures produce vastly different narratives. It is worth asking, however, if the practice of storytelling reflects something beyond ordinary cultural diversity. We now take it for granted that language is not merely a cultural practice but the result of biological processes genetically coded through the process of evolution. Narrative, I want to speculate, is not just a special use of language—like making lists or writing sonnets—but a form of human behavior as biological as the capacity for speech. Neuroscience has only started to explore the specific structures in the brain that make narrative (and other forms of cognition) possible, such as cerebral locales governing the ability to grasp temporal sequence and causal relations. For several decades, however, we have possessed powerful indirect evidence (not proof but evidence) that the construction of narrative is something the human brain seems biologically driven to do. We tell stories driven by the same biological imperative that drives us to adopt upright posture. The creature that Nietzsche called "*the* sick animal" is also, inescapably, the narrative animal.

Vivid evidence for a biocultural view of narrative comes from a well-known inquiry ("the chicken and snow shovel experiment") into split-brain perception.[10] Researchers divided the individual's field of vision so that the two hemispheres of the brain each received a different visual stimulus (figure 6). The language-rich left hemisphere saw a chicken claw, while the nearly mute right hemisphere saw a snow scene. The individual was then asked to select an image corresponding to the visual stimulus, and there were two easy cor-

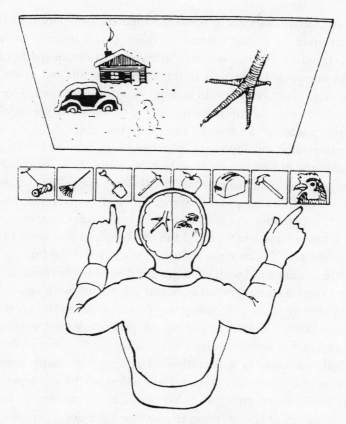

Figure 6. The Chicken and Snow Shovel Experiment. Reprinted by permission from Michael S. Gazzaniga and Joseph E. LeDoux, *The Integrated Mind* (New York: Plenum Press, 1978).

rect choices: the head of a chicken and a snow shovel. This part of the experiment caused no problem. The difficulty arose when researchers asked the individual to explain the choices. An explanation for the chicken head was obvious: the left brain had simply matched two parts of the same fowl. There is no way, however, that the left brain could understand the choice of the snow shovel. Only the right brain saw the snow scene, and it was the right brain that picked the snow shovel. What makes the experiment so fascinating is that the right brain, of course, does not possess the capacity for speech, so that it cannot provide a verbal account explaining why it chose the snow shovel. In effect, the researchers contrived to confront the left brain with an inexplicable mystery. In this impasse, again and again, they observed variants on a single strange and consistent behavior. The left brain, despite its complete ignorance of the snow scene, almost instantly "made up" an account to explain the inexplicable shovel.

The fabricated or made-up explanation was delivered with an air of confidence. Never, when asked to explain the choice of the shovel, did the individual say something like "I don't know" or "I don't understand" or "It's all a mystery to me." Instead, bogus but apparently plausible explanations poured forth. In a typical instance, one person said: "I saw a claw and I picked the chicken, and you have to clean out the chicken shed with a shovel." This is what the human brain does when confronted with something it cannot understand.

The experiment suggests that, when confronted with situations of inexplicable impasse, our brains are predisposed to the creation of narrative. They are built, in effect, to produce verbal explanatory structures that in some way resolve the impasse. Not every verbal explanatory structure is a narrative, of course, but many constitute miniature or fragmentary stories. The earliest myths and legends are verbal explanatory structures that account for mysteries ranging from the origin of the universe to how the tiger got its stripes. Such storytelling seems as inescapably human, consistent across cultures and times, as singing and dancing. It is behavior that takes the particular shape given to it by a specific culture, but the behavior is not, strictly speaking, a product of culture: it is the cultural manifestation of an underlying biological drive. The impulse toward narrative, like the drive behind the colorful varieties of human sexual behavior, is ultimately biological.

Narrative, according to this line of thought, is not simply a possibility inherent in human biology, like bungee jumping. It is not just something we *can* do but something we cannot *help* doing. It is as if the human brain cannot rest until it has produced a verbal explanatory structure—employing whatever resources are available in the culture—to account for what it cannot know. Telling stories is, quite simply, what human beings have done for thousands of years, as stories helped knit together the fabric of social life on which group survival depended. This connection between storytelling and group survival is quite clear in the Native American oral tradition, where a knowledge of theology, education, medicine, kinship relations, and every crucial aspect of community life is experienced through ritual and story. Contemporary Native American author Leslie Marmon Silko alludes to this tradition in a poem contained in her novel *Ceremony* (1977):

> I will tell you something about stories,
> [he said]
> They aren't just entertainment.
> Don't be fooled.
> They are all we have, you see,
> all we have to fight off
> illness and death.
>
> You don't have anything
> if you don't have the stories.[11]

In the Native American tradition, stories (especially in their kinetic form as ritual) bind the individual within the sacred web of life that includes not only clan and tribe but also ancestor spirits, animals, and the earth itself. The web (like its variant, the sacred hoop) constitutes a powerful narrative image of wholeness. Within Native American thought, illness can have many specific sources, from a snake bite to a failed duty, but health and wholeness always involve the individual's restoration to a place of harmony within the narrative web of life.

In the biomedical tradition, stories, of course, are a poor substitute for scientific knowledge. From a postmodern point of view, however, with its pluralistic respect for the wisdom of various traditions, the stories we tell as individuals and as cultures have a significant impact upon illness and health. Case histories and statistical instruments cannot possibly capture the complex dimensions of the individual experience of illness illuminated by narrative. It is stories, not randomized, double-blind studies, that convey such hard-to-grasp variables as the personal beliefs, emotional histories, and cultural contexts that make every experience of illness both individual and social.[12] Even stories with wide circulation inside a culture—such as stories of victimization—take on a revealing individual slant as they are retold by specific persons. Tod Chambers, a bioethicist, makes the crucial point that even case histories used in textbooks of ethics are not transparent reports of fact but "constructed" artifacts. As he explains, "Every telling of a story—real or imagined—encompasses a series of choices about what will be revealed, what will be privileged, and what will be omitted; there are no artless narrations."[13] A biocultural perspective implies a need to understand both the stories that shape the individual experience of illness and the art that shapes the stories we tell. This new understanding of narrative is beginning to have an impact upon the day-to-day practice of bioethics.[14]

NARRATIVE AND MORAL KNOWLEDGE

The role of narrative in medical ethics finds two exceptional analysts in Kathryn Montgomery Hunter and Arthur W. Frank, whose valuable work provides the basis for my brief excursion here, an excursion that pushes a little further into the territory that they and others (such as physicians Rita Charon and Howard Brody) have opened up.[15] Hunter's article "Narrative" in the *Encyclopedia of Bioethics* emphasizes that ethics concerns not only general principles but also their application to particular cases. Narrative, she argues convincingly, is what encourages and permits us to examine the detailed circumstances that interpenetrate each particular case and make it, if not unique, distinctive. Stories, further, refine our moral vision by helping to uncover the meanings that always cluster around illness, especially "the meaning of illness in the life of the patient" and the "meaning of a patient-doctor interaction in the life of the physician." Narrative, she reminds us, has been recognized as a medium of moral knowledge since the ancient Greeks, and in her account (updated with reference to structural linguistics and cognitive psychology) narrative remains "central" to contemporary bioethics.[16]

One assumption in the impressive case for narrative that Hunter makes in the *Encyclopedia of Bioethics* is so basic to most thinking about bioethics that it nearly slips from sight and thus needs to be made visible. Bioethics for Hunter is preeminently an arena of "moral *reasoning*." She finds narrative especially valuable because it develops the "interpretive reasoning" that finds a close parallel in the "clinical reasoning" basic to medicine. No one would disagree with her emphasis on the place of reason in bioethics. It is fair to suggest, however, that behind Hunter's analysis, offstage but influential, stands one of her favorite narrative heroes: the archreasoner Sherlock Holmes. Holmes is an appropriate figure in an account of medical reasoning, since he is not only the fictive creation of a doctor (Arthur Conan Doyle) but also a creation based on Doyle's medical school professor of pathology. The question for narrative bioethics—a question to which I will return shortly—is how far the privilege quite properly accorded to reason leaves open a space for a complementary moral knowledge based on or enlightened by feeling.

Arthur W. Frank—a sociologist whose own serious illness deeply informs his writing—offers a perspective that differs sharply from Hunter's emphasis on moral reasoning. The basis for narrative ethics that Frank develops in *The Wounded Storyteller* (1995) is what he calls thinking *with* stories.[17] Such thinking has little to do with reason or medical decision making. It centers, instead, on the related processes of moral reflection and of personal change that combine for Frank in the philosophical term "becoming." This moral process of "becoming" applies both to the teller and to the listener. Telling the stories of their illnesses constitutes a moral action by which the ill negotiate the reshaping of their own lives. Listening to such stories and responding to them with empathy constitutes for the listener an equally important moral act that also contains a possibility for significant life changes. For Frank, the source of illness stories lies ultimately in the wounded body and its suffering. Once we truly attend to illness stories and their bodily sources—rather than ignore them, translate them into biomedical dialects, or reject them in favor of various discourses of philosophical reason—we have for Frank entered an arena of moral "becoming."

It is moral reflection and personal change set in motion by stories of illness—not the conventional quest in bioethics to determine "clear guidelines or principles for making decisions" (160)—that constitute for Frank the goal of narrative ethics. This attractive program, however, also has its limitation. Primarily, it evades the troubling indeterminacy that postmodern theorists find inherent in narratives and in our attempts to make sense of them. "In narrative ethics, if the point of a story is not clear," Frank writes in his conclusion, "don't explain, tell another story" (183). This is a revealing moment that honors—but does not quite come to terms with—the opacity of narrative. On one hand, Frank implies that some illness stories carry a clear "point," although it is unclear from a postmodern perspective how we can know or agree exactly what it is. On the other hand, stories whose point is unclear invite an infinite regress of additional stories that equally resist full explanation. Busy medical staffs simply do not have time to hear a potentially endless sequence of indeterminate illness narratives. Narrative is a beast that resists all our efforts to domesticate it. It is *Tristram Shandy*, *Finnegan's Wake*, and the complete writings of the Marquis de Sade. In fact, our resistance to the specific class of narratives that Frank calls "chaos" stories helps explain why (as he indicates) society is happy to have medicine interpret them as diagnostic of depression: the narrative threat is contained and domesticated with medication. The official antinarrative stance in medicine stems partly from a strategic choice to keep the camel outside the tent, since narrative can unsettle and damage as well as heal. It reminds us that "becoming" has limits as a goal of narrative ethics—limits implicit in its evident merits and in the nature of narrative—that are as significant as limitations in the equally valuable goal of moral reasoning.

Limitations implicit in Frank's emphasis on becoming and in Hunter's emphasis on moral reasoning, I want to emphasize, do not subvert the value of a narrative bioethics that develops both finer reasoning about illness and deeper possibilities for moral growth and action. All useful standards—even the bedrock biomedical principle of patient autonomy—have limits.[18] From a postmodern perspective, limitations do not constitute grounds for rejecting a useful standard, since no standards can escape them. My appendix to the work of Hunter and Frank, which continues to draw upon their insights, consists in an initial sketch of three concepts foreign to most medical literature—foreign to most writing on ethics—that deserve consideration in any future narrative bioethics: emotion, dialogue, and the everyday.

EMOTION, DIALOGUE, AND THE EVERYDAY

Emotion currently holds a marginal place in bioethics, smuggled in (if it enters at all) through routine calls for empathy, a virtue few dispute and fewer seem to practice.[19] Unfortunately, a bioethics based on empathy tends to overlook our remarkable powers to turn away from suffering, especially when suffering occurs in hospitals or other remote places, like Bosnia. It is unclear, further, why an ethical response to suffering should be based on empathy rather than on the principle that—no matter what we feel or do not feel—suffering is intolerable, that we have an absolute obligation to prevent and to relieve it. Empathy, in any case, is an overworked, undervalued, and poorly understood standard that does not exhaust the advantages of emotion in bioethics. A narrative bioethics offers the chance to explore a variety of contexts in which feeling can play a valuable, even crucial, role in moral thought and action, supplementing and perhaps even modifying the power of reason.

The postmodern philosopher who writes most persuasively about the role of emotion in moral knowledge is Martha Nussbaum. Nussbaum takes the controversial but increasingly respected position that the practice and explanation of moral philosophy extends beyond the work of philosophers to include novels, drama, and other writing usually described as literature.[20] This position makes particular sense when postmodernism questions the arbitrary boundaries that traditionally separate literature from philosophy, but Nussbaum also brings to her analysis of literary works a classicist's knowledge of ancient Greek and Roman writing, where philosophy took numerous forms, including fables, letters, poems, and the oral dialogues that Socrates conducted as (on at least one famous occasion) he sat drinking long into the night. Nussbaum explores, for example, how Sophocles, Aeschylus, and Euripides deal with questions about the good life that also constitute a pressing topic for Aristotle and Plato.[21] Turning to the modern world, she examines in Henry James's novel *The Golden Bowl* the moral implications flowing not only from the choices and values of individual characters but also from their minor self-deceptions, tacit social conflicts, and almost invisible domestic habits (such as their relation to artifacts and works of art). She does not deny or elide the differences between philosophers and novelists but rather demonstrates that the exploration of moral knowledge takes many forms that most people regard as literary. Her concern with moral knowledge distinguishes her from various contemporary writers who—similarly following the "linguistic turn" of postanalytic philosophy—focus on the philosophical implications of metaphor, language, and narrative.[22] Even more audacious than her demonstration that literature constitutes a way of "doing" philosophy, however, is Nussbaum's argument that emotion holds an important place in the constitution of moral knowledge.

Greek tragedy provides the occasion for Nussbaum's argument. No one—least of all Plato and Aristotle—would deny that tragedy invites an emotional response from the audience. But what is emotion? How should we understand its place? Plato banned the dramatic poets from his ideal republic because among other transgressions, such as telling lies about the gods, they stirred up unruly and possibly dangerous emotions in the audience. Aristotle sought to redeem tragedy from this pejorative Platonic interpretation of feeling with the argument that what tragedy provoked in the audience was a "catharsis" of emotion—especially a catharsis of pity and fear. Although classicists dispute the meaning of "catharsis" (some defining it as purgation, others as clarification, others as purification), they do not dispute that Aristotle finds a productive role for emotion in tragedy. Nussbaum's contribution is to argue that the process of moral understanding in tragedy is inseparable from the experience of emotion. She writes: "Our cognitive activity, as we explore the ethical conception embodied in the text, centrally involves emotional response. We discover what we think about these events partly by noticing how we feel; our investigation of our emotional geography is a major part of our search for self-knowledge." Self-knowledge is indispensable for moral action, but Nussbaum is not satisfied with describing emotion as a mere adjunct to cognitive processes. "[E]motional response can sometimes be not just a *means* to practical knowledge," she clarifies, "but a constituent part of the best sort of recognition or knowledge of one's practical situation."[23] Emotion is woven into the fabric of moral knowledge.

Nussbaum has her critics, but the skirmishing of professional philosophers need not delay us here.[24] What Nussbaum offers to narrative bioethics is an argument and a tradition for rethinking the role of emotion in moral knowledge. Her approach parallels a recent rethinking of emotion in psychology, where feelings are understood not as states called forth or caused by events but rather as states we create through our *interpretation* of events, as, in effect, biological products of the limbic system that are also cultural (and hence potentially moral) constructions.[25] Such a biocultural view of emotion holds obvious attractions as a contribution to our understanding of postmodern illness. How far might we strengthen both the "moral reasoning" invoked by Hunter and the process of "becoming" invoked by Frank if we acknowledge and openly explore the role that Nussbaum proposes for emotion in ethics?

The discussion of emotion in bioethics has not really begun, and it cannot begin until we overcome the philosophical prejudice against emotion at least as old as the pre-Socratics and ossified in the Cartesian split between bodies and minds. Emotion in this traditional prejudice is most often depicted as the hazardous opponent of reason:

we regularly encounter metaphors of a disreputable lower force (animal or body) that threatens to disturb the serene and noble function of intellect. Metaphors deeply imbued with sexual politics often portray it as female—unreliable, unstable, prone to hysterical excess (as if "masculine" reason never attained its own wildly unstable states). A corrective, biocultural perspective would require us to consider the social origin of such metaphors and their influence on our knowledge of feeling. It would propose that emotion is as valuable a legacy of our evolutionary heritage as are binocular vision and opposable thumbs. Neuroscientist Antonio R. Damasio recounts a case in which a localized brain injury impaired a man's ability to experience emotion, while leaving intact the ability to reason. The injured man's predicament, says Damasio, was a capacity *"to know but not to feel."* [26] This emotionless reasoner had, significantly, completely lost the power to make decisions (a power implicit in the idea of moral knowledge). Obviously, under certain circumstances emotion can disrupt reason, but we ignore the many occasions when emotion is crucial to effective reasoning. Emotion, as the Star Trek crew keeps trying to persuade the cold-blooded Vulcan reasoner, Mr. Spock, is what makes us human. Why should we try so hard to cleanse bioethics of feeling? Exploring the role that emotion plays in moral knowledge offers the possibility for more human-scale and less abstract discussion of ethical issues. Everyone knows that hospitals are scenes of wrenching emotional drama. Narrative bioethics offers a principle that respects—rather than a prejudice that automatically mistrusts or excludes—the evidence derived from human emotional experience. A narrative bioethics unable to deal openly and effectively with emotion is simply a contradiction in terms.

Dialogue, like emotion, is an everyday affair that narrative bioethics places in a new light. Narrative most often includes dialogue, directly or indirectly, but dialogue in postmodern analysis refers to something far more significant than conversational exchange: it has become, especially in the work of Mikhail Bakhtin, fundamental to an understanding of what narrative is and does. Bakhtin is a postmodernist by adoption—his writings were first translated

into English during the 1970s—and dialogue in his hands under-
writes an entire theory of the novel. Novels for Bakhtin respect the
basic truth that language is always saturated with what he calls "the
discourse of the other." [27] Simply put, he means that our utterances
(even if we are just talking to ourselves) necessarily bear the traces of
previous usage, much as our speech and writing always incorporate
the words of other people or anticipate another person's response.
They are directed *to* a particular audience, in a specific context, continuing or opening an exchange rooted in its own social and historical locale. "Every word," Bakhtin wrote, "gives off the scent of a profession, a genre, a current, a party, a particular work, a particular
man, a generation, an era, a day, and an hour. Every word smells of
the context and contexts in which it has lived its intense social life." [28]
After Bakhtin, a narrative bioethics attentive to dialogue must be
equally attentive to the social life of language as carrying within it—
like most things interpersonal—serious if latent moral implications.

One moral implication of dialogue concerns the simple act of listening. There are few clearer ways to express disrespect for other
people than not to listen to what they say. The decision not to listen
contains an implicit judgment about value—not just the value of
what you anticipate will be said but, ultimately, or so it will be con-
strued, the value that you attribute to the person you judge not worth
listening to. When we turn a deaf ear to someone, we reject any claim
upon us, we sever communion, we eliminate the speaker from our
field of action. Listening, Arthur Frank concurs, is a moral act, especially when what we hear may prove disturbing. "One of our most
difficult duties as human beings," he writes, "is to listen to the voices
of those who suffer." [29] Such listening is deeply relevant to medicine
because a new emphasis on patients' speech began to transform illness, around the 1950s, from something almost exclusively seen to
something heard: the nineteenth-century clinical gaze (with its emphasis on what is visible) gained a powerful ally in the act of listening, through which invisible symptoms become audible. The danger
today is that clinical investigation of a patient's speech will focus
only on what is *heard*, not on what is *said*.[30] What the physician does

not hear (or what the patient is unable to communicate) simply evaporates from the diagnostic scene. Thus the implicit moral dimensions of skilled listening—which almost require a knowledge of dialogue—coincide with important clinical acts and decisions.

A narrative bioethics would insist that effective listening—as an indispensable part of the doctor-patient dialogue—is a necessary skill for physicians, as some within medicine have explicitly argued.[31] It may sound strange to describe effective listening as a skill, since for most people listening is as automatic as drawing breath, but listening matters for bioethics because various studies demonstrate that doctors are in general poor listeners. In one famous 1984 study, patients responding to the initial inquiry about their complaint were allowed to speak for eighteen seconds, on average, before the physician interrupted to take control.[32] This is not dialogue but medical monologue punctuated by the patient's desperate efforts to be heard. Ten years later, the situation did not look quite so bleak: a study of physicians in private practice showed that patients initiated at least half of the interruptions and that two-thirds of such interruptions brought new information to light.[33] Maybe patients are getting more aggressive and doctors more receptive (among other possibilities). Still, there is no doubt that medical communication needs improvement. Moreover, empathetic listening that values the speaker, while crucial, is not identical with clinically effective listening which leads to accurate diagnosis. It is clearly unethical to practice medicine without the necessary skills. Surgeons who lack the skills needed for surgery are not merely unskilled surgeons; they are frauds who put their patients in jeopardy. Doctors who neglect to gain the skills and knowledge required for clinically effective listening—although this idea is absolutely foreign to Western medicine—are engaged in unethical medical practice.

An engagement with dialogue—in the comprehensive and detailed sense that Bakhtin intends—offers a means to develop skills in clinically effective listening. Competitive swimmers and runners must relearn how to breathe, and physicians must relearn how to listen. Thus it is not enough to declare listening a virtue, as if its value were self-evident or context-free; physicians must know *why* to listen, *how* to listen, and what to listen *for*. A skill in dialogue complements the related skills that are coming to be known inside medical education as narrative competencies: "the capacity to adopt others' perspectives, to follow the narrative thread of complex and chaotic stories, to tolerate ambiguity, and to recognize the multiple, often contradictory meanings of events."[34] These are skills almost inconceivable without some knowledge, intuitive or learned, of dialogics. Several specialties within medicine already recognize the value of such knowledge. The American Board of Internal Medicine, in its 1995 publication on physician competency in end-of-life patient care, includes an entire section dedicated to the use of narratives. Such skills in listening effectively are especially crucial at the end of life, when curative intervention is often inappropriate and when suffering may be less responsive to drugs than to insights that come mainly through skillful attention to the patient's speech. Dialogue is not an easy answer to all the questions raised by the need for effective listening, but it is one important tool with which narrative bioethics can begin to make a difference in the practice of clinical medicine.

A third major contribution of narrative bioethics might come in its shift of focus away from abstract principles and away from megawatt, life-and-death, technology-driven emergencies onto the ordinary and the everyday. Bioethics is increasingly asked to address issues so big, so complex, and so hot that they routinely make the evening news: issues such as physician-assisted suicide, cloning, organ harvests, fetal-tissue implants, brain death, and abortion, to name a few. These are important problems, but it is doubtful whether narrative bioethics will help us solve them. What narrative bioethics can do well, however, is to focus on smaller, more manageable questions that the media preoccupation with megawatt issues tends to render invisible. It can thus help reclaim for moral knowledge an entire area of medical practice that, because it is invisible, seems almost devoid of ethical implications. It can offer us an ethical understanding of the everyday world that may prove crucial in the experience of illness.

There is no better guide to the philosophical implications of ordinary experience than Stanley Cavell. The Harvard philosopher has spent his career in the unorthodox project of rethinking what it means to focus on ordinary language and on the everyday world. The motive for this rethinking has been his lifelong engagement with the threat posed by philosophical skepticism. To most people, skepticism implies simply a passing mood of ironic detachment or incredulity, but it means something very different to philosophers. Philosophical skepticism implies a radical and systematic doubt about the possibilities of reason. Skepticism is an ancient philosophical position with numerous variants—closely allied, in its distrust of abstract systems, with the development of empirical medicine as early as the third century B.C. Today it tends to center on the power of reason to provide a doubt to match and cancel every affirmation. For a skeptical postmodern philosopher, reason is its own most formidable opponent, a grand master sitting opposite itself in a chess game that cannot be won, the carrier of radical doubt that prevents us from enjoying a firm possession of cherished principles and familiar certainties for which we commonly invoke reason as our guarantor.

A philosopher who takes skepticism seriously, as Cavell does, faces the threat of a world utterly drained of the rational assumptions that supply so much of its comfort and value. Under the steely gaze of skepticism, rational principles of bioethics such as patient autonomy and physician beneficence melt away into groundless local standards that merely allow the big business of Western medicine to proceed without perpetual crisis. Human life, not bioethics alone, threatens to crumble under the assault of unrelenting doubt into a bleak scene of loss where we wander in the dark, without consolation or reasonable hope, waiting like Beckett's forlorn protagonists for a principle of meaning that never appears. Cavell's response to skepticism is not a super-defense of reason—not the construction of a rational system impregnable to the doubts of reason—but rather a return to the realm of the ordinary and the everyday: a realm that philosophers normally flee or neglect in their quest for something more elevated, abstract, and profound.

"The answer to skepticism," Cavell writes, attributing his answer to the tradition of modernist and postmodern thought known as ordinary language philosophy, "must take the form not of philosophical construction but of the reconstruction or resettlement of the everyday."[35] The answer to skepticism, in other words, is not to construct a new philosophical argument or system but to transform philosophy into an engagement with the neglected everydayness of human life. Although Cavell's recent work does not explicitly concern moral knowledge, a philosophical engagement with the everyday has profound ethical implications as it affects the way we live and the possibilities for "becoming."[36] It also finds in narrative a central resource for exploring such ethical implications, since narrative (from the novel to the television sitcom) has provided a privileged site for the representation of everyday life. Cavell, in fact, bases much of his own analysis on narrative, lately focusing on movies and plays, where he finds a rich exfoliation of materials that open up our engagement with the everyday world.[37] One central text in his ongoing philosophical resettlement of the everyday, as his readers cannot miss, is *Walden*. Cavell reads *Walden* as a story about the rediscovery of the ordinary world in the basic human act—which involves ethics rather than carpentry—of building of a house: "that is, the finding of one's habitation, of where it is one is at home."[38]

Isn't this resettlement of the everyday, this finding or building of one's habitation, what most people must do under the condition of serious illness? Emerson, no less cannily narrative in his writing than Thoreau, provides another main source for Cavell's reflections on the power of the everyday to give a mooring to human life. It is his engagement with Emerson and Thoreau (an engagement enriched by the work of Wittgenstein and ordinary language philosophy) that ultimately allows Cavell to work out an implicit ethics of everyday life that he can set against the still unvanquished threat of radical doubt and skeptical nihilism. Cavell allows us to see how moral knowledge can take shape less through reasoning about abstract principles than through reawakening our lives to the everyday world that narrative—in its concern with the here and now, with what Bakhtin calls the unfinished flow of contemporary time—permits us to recognize, to appreciate, and to infuse with value.

Cavell helps us imagine a kind of bioethics—narrative at the core—that opens up a reengagement with the ordinary and everyday world of illness and medicine. Such an ethics would not occupy its time in searching for unshakable principles to govern organ transplants, say, or in reasoning out the dangers of biotechnology. It would not lust after the great events of our time, but rather would undertake the difficult task of keeping its focus on what Cavell calls the "uneventful," that which is *not* out of the ordinary.[39] It would necessarily pose different questions than a bioethics based on great events. It would ask doctors how they treat their secretaries. It would ask if they leave patients stranded for hours in waiting rooms. It would ask why nurses' aides are badly underpaid and if their underpayment has anything to do with race or gender. It would ask whether a doctor listens carefully—or brushes off a complaint. It would ask what rights and courtesies are owed to a patient's family. It would ask what words a doctor uses to describe a patient. Are they words that regard the patient as a person—an ethical and moral agent—or as a collection of organ systems?

The questions that narrative bioethics brings to light are certainly less glamorous than the hot-button issues that television networks love. We might consider them—to cite a term used by ethicist Paul A. Komesaroff—a kind of "microethics."[40] The value of these questions, however, should not be judged on a conventional scale of large versus small. One benefit flowing from a microethics of the everyday would lie in helping us to recognize that significance is unrelated to size and glamour. Another benefit would lie in helping us to ground more glamorous issues in the mundane facts of everyday life, in the ordinary lives of ordinary people. In reawakening us to the everyday, the questions raised by a narrative bioethics not only hold the promise of opening up to ethical inquiry an often ignored area of medical practice and thereby extending the range of moral knowledge and action, but also might just reawaken a passion for medicine in doctors weary of insurance providers and worn down by conflict over intractable, big-ticket issues. They might give back to medical staffs the gift with which many of them began: a recognition of the immense power and reward contained in the most ordinary acts that involve the care of patients. The benefits would not stop at improvements in medical practice that trickle down, slowly and indirectly, to patients. There are also more direct benefits implied or contained within a narrative bioethics reawakened to the ordinary and the everyday.

MYTH, METAPHOR, AND NARRATIVE

It is Nietzsche, a philosopher greatly favored by postmodern thinkers, whom Susan Sontag credits with formulating the thought behind her groundbreaking book *Illness as Metaphor* (1978), which she wrote in the grip of anxieties created both by her diagnosis with cancer and by a subsequent struggle against cultural "mystifications" that surrounded her condition. Her aim, she says, was to "alleviate unnecessary suffering" for others by examining the harmful myths and metaphors that interpenetrate the experience of cancer. She quotes directly from Nietzsche: *"Thinking about illness!*—To calm the imagination of the invalid, so that at least he should not, as hitherto, have to suffer more from thinking about his illness than from the illness itself—that, I think, would be something!" Sontag goes on to explain: "The purpose of my book was to calm the imagination, not to incite it. Not to confer meaning, which is the traditional purpose of literary endeavor, but to deprive something of meaning."[41]

It is hard to overstate the importance of *Illness as Metaphor* in directing attention to the meanings that surround and interpenetrate the experience of illness. There is practical, therapeutic value in an effort to "calm the imagination" of patients gripped by harmful myths. Yet, in her intention to deprive it of harmful meaning, Sontag wants to reduce illness to a scientific, biological fact. Unfortunately, returning illness to science does not deprive it of meaning but simply leaves it in the grip of a reductive, positivist, biomedical narrative that focuses solely on bodily processes. Although her goal is praise-worthy and her research brilliant, the effort to cleanse illness of *all* meaning discounts the therapeutic benefit that positive myths and meanings can supply. It ignores the healing role that stories play in non-Western cultures. It forgets that military metaphors sometimes harmful in our thinking about disease (as when doctors feel justified in combating a disease with therapies that eventually destroy the pa-tient) may also be employed to empower AIDS activists in the fight against an unjust and unresponsive health care system. The slipperi-ness of metaphor can be turned to good use as well as to ill, much as racist taunts can be transformed into tools of resistance. Science has a hard time operating in the absence of metaphor. Even the biomedical model is a kind of bare-bones scientific narrative. The influence of mind and culture upon illness—not sweeping mistrust of inherently deceptive or harmful qualities in metaphor—is what ultimately mat-ters to a postmodern medicine attuned to a new narrative of illness as biocultural.

The positive impact of mind and culture is captured—in ways that the biomedical model cannot predict—in two illnesses that play a significant role in traditional nomadic Apache life, although they are unknown to Western medicine: bear-sickness and snake-sickness.[42] Apaches who encounter bears or snakes often come down with illnesses severe enough to require healing ceremonies. Merely crossing the path left by a snake can bring on loathsome facial sores, while bear fur snagged on a tree can produce physical deformities re-quiring the skills of a shaman. Such illness and healing, from the per-spective of scientific biomedicine, look like sheer superstition akin to the vision of Black Elk as he lay motionless in his parents' tipi. The grounding of these unusual maladies in everyday Apache life, how-ever, seems quite clear on reflection. Apache shamans possessed herbal remedies effective against most of the injuries and afflictions common to their people. (Colonial and frontier American medicine borrowed copiously from this native lore.) What Apache medicine could not cure was the venom from a southwestern prairie rattler (in-variably fatal) or the terrible flesh wounds inflicted by a bear. It seems likely that Apache culture included a bred-in-the-bone biocultural wisdom that strongly persuaded and predisposed Apaches to avoid bears and rattlesnakes. Sickness is an effective means of persuading us to avoid what is more harmful than a temporary sickness.

Sontag's work to explode the harmful myths surrounding cancer is a marvelous example of the good that can flow from an attention to narrative. Finally, however, despite the importance of calming patients who are agitated by baseless and harmful myths, the effort to strip illness of all meaning and to expose it (underneath the rags of metaphor) as nothing more than unvarnished biological fact ultimately cannot succeed. It cannot succeed because illness is so often biocultural. Imagination, narrative, and other human meaning-making activities have an inescapable role in constructing the experience of someone who is ill. Microbes and cells—within the body or studied in a laboratory—do not by themselves constitute illness; they are instead the biological ground on which illness comes to be set in motion. Contrariwise, culture constitutes the ground on which microbes and cells are re-set in motion: biocultural interdependencies create ever new relations between the microscopic and the interpersonal realms. Cultural contexts are thus not something we can wash out of illness in order to view it as isolated, pure, elemental, and scientific. A narrative bioethics that returns us to the ordinary and the everyday also returns us to the cultural contexts in which the great bulk of our experience of illness occurs. It returns us to the arena where we construct not only bear-sickness or snake-sickness but also AIDS, cancer, and Alzheimer's disease, offering us tools to investigate both the harm and the benefits implicit in a new, biocultural narrative of illness.

Stanley Cavell quotes renowned skeptical philosopher David Hume as writing that skepticism is an incurable malady.[43] The implication, for Cavell, is that the threat of skepticism is not something we vanquish, overcoming it once and for all, but rather a condition (possibly fatal and always an experience of loss) that we must learn to live with. One role of narrative bioethics is to help us learn how to live with illness and with its losses as they shape and reshape our lives. It helps us see illness, despite the unfamiliar country it opens upon, as possessing an everydayness that invites our discoveries, even when such discoveries include a bleakness and loss that few would willingly choose to experience. Despite its losses, illness is a state in which we are not wholly shut out from something so mundane and everyday as, for example, the experience of pleasure.

Pleasure, like emotion, belongs securely to the everydayness that narrative bioethics takes as its special province. Cavell reminds us how extraordinary it is that we can receive enjoyment from something as familiar and unremarkable as reading a book or looking at a picture.[44] In this sense, he articulates what Don DeLillo described as an underlying motif amid the randomness, chaos, and consumerism of *White Noise:* "a sense of the importance of daily life and of ordinary moments." ("I tried to find a kind of radiance in dailiness," he has said of the novel.)[45] Inseparable from its trials and its sometimes permanent losses, illness fills our lives with everyday routines and experiences—a kind of altered but inescapable dailiness—that narrative bioethics invites us to rethink. In threatening to undo or unfix the self, in showing us a picture of ourselves that we desperately do not wish to see, illness also holds the potential to reveal the everyday world in a new light, to show us a beauty or truth or mystery inscribed in ordinary events whose everydayness we dismiss in the quest for something far better. Illness can show us almost for the first time the ordinary (incredible) stars overhead—the contours of our own shining world—when, like Dante trudging upward out of the inferno or like William Styron recovering from depression, we regain the power to sense a kind of radiance within the everyday.

"I feel like I'm counting my days in milliseconds, never mind hours," writes Audre Lorde (in an italics of excitement) about the outcome of her mastectomy for breast cancer. *"And it's a good thing, that particular consciousness of the way in which each hour passes, even if it is a boring hour. I want it to become permanent."* [46] Lorde's new appreciation of the everyday and even the boring, while it comes at great cost, has at least something in common with the impulse that encouraged Andy Warhol to make an eight-hour film that focused solely on the exterior

of the Empire State Building, a film in which the camera remains motionless. "Sometimes the little times you don't think are anything
while they're happening," Warhol wrote, "turn out to be what marks
a whole period of your life."[47] Pillows and wallpaper, transformed
with his postmodern touch, are among the invisible household items
that, like his early soup cans, Warhol invited us to reexperience freed
from their normal invisibility. Anatole Broyard—one among 350,000
American men diagnosed each year with prostate cancer—found a
kind of intoxication in the medical routines that eventually enclose
even a fatal illness. Illness in the postmodern era, because we are
coming to recognize how culture helps shape it in convergence with
biology, includes within it a flexible space where, except during the
most dire emergencies, we still retain access to the resources of the
ordinary, the everyday, and the uneventful, if we can learn how
to recognize and to recover them. This recovery—the word carries
potent medical connotations—may involve an act much like the
process of healing.

FINAL REPRESENTATIONS

Narrative bioethics offers one example of the changes possible when
we take seriously the idea that illness is biocultural. It is not likely
that every medical specialty will find a significant role for narrative,
although even surgeons—a group notably cavalier about the pain of
postoperative patients—could benefit from the skills in listening that
attention to narrative develops. X rays and CT scans, it is well worth
remembering, are not self-explanatory, not facts, but visual representations of the body, images that are often deeply ambiguous and that
demand interpretation, creating the occasions for complex and not
wholly scientific narratives. It matters greatly what details such mininarratives include and what details they omit or deliberately exclude.
The biomedical model, like an X ray, is ultimately a representation,
one so powerful and persuasive that we often mistake it for fact. No
matter how factual we consider it, the biomedical model also gener-

ates a flow of related narrative images—the body as a machine, for example, and disease as a mechanical defect—that profoundly influence how we think about our illnesses. One important role of disciplines outside medicine is to help us recognize the nature and limits of the representations without which medicine cannot do its work.

There is no getting away from representations in postmodern theory. At times it seems as if reality has wholly disappeared behind a layer of models and discourses, but postmodernism does not see things quite that way. Rather, it argues that we know and experience the world only *through* the representations we create. Thus death is an ineluctable biological fact, a brute fragment of reality, but our personal attitude toward death and dying has much to do with how our culture *represents* them. As French historian Philippe Ariès has shown, the so-called tame death of the Middle Ages—a death rendered familiar, nonthreatening, and so dependable that people accurately predicted the exact day when they would die—owes its distinctive character not only to the abstract structures of scholastic theology but also to medieval culture and its burial customs that covered over the face of the cadaver with successive masklike structures: "the sewn shroud, the coffin, and the catafalque or [pictorial] representation." [48] Ariès sees a revival today of the "wild" or "savage" deaths of premedieval times—expressing a terror in the face of unmediated nature—reflected in the new fears of machine-prolonged dying that typify our time. Unlike medieval tales, our distinctive narratives focus on people trapped in liminal, vegetative states where living and dying obscenely commingle: a contemporary version of live burial. The goal for postmodern theory is not an escape from representation—not the futile quest for an unmediated relation to facts—but rather a struggle to understand in what ways our lives are always shaped, for better or worse, by cultural narratives and representations.

A biocultural model, of course, must include whatever we can learn about the science of disease. Yet science will never encompass the whole event. An adequate representation must acknowledge ways in which human biology is altered by the influence of mind and culture. At present, the extensive interactions among body, mind, and

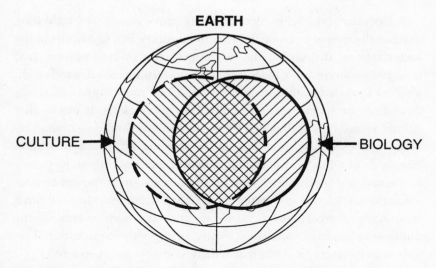

Figure 7. A Biocultural Model. From *The Placebo Effect: An Interdisciplinary Exploration,* edited by Anne Harrington. Copyright © 1997 by the President and Fellows of Harvard College. Reprinted by permission of Harvard University Press.

culture remain unexplored. (Demonstrable immune-system links to psychological stress have provided a ground for initial study.) This uncomfortable point, however, is exactly where we need a model that looks beyond solely biological explanations toward a comprehensive biocultural vision. This new postmodern vision does not hold all the answers, since it represents complex human events like health and illness as surrounded by unknown, even unknowable dimensions. As distinct from the human-centered world that we scratch upon its surface, the earth contains much that eludes us, in the same way that frequencies audible to elephants and dogs remain inaudible to the human ear, and illness never completely loses contact with this inaudible, unknowable portion of the earth that resists full explanation. Diagrams are designed to simplify—the one in figure 7 should be four-dimensional, spinning, and in continuous flux—but it is worth looking briefly at the implications contained in even a drastically simplified sketch.

A biocultural model in medicine may prove exactly the right tool, granted the power of medicine in contemporary life, to help us in the wider task of dislodging the ongoing Cartesian assumptions that treat bodies as complex machines. Postmodern illness demands a dialogical knowledge that cannot resemble the monologues of single disciplines or specialties, no matter how prestigious. It insists that culture is indelibly influenced by human biology and that human biology is consistently modified by the shaping influence of culture. The value of a biocultural model, however, lies not only in its power to dismantle a mechanistic view of life but also in its power to subsume the knowledge generated by mechanistic assumptions within a more comprehensive vision. As for most postmodern endeavors, the ultimate measure of soundness is not correspondence to external reality—as if we could claim that we know reality independent of our theories and representations—but rather how well a concept works, what it allows us to do, whether it changes our experience for the better. This measure of a theory or representation is what the pragmatist philosopher William James called its "cash-value."[49] How, James might ask bluntly, can we sum up the cash-value of a belief that illness is biocultural?

Narrative will never replace lasers, but a twenty-first-century biocultural medicine attuned to the influence of mind, emotion, and culture can help greatly in addressing illnesses that, like AIDS, involve not only the life cycle of a virus or pathogen but also issues of personal behavior and of public health. It can help us see how cultural activities like the destruction of rain forests and the disposal of toxic waste have a direct impact on individual well-being. It can give us additional resources to help the increasing numbers of people who suffer from chronic incurable illnesses, where medication alone is not the answer. It can offer knowledge about the social and iatrogenic sources of illness, knowledge that would encourage millions of people to avoid unnecessary surgeries, to deal effectively with their impairments, and to enjoy healthy lives despite the presence of illness. It can utilize human spiritual experience to maximize health in ways that mainline biomedicine cannot comprehend. In respecting rather than dismissing the patient's narrative, it can offer a means of healing where cure may be impossible and can provide dying patients with compassionate, palliative care replacing the aggressive, machine-assisted, six-figure, cure-based medicine common in American hospitals during the patient's last weeks of life.[50] At its most revolutionary, it can spark a major reallocation of financial resources toward prevention, as we seriously begin to address the cultural causes and contexts of illness rather than continue to pour endless funds into stopgap measures and half-way technologies, like the ruinously expensive organ-transplant and drug-treatment programs that mostly end up subsidizing doctors and hospitals. Expect that organized opposition to a biocultural model will intensify overnight when incomes, not just ideas of illness, are at stake.

A biocultural model—no matter what its eventual cash-value—cannot logically take a dismissive attitude toward stories because it too, like the mechanistic biomedical model it challenges, is finally another narrative. It offers us a more accurate and useful story—but not a lock on truth with a capital *T*. Its advantage lies in understanding stories not only as possible clinical tools but also as forms of cultural knowledge and power. Look around any crowded cinema: why have all these people—with dozens of ways to entertain themselves—bought tickets to see a story played out against a silver screen? Stories, as Leslie Marmon Silko insists, are not just entertainment. They are the materials with which a culture redefines its own image and self-understanding. This process has an inescapable, if indirect, influence upon well-being. The stories we tell, as Silko implies, do more than describe or represent health and illness: they ultimately give them the shapes we will re-create and rediscover in our own lives. From this point of view, postmodern illness is illness as reconstructed through the distinctive stories we tell at a time when the major cultural narratives of illness are seriously in conflict.

The modernist narrative of biomedicine, with its heroic doctors and researchers struggling to find a cure in time to stop the epidemic and rescue the patient or save the world, has begun to give way to a far more complicated and confusing narrative that contains painful moments of breakdown and failure. It is a fragmentary narrative that reaches us in news flashes and infomercials, a still unfolding story in which the heroes are often faceless teams rather than individual scientists or doctors, in which—despite lasers, gene therapies, and synthetic drugs—the systematic overuse of antibiotics creates ever more powerful pathogens, in which a popular laxative turns out to contain a dangerous carcinogen, in which trendy diet pills are shown to damage heart valves (although a later study disputes this finding), in which our local food supplies (now increasingly drawn from international markets and remote packaging plants) provide meat, fruit, and vegetables contaminated with life-threatening *E. coli* bacteria, in which (maybe the ultimate sign of things to come) more than seven hundred people in Japan are taken to hospitals—some had seizures, vomited blood, or blacked out—after watching a popular animated television cartoon that concluded with an explosion of flashing lights. It is an untold, unnoticed story in which the cultural fantasy of living forever—or at least pushing back death through an unending series of medical purchases—creates sickly lives obsessed with heartburn, bowels, megavitamins, and miracle cures. This new postmodern narrative, in short, represents for us the confusing historical moment we are living through when the biomedical model has begun to reveal its inherent limitations but when a biocultural model (or whatever we come to call it) has not yet proven its power to constitute a satisfying and coherent replacement.

This new postmodern narrative certainly immerses us in confusion, as befits a transitional moment when ideas about health and illness are in flux. It also points to important and promising changes ahead. We would need a crystal ball to foretell the ending. There seems little doubt, however, that the full story of postmodern illness, whenever it comes to be told, will be a tale in which we recognize for the first time just how thoroughly our lives—and especially our illnesses—take shape every day at the crossroads of biology and culture.

Notes

INTRODUCTION: HOW TO LIVE FOREVER

1.   In Friedrich Nietzsche, *On the Genealogy of Morals* (1887), in *On the Genealogy of Morals and Ecce Homo*, trans. Walter Kaufmann and R. J. Hollingdale (New York: Random House, 1967), 121: "der Mensch ist kränker, unsicherer, wechselnder, unfestgestellter als irgendein Tier sonst, daran ist kein Zweifel—er ist *das* kranke Tier." On the complications in Nietzsche's understanding of illness, including its relation to genius, see David Farrell Krell, *Infectious Nietzsche* (Bloomington: Indiana University Press, 1996).

2.   John G. Neihardt, *Black Elk Speaks: Being the Life Story of a Holy Man of the Oglala Sioux* (1932; reprint, Lincoln: University of Nebraska Press, 1988), 22.

3.   Ibid., 180.

4.   See, among others cited later, Linda Nicholson and Steven Seidman, eds., *Social Postmodernism: Beyond Identity Politics* (Cambridge: Cambridge

University Press, 1995); Thomas Docherty, ed., *Postmodernism: A Reader* (New York: Columbia University Press, 1993); Fredric Jameson, *Postmodernism, or, The Cultural Logic of Late Capitalism* (Durham, N.C.: Duke University Press, 1991); Steven Best and Douglas Kellner, *Postmodern Theory: Critical Interrogations* (New York: Guilford Press, 1991); Bryan S. Turner, ed., *Theories of Modernity and Postmodernity* (Newbury Park, Calif.: Sage Publications, 1990); David Harvey, *The Condition of Postmodernity: An Enquiry into the Origins of Cultural Change* (Oxford: Basil Blackwell, 1989); and Jean-François Lyotard, *The Postmodern Condition: A Report on Knowledge* (1979), trans. Geoff Bennington and Brian Massumi (Minneapolis: University of Minnesota Press, 1984).

5.   For some representative texts, see René J. Dubos, *The White Plague: Tuberculosis, Man, and Society* (Boston: Little, Brown, 1952); Michel Foucault, *Madness and Civilization: A History of Insanity in the Age of Reason* (1961), trans. Richard Howard (New York: Random House, 1965); George L. Engel, "The Need for a New Medical Model: A Challenge for Biomedicine," *Science* 196, no. 4286 (1977): 129–36; Melvin Konner, *The Tangled Wing: Biological Constraints on the Human Spirit* (New York: Harper and Row, 1982); Oliver Sacks, *The Man Who Mistook His Wife for a Hat and Other Clinical Tales* (New York: Summit Books, 1985); and Arthur Kleinman, *The Illness Narratives: Suffering, Healing, and the Human Condition* (New York: Basic Books, 1988).

6.   See René Dubos, "Determinants of Health and Illness" (1968), in *Culture, Disease, and Healing: Studies in Medical Anthropology*, ed. David Landy (New York: Macmillan, 1977), 31–41; Elliot G. Mishler et al., *Social Contexts of Health, Illness, and Patient Care* (Cambridge: Cambridge University Press, 1981); Howard Waitzkin, "The Social Origins of Illness: A Neglected History," in *The Second Sickness: Contradictions of Capitalist Health Care* (New York: Free Press, 1983), 65–85; Sander L. Gilman, *Disease and Representation: Images of Illness from Madness to AIDS* (Ithaca, N.Y.: Cornell University Press, 1988); Charles E. Rosenberg and Janet Golden, eds., *Framing Disease: Studies in Cultural History* (New Brunswick, N.J.: Rutgers University Press, 1992); Shirley Lindenbaum and Margaret M. Lock, eds., *Knowledge, Power, and Practice: The Anthropology of Medicine and Everyday Life* (Berkeley: University of California Press, 1993); Cecil G. Helman, *Culture, Health, and Illness: An Introduction for Health Professionals*, 3d ed. (Oxford: Butterworth-Heineman, 1994); Peter Conrad and Rochelle Kern, eds., *The Sociology of Health and Illness: Critical Perspectives*, 4th ed. (New York: St. Martin's Press, 1994); Robert A. Hahn, *Sickness and Healing: An Anthropological Perspective* (New Haven: Yale University Press, 1995); Roy Porter, *Disease, Medicine, and Society in England, 1550–1860*, 2d ed. (Cambridge: Cambridge University Press, 1995); Allan Young, *The Harmony of Illusions: Inventing Post-Traumatic Stress Disorder*

(Princeton: Princeton University Press, 1995); and Margaret M. Lock, *Encounters with Aging: Mythologies of Menopause in Japan and North America* (Berkeley: University of California Press, 1995).

7.   See Zygmunt Bauman, *Mortality, Immortality, and Other Life Strategies* (Stanford: Stanford University Press, 1992); Nicholas J. Fox, *Postmodernism, Sociology, and Health* (Toronto: University of Toronto Press, 1994); Arthur W. Frank, *The Wounded Storyteller: Body, Illness, and Ethics* (Chicago: University of Chicago Press, 1996); and Elaine Showalter, *Hystories: Hysterical Epidemics and Modern Media* (New York: Columbia University Press, 1997). Showalter does not mention postmodernism, but her discussion centers on illnesses that have emerged since World War II.

8.   Theodor Landis and Marianne Regard, "'Gourmand Syndrome': Eating Passion Associated with Right Anterior Lesions," *Neurology* 48, no. 5 (1997): 1185–90.

9.   Nardos Lijam et al., "Social Interaction and Sensorimotor Gating Abnormalities in Mice Lacking Dvl1," *Cell* 90, no. 5 (1997): 895–905; Deborah Blum, *Sex on the Brain: The Biological Differences between Men and Women* (New York: Viking, 1997).

10.   Lyotard, *The Postmodern Condition*, 37. For an American philosopher's view of the debate between Lyotard and German philosopher Jürgen Habermas, see Richard Rorty, "Habermas and Lyotard on Postmodernity," in *Habermas and Modernity*, ed. Richard J. Bernstein (Cambridge: MIT Press, 1985), 161–75.

11.   See Fritjof Capra, *The Turning Point: Science, Society, and the Rising Culture* (New York: Simon and Schuster, 1982), 93–94. Fritjof here is expanding on ideas developed in the 1960s by Berkeley physicist Geoffrey Chew.

12.   The term *biocultural*, too, is unoriginal although not today in wide circulation. See, for example, Lorna G. Moore et al., eds., *The Biocultural Basis of Health: Expanding Views of Medical Anthropology* (St. Louis: Mosby, 1980).

13.   Jonathan Knowles, "Hunting Down Disease," *Odyssey* 3, no. 1 (1997): 22.

14.   Barry D. Jordan et al., "Apolipoprotein E epsilon 4 Associated with Chronic Traumatic Brain Injury in Boxing," *JAMA* 278, no. 2 (1997): 136–40; Gretchen Vogel, "Gene Discovery Offers Tentative Clues to Parkinson's," *Science* 276, no. 5321 (1997): 2405–7. The gene is thought to account for only a small fraction of the cases of Parkinson's, but researchers hope it may shed light on nonhereditary forms of the disease.

15.   See George Anders, *Health against Wealth: HMOs and the Breakdown of Medical Trust* (New York: Houghton Mifflin, 1996). For an early analytic overview of HMOs, see Harold S. Luft, *Health Maintenance Organizations: Dimensions of Performance* (New York: John Wiley and Sons, 1981).

16.   Robert H. Blank, *The Price of Life: The Future of American Health Care* (New York: Columbia University Press, 1997), 128, vii. For other changes in the structure of American health care, see David J. Rothman, *Beginnings Count: The Technological Imperative in American Health Care* (New York: Oxford University Press, 1997).

17.   Ira Byock, *Dying Well: The Prospect for Growth at the End of Life* (New York: Riverhead Books, 1997), 26.

18.   Sherwin B. Nuland, *How We Die: Reflections on Life's Final Chapter* (New York: Alfred A. Knopf, 1994), 72.

19.   For a fine study detailing the contributions of nurses' aides, see Timothy Diamond, *Making Gray Gold: Narratives of Nursing Home Care* (Chicago: University of Chicago Press, 1992).

20.   James Gleick, *Chaos: Making a New Science* (New York: Viking, 1987), 79; Nina Hall, ed., *Exploring Chaos: A Guide to the New Science of Disorder* (1992; reprint, New York: W. W. Norton, 1993); and Robin Robertson and Allan Combs, *Chaos Theory in Psychology and the Life Sciences* (Mahwah, N.J.: Lawrence Erlbaum Associates, 1995). N. Katherine Hales has written several excellent studies exploring relations between chaos theory and contemporary, or postmodern, literature: *The Cosmic Web: Scientific Field Models and Literary Strategies in the Twentieth Century* (Ithaca, N.Y.: Cornell University Press, 1984); *Chaos Bound: Orderly Disorder in Contemporary Literature and Science* (Ithaca, N.Y.: Cornell University Press, 1990); and *Chaos and Order: Complex Dynamics in Literature and Science* (Chicago: University of Chicago Press, 1991).

21.   James S. Goodwin, "Chaos, and the Limits of Modern Medicine," *JAMA* 278, no. 17 (1997): 1400.

CHAPTER ONE: THE COUNTRY OF THE ILL

1.   Anatole Broyard, *Intoxicated by My Illness and Other Writings on Life and Death,* ed. Alexandra Broyard (New York: Clarkson Potter, 1992), 39, 68.

2.   Reynolds Price, interview by Francis J. Keefe, videotape, 1997, Department of Medical Psychology, Duke University Medical Center, Durham, North Carolina.

3.   Marian E. Gornick et al., "Effects of Race and Income on Mortality and Use of Services among Medicare Beneficiaries," *New England Journal of Medicine* 335, no. 11 (1996): 791–99; David S. Strogatz, "Use of Medical Care for Chest Pain: Differences between Blacks and Whites," *American Journal of Public Health* 80, no. 3 (1990): 290–94; and Michelle D. Holmes et al., "Racial Inequalities in the Use of Procedures for Ischemic Heart Disease," *JAMA* 261, no. 22 (1989): 3242–43.

4.   Eugene Schwartz et al., "Black/White Comparisons of Deaths Preventable by Medical Intervention: United States and the District of Columbia, 1980–1986," *International Journal of Epidemiology* 19, no. 3 (1990): 591–98. For a review of various statistics comparing the health of blacks and whites, see Robert A. Hahn, *Sickness and Healing: An Anthropological Perspective* (New Haven: Yale University Press, 1995), 82–89.

5.   Robert Goldman and Steven Papson, "The Postmodernism That Failed," in *Postmodernism and Social Inquiry,* ed. David R. Dickens and Andrea Fontana (New York: Guilford Press, 1994), 224.

6.   For a good introduction to the difficulties of definition, see Ihab Hassan, "Toward a Concept of Postmodernism," in *The Postmodern Turn: Essays in Postmodern Theory and Culture* (Columbus: Ohio State University Press, 1987), 84–96. Hassan's useful list of contrasts between modern and postmodern (91–92) ignores equally crucial continuities that make their relation more than a simple polarity of opposites.

7.   Anthony Cronin (in *Samuel Beckett: The Last Modernist* [London: Harper Collins Publishers, 1996]) places Beckett with the moderns, but Beckett could also be placed among the first postmoderns: quintessential postmodern thinker Michel Foucault, for example, says that *Waiting for Godot* (1952) marked a turning point in his own development (James Miller, *The Passion of Michel Foucault* [New York: Doubleday, 1993], 64–65).

8.   Charles Jencks defines postmodernism in architecture (where the concept originated and retains a quite specific meaning) as *"double-coding: the combination of Modern techniques with something else (usually traditional building)"*—and he distinguishes double-coded postmodernism from the related styles that he calls "late-Modern" and "schismatic postmodernism" (*What Is Post-Modernism?* 2d ed. [London: Academy Editions, 1987], 14). Yet double-coding, while a useful concept when applied to architecture, will not help us distinguish modern from postmodern literary texts.

9.   In her helpful exposition of various divergent positions, Pauline Marie Rosenau distinguishes between "affirmative" and "skeptical" orientations within postmodernism (*Post-Modernism and the Social Sciences: Insights, Inroads, and Intrusions* [Princeton: Princeton University Press, 1992], 14–17). On the conflict endemic to postmodern life, see James Davison Hunter, *Culture Wars: The Struggle to Define America* (New York: Basic Books, 1991).

10.   Arthur W. Frank, *The Wounded Storyteller: Body, Illness, and Ethics* (Chicago: University of Chicago Press, 1996), 6. I will return to Frank's valuable emphasis on storytelling in the conclusion.

11.   For a discussion of images and their power, see Goldman and Papson, "The Postmodernism That Failed," 224; and two books by Jim Collins, *Uncommon Cultures: Popular Culture and Post-Modernism* (New York: Routledge,

1989) and *Architectures of Excess: Cultural Life in the Information Age* (New York: Routledge, 1995).

12.   Jean Baudrillard, "Simulacra and Simulations" (1981), reprinted in *Selected Writings*, ed. Mark Poster (New York: Polity Press, 1988), 172. See also Hillel Schwartz, *The Culture of the Copy: Striking Likenesses, Unreasonable Facsimiles* (New York: Zone Books, 1996).

13.   Victor Bockris, *The Life and Death of Andy Warhol* (New York: Bantam Books, 1989), 348–49.

14.   Lucian L. Leape, "Error in Medicine," *JAMA* 272, no. 23 (1994): 1851–57; Jean-François Timsit et al., "Mortality of Nosocomial Pneumonia in Ventilated Patients: Influence of Diagnostic Tools," *American Journal of Respiratory and Critical Care Medicine* 154, no. 1 (1996): 116–23; and M. Hussain et al., "Prospective Survey of the Incidence, Risk Factors, and Outcome of Hospital-Acquired Infections in the Elderly," *Journal of Hospital Infection* 32, no. 2 (1996): 117–26.

15.   On "the aestheticization of everyday life," see Mike Featherstone, *Consumer Culture and Postmodernism* (Newbury Park, Calif.: Sage Publications, 1991), 65–82.

16.   Ranier Crone, "Form and Ideology: Warhol's Techniques from Blotted Line to Film," in *The Work of Andy Warhol*, ed. Gary Garrels, Dia Art Foundation Discussions in Contemporary Culture, no. 3 (Seattle: Bay Press, 1989), 70–92.

17.   Andy Warhol, *The Philosophy of Andy Warhol (From A to B and Back Again)* (New York: Harcourt Brace Jovanovich, 1975), 150.

18.   Paul Crowther, "Postmodernism in the Visual Arts: A Question of Ends," in *Postmodernism and Society*, ed. Roy Boyne and Ali Rattansi (New York: St. Martin's Press, 1990), 252.

19.   For a brief but illuminating discussion of Warhol in the context of postmodernism, see Fredric Jameson, *Postmodernism, or, The Cultural Logic of Late Capitalism* (Durham, N.C.: Duke University Press, 1991), 8–10.

20.   See Terry Eagleton, "Capitalism, Modernism, and Postmodernism" (1985), in *Modern Criticism and Theory: A Reader*, ed. David Lodge (New York: Longman, 1988), 385–98. Eagleton sees Warhol as emptying art of political content, surrendering to forces that transform art into a commodity, betraying the revolutionary impulse of modernism. While no political revolutionary, Warhol has a more complex relation to modernism than is suggested by metaphors of emptying, surrender, and betrayal. "An artist," he wrote, "is somebody who produces things that people don't need to have but that he—for *some reason*—thinks it would be a good idea to give them" (*The Philosophy of Andy Warhol*, 144).

21.   Warhol, *The Philosophy of Andy Warhol*, 54. Warhol explores visually what postmodern philosopher Jacques Derrida explored in language: the perception that everything is a text. For an excellent discussion of the philo-

sophical implications of Warhol's work, see Arthur C. Danto, "The Philosopher as Andy Warhol," in *The Andy Warhol Museum* (New York: Distributed Art Publishers, 1994), 73–92.

22.   For a fascinating study of the relations between biography and art, see Robert Rosenblum, "Picasso's Blond Muse: The Reign of Marie-Thérèse Walter," in *Picasso and Portraiture: Representation and Transformation,* ed. William Rubin (New York: Museum of Modern Art, 1996), 337–83. Emphasizing Picasso's "multiplicity of invention" (364), Rosenblum notes that Picasso "continued to create more familiar and tranquil images of Marie-Thérèse until the end of the decade" (370).

23.   See Bettyann Kevles, "The Transparent Body in Late Twentieth-Century Culture," in *Naked to the Bone: Medical Imaging in the Twentieth Century* (New Brunswick, N.J.: Rutgers University Press, 1997), 261–96. Kevles notes that at the end of World War II, the X ray alone defined the inside of the body (261). Postmodern inventions to scan interior structures—such as CT, MRI, PET, and ultrasound—extend the modernist fragmentation of the body, adding the computerized cinematic possibilities of motion and three-dimensional pictures.

24.   Peter Schjeldahl, quoted in Bockris, *The Life and Death of Andy Warhol,* 167.

25.   On the sexual, erotic, and gay side of Warhol, see Jennifer Doyle, Jonathan Flatley, and José Esteban Muñoz, eds., *Pop Out: Queer Warhol* (Durham, N.C.: Duke University Press, 1996).

26.   See Eric J. Cassell, "Illness and Disease," *Hastings Center Report* 6, no. 2 (1976): 27–37; K. W. M. Fulford, *Moral Theory and Practice* (Cambridge: Cambridge University Press, 1989), 57–86; Uta Gerhardt, *Ideas about Illness: An Intellectual and Political History of Medical Sociology* (New York: New York University Press, 1989); and Robert P. Hudson, "Concepts of Disease in the West," in *The Cambridge World History of Human Disease,* ed. Kenneth F. Kiple (New York: Cambridge University Press, 1993), 45–52.

27.   See S. Kay Toombs, *The Meaning of Illness: A Phenomenological Account of the Different Perspectives of Physician and Patient* (Boston: Kluwer Academic Publishers, 1992).

28.   Kathryn Montgomery Hunter, *Doctors' Stories: The Narrative Structure of Medical Knowledge* (Princeton: Princeton University Press, 1991), 18. Hunter's entire section "Medicine and Science" is a valuable caution against misconstruing the (science-based) practice of medicine as a science.

29.   Julia Epstein, *Altered Conditions: Disease, Medicine, and Storytelling* (New York: Routledge, 1995), 9.

30.   On problems with the current understanding of alcoholism, see Herbert Fingarette, *Heavy Drinking: The Myth of Alcoholism as a Disease* (Berkeley: University of California Press, 1988).

31.   See Darrell L. Tanelian, "Reflex Sympathetic Dystrophy: A Reevaluation of the Literature," *Pain Forum* 5, no. 4 (1996): 247–56: "I have seen numerous patients referred to pain clinics and labeled with the diagnosis of RSD when their only clinical symptomatology is the report of pain in an upper or lower extremity" (247).

32.   On the social "framing" or "construction" of changing medical categories, see, for example, Henry Cohen, "The Evolution of the Concept of Disease," in *Concepts of Medicine: A Collection of Essays on Aspects of Medicine*, ed. Brandon Lush (Oxford: Pergamon Press, 1961), 159–69; Charles E. Rosenberg and Janet Golden, eds., *Framing Disease: Studies in Cultural History* (New Brunswick, N.J.: Rutgers University Press, 1992); and, especially relevant for postmodern illness, Paula A. Treichler, "AIDS, HIV, and the Cultural Construction of Reality," in *The Time of AIDS: Social Analysis, Theory, and Method*, ed. Gilbert Herdt and Shirley Lindenbaum (Newbury Park, Calif.: Sage Publications, 1992), 65–98.

33.   See Paula A. Treichler, "AIDS, Homophobia, and Biomedical Discourse: An Epidemic of Signification" (1987), reprinted in *AIDS: Cultural Analysis/Cultural Activism*, ed. Douglas Crimp (Cambridge: MIT Press, 1987), 31–70.

34.   See, for example, Steven Feierman and John M. Janzen, eds., *The Social Basis of Health and Healing in Africa* (Berkeley: University of California Press, 1992); and Emiko Ohnuki-Tierney, *Illness and Culture in Contemporary Japan: An Anthropological View* (Cambridge: Cambridge University Press, 1984).

35.   Talcott Parsons, *The Social System* (New York: Free Press, 1951); "Definitions of Health and Illness in the Light of American Values and Social Structure," in *Patients, Physicians, and Illness: A Sourcebook in Behavioral Science and Health*, ed. E. Gartly Jaco (New York: Free Press, 1958), 121–44; and *Action Theory and the Human Condition* (New York: Free Press, 1978). Medicine, of course, is a powerful presence that helps shape modern and postmodern cultures, which, in turn, help to reshape and to reinforce various sick roles.

36.   Khari LaMarca et al., "A Progress Report of Cancer Centers and Tribal Communities: Building a Partnership Based on Trust," *Cancer* 78, no. 7 (1996): 1633–37.

37.   See the two studies by Lynn Payer, *Medicine and Culture: Varieties of Treatment in the United States, England, West Germany, and France* (New York: Henry Holt, 1988) and *Medicine and Culture: Notions of Health and Sickness in Britain, the U.S., France, and West Germany* (London: Gollancz, 1988).

38.   William James, *Pragmatism* (1907), ed. Fredson Bowers and Ignas K. Skrupskelis (Cambridge: Harvard University Press, 1975), 117.

39.   On postmodern interest in culture (which, from its traditional home in anthropology, now spills over into far-flung enterprises associated with the new field of cultural studies), see Clifford Geertz, *The Interpretation of Cultures* (New York: Basic Books, 1973); James Clifford and George E. Marcus, eds., *Writing Culture: The Poetics and Politics of Ethnography* (Berkeley: University of California Press, 1986); Lawrence Grossberg, Cary Nelson, and Paula A. Treichler, eds., *Cultural Studies* (New York: Routledge, 1992); Fredric Jameson, "On 'Cultural Studies,'" *Social Text* 34, no. 1 (1993): 17–52; and Cary Nelson and Dilip Parameshwar Gaonkar, eds., *Disciplinarity and Dissent in Cultural Studies* (New York: Routledge, 1996).

40.   On foundations, see David Ashley, "Postmodernism and Antifoundationalism," in *Postmodernism and Social Inquiry*, ed. David R. Dickens and Andrea Fontana (New York: Guilford Press, 1994), 53–75.

41.   Stephen Greenblatt, "Towards a Poetics of Culture," in *The New Historicism*, ed. H. Aram Veeser (New York: Routledge, 1989), 1–14.

42.   Jean-François Lyotard, *The Postmodern Condition: A Report on Knowledge* (1979), trans. Geoff Bennington and Brian Massumi (Minneapolis: University of Minnesota Press, 1984), 76.

43.   Cornel West, "Black Culture and Postmodernism," in *Remaking History*, ed. Barbara Kruger and Phil Mariani, Dia Art Foundation Discussions in Contemporary Culture, no. 4 (Seattle: Bay Press, 1989), 87–96.

44.   Faith McLellan, "'A Whole Other Story': The Electronic Narrative of Illness," *Literature and Medicine* 16, no. 1 (1997): 88–107.

45.   Broyard, *Intoxicated by My Illness*, 42. Subsequent quotations will be documented within the text.

46.   Henry Louis Gates Jr., *Thirteen Ways of Looking at a Black Man* (New York: Random House, 1997), 181.

47.   See, for example, Jerome Bruner, *Acts of Meaning* (Cambridge: Harvard University Press, 1990); and Paul Ricoeur, *Time and Narrative* (1983), trans. Kathleen McLaughlin/Blamey and David Pellauer, 3 vols. (Chicago: University of Chicago Press, 1984–88).

CHAPTER TWO: WHAT IS POSTMODERN ILLNESS?

1.   Katharine Park, "Black Death," in *The Cambridge World History of Human Disease*, ed. Kenneth F. Kiple (Cambridge: Cambridge University Press, 1993), 614.

2.   See Eric J. Cassell, "Illness and Disease," *Hastings Center Report* 6, no. 2 (1976): 27–37. My discussion is indebted to Cassell's analysis.

3.   Stephen J. Kunitz, "Diseases and Mortality in the Americas since 1700,"

in *The Cambridge World History of Human Disease,* ed. Kenneth F. Kiple (Cambridge: Cambridge University Press, 1993), 328–34.

4. Thomas McKeown, *The Origins of Human Disease* (Oxford: Basil Blackwell, 1988), 91.

5. René Leriche, quoted in Georges Canguilhem, *The Normal and the Pathological* (1966), trans. Carolyn R. Fawcett (New York: Zone Books, 1989), 91.

6. Hans-Georg Gadamer, *The Enigma of Health: The Art of Healing in a Scientific Age* (1993), trans. Jason Gaiger and Nicholas Walker (Stanford: Stanford University Press, 1996), 20.

7. There are really three types of plague—bubonic, septicemic, and pneumonic—each with a different means of transmission, and all three were present during the Black Plague of the Middle Ages. The pneumonic type represented about 4 percent, septicemic about 19 percent, and bubonic about 77 percent (Ynez Violé O'Neill, "Diseases of the Middle Ages," in *The Cambridge World History of Human Disease,* ed. Kenneth F. Kiple [Cambridge: Cambridge University Press, 1993], 276).

8. Strong evidence of syphilis in the pre-Columbian New World comes from recent work on skeletal remains ("The Origin of Syphilis," *Discover* 17, no. 10 [1996]: 23). See also James B. Wyngaarden and William N. Kelley, *Gout and Hyperuricemia* (New York: Grune and Stratton, 1976).

9. See Linda Hutcheson and Michael Hutcheson, *Opera: Desire, Disease, Death* (Lincoln: University of Nebraska Press, 1996).

10. Frank W. Putnam, *Diagnosis and Treatment of Multiple Personality Disorder* (New York: Guilford Press, 1989), 26–44. On various postmodern and poststructuralist concepts of subjectivity, see Paul Smith, *Discerning the Subject* (Minneapolis: University of Minnesota Press, 1988), and Eduardo Cadava, Peter Connor, and Jen-Luc Nancy, eds., *Who Comes After the Subject?* (New York: Routledge, 1991).

11. Ian Hacking, *Rewriting the Soul: Multiple Personality and the Sciences of Memory* (Princeton: Princeton University Press, 1995).

12. See, for example, Michael Weissberg, *The First Sin of Ross Michael Carlson: A Psychiatrist's Personal Account of Murder, Multiple Personality Disorder, and Modern Justice* (New York: Delacorte Press, 1992).

13. Elaine Showalter, *Hystories: Hysterical Epidemics and Modern Media* (New York: Columbia University Press, 1997). Showalter includes MPD, Gulf War syndrome (GWS), and chronic fatigue syndrome (CFS) along with claims of alien abduction and of satanic ritual abuse as examples of contemporary hysteria. She may be correct—although I think her conclusions on MPD, GWS, and CFS are premature. In any case she is concerned solely with the cultural dimensions of illness. All illnesses, in my view, including illnesses with no known organic cause, possess a biological dimension, and it is the convergence of biology with culture that produces illness.

14. On "spinal irritation" and other vanishing illnesses, see Edward Shorter, *From Paralysis to Fatigue: A History of Psychosomatic Illness in the Modern Era* (New York: Free Press, 1992). Shorter, like Showalter, regards CFS as a psychosomatic illness, as does Simon Wesseley, who traces its parallels with neurasthenia ("The History of Chronic Fatigue Syndrome," in *Chronic Fatigue Syndrome*, ed. Stephen E. Straus [New York: Marcel Dekker, 1994], 3–44). For a thorough journalistic account convinced that CFS is an organic disease, see Hillary Johnson, *Ostler's Web: Inside the Labyrinth of the Chronic Fatigue Syndrome Epidemic* (New York: Crown Publishers, 1996). For varying biomedical perspectives, see the published proceedings of the 1992 CIBA conference, *Chronic Fatigue Syndrome* (London: Wiley, 1993); Mark A. Demitrack and Susan E. Abbey, *Chronic Fatigue Syndrome: An Integrative Approach to Evaluation and Treatment* (New York: Guilford Press, 1996); and Jay A. Goldstein, *Betrayal by the Brain: The Neurologic Basis of Chronic Fatigue Syndrome, Fibromyalgia Syndrome, and Related Neural Network Disorders* (New York: Hayworth Medical Press, 1996).

15. Robert W. Haley, Thomas L. Kurt, and Jim Horn, "Is There a Gulf War Syndrome?" *JAMA* 277, no. 3 (1997): 215–30. Gulf War veterans undoubtedly show a higher incidence of self-reported medical and psychiatric conditions than do military personnel not deployed to the Persian Gulf, and most scientific studies end by calling for additional study. See the Iowa Persian Gulf Study Group, "Self-Reported Illness and Health Status among Gulf War Veterans: A Population-Based Study," *JAMA* 277, no. 3 (1997): 238–45; and Robert W. Haley and Thomas L. Kurt, "Self-Reported Exposure to Neurotoxic Chemical Combinations in the Gulf War," *JAMA* 277, no. 3 (1977): 231–37. Government delays in admitting the danger from chemical weapons and the extent of troop exposure to these chemicals—including exposure to the defoliant Agent Orange during the Vietnam War—simply feeds doubt (Warren E. Leary, "Experts Urge Broader Study of Chemical Weapons Exposure," *New York Times*, 8 September 1996, sec. 1, 38).

16. Robert A. Aronowitz, "From Myalgic Encephalitis to Yuppie Flu: A History of Chronic Fatigue Syndromes," in *Framing Disease: Studies in Cultural History*, ed. Charles E. Rosenberg and Janet Golden (New Brunswick, N.J.: Rutgers University Press, 1992), 155–81.

17. Mirko D. Grmek, *History of AIDS: Emergence and Origin of a Modern Epidemic* (1989), trans. Russell C. Maulitz and Jacalyn Duffin (Princeton: Princeton University Press, 1990), xi.

18. Rose Weitz, "Uncertainty and the Lives of Persons with AIDS," *Journal of Health and Social Behavior* 30, no. 3 (1989): 270–81.

19. Jeffrey Weeks, "Post-Modern AIDS?" in *Ecstatic Antibodies: Resisting the AIDS Mythology*, ed. Tessa Boffin and Sunil Gupta (London: Rivers Oram Press, 1990), 133–41.

20.   Grmek, *History of AIDS*, 109.

21.   Andrew Purvis, "The Global Epidemic," *Time*, 30 December 1996–6 January 1997, 77–78.

22.   Grmek, *History of AIDS*, 109. As Grmek notes, because AIDS attacks the immune system, it produces symptoms indirectly, by opportunistic infection and malignancy; even when considered as a disease in the classical sense, AIDS in its effect on individual cells creates lesions at a level undetectable before the advent of postmodern medical technology.

23.   Karen J. Carlson, Stephanie A. Eisenstat, and Terra Ziporyn, *The Harvard Guide to Women's Health* (Cambridge: Harvard University Press, 1996). On the social and biological issues affecting women's health, see Lesley Doyal, *What Makes Women Sick: Gender and the Political Economy of Health* (New Brunswick, N.J.: Rutgers University Press, 1995).

24.   Wayne Katon and Herbert Schulberg, "Epidemiology of Depression in Primary Care," *General Hospital Psychiatry* 14, no. 4 (1992): 237–47. See also J. Angst, "Epidemiology of Depression," *Psychopharmacology* 106, suppl. (1992): S71–S74.

25.   Myrna M. Weissman and Gerald L. Klerman, "Sex Differences and the Epidemiology of Depression," *Archives of General Psychiatry* 34, no. 1 (1977): 98–111; Olympia J. Snowe, "Women's Health Research and Women's Mental Health and Substance Abuse Acts," *Congressional Record* 137, no. 38 (6 March 1991): E770–E771. Depression is a malleable category, reshaped by cultures; and quantitative measures must be interpreted cautiously. See Arthur Kleinman and Byron Good, eds., *Culture and Depression: Studies in the Anthropology and Cross-Cultural Psychiatry of Affect and Disorder* (Berkeley: University of California Press, 1985).

26.   See Anne Hunsaker Hawkins, *Reconstructing Illness: Studies in Pathography* (West Lafayette, Ind.: Purdue University Press, 1993); and Carl H. Klaus, "Embodying the Self: Malady and the Personal Essay," *Iowa Review* 25, no. 2 (1995): 177–92.

27.   Patrick D. Wall and Mervyn Jones, *Defeating Pain: The War against a Silent Epidemic* (New York: Plenum Press, 1991), 15. Patrick Wall, professor of anatomy at University College (London), in 1965 coauthored with psychologist Ronald Melzack the pioneering gate-control theory of pain. On the limitations of the theory, see Ronald Melzack, "Gate Control Theory: On the Evolution of Pain Concepts," *Pain Forum* 5, no. 2 (1996): 128–38.

28.   Ernest Volinn, "Back Pain and Associated Disability in the United States," *American Pain Society Bulletin* 6, no. 6 (1996): 8.

29.   Health Agencies Update, "Latex Allergy Alert," *JAMA* 277, no. 3 (1997): 194; Gregory R. Wagner, "Asbestosis and Silicosis," *Lancet* 349, no. 9061

(1997): 1311–15; and Myrna L. Armstrong, "You Pierced What?" *Pediatric Nursing* 22, no. 3 (1996): 236–38.

30.   On Foucault's contributions, see Nikolas Rose, "Medicine, History, and the Present," in *Reassessing Foucault: Power, Medicine, and the Body*, ed. Colin Jones and Roy Porter (New York: Routledge, 1994), 48–72.

31.   See *The Wellness Encyclopedia* (Boston: Houghton-Mifflin, 1991); and James Marti and Andrea Hine, *The Alternative Health and Medicine Encyclopedia* (Detroit: Gale Research Company, 1995).

32.   Bill Moyers, *Healing and the Mind*, ed. Betty Sue Flowers (New York: Doubleday, 1993), 323–63. The interviews are with Michael Lerner ("Healing") and Rachel Naomi Remen ("Wholeness"). See also, for example, Daniel Goleman and Joel Gurin, eds., *Mind/Body Medicine: How to Use Your Mind for Better Health* (Yonkers, N.Y.: Consumer Reports Books, 1993).

33.   Papers from the workshop are included in Anne Harrington, ed., *The Placebo Effect: An Interdisciplinary Exploration* (Cambridge: Harvard University Press, 1997).

34.   Patrick D. Wall, "The Placebo Effect: An Unpopular Topic," *Pain* 51, no. 1 (1992): 1–3.

35.   Joseph T. Shipley, *The Origins of English Words: A Discursive Dictionary of Indo-European Roots* (Baltimore: Johns Hopkins University Press, 1984), 154.

36.   Robert G. Jahn, "Information, Consciousness, and Health," *Alternative Therapies in Health and Medicine* 2, no. 3 (1996): 37. See also the earlier report on PEAR's research, Robert G. Jahn and B. J. Dunne, *Margins of Reality: The Role of Consciousness in the Physical World* (New York: Harcourt Brace Jovanovich, 1987).

37.   Joseph J. Jacobs, "Building Bridges between Two Worlds: The NIH's Office of Alternative Medicine," *Academic Medicine* 70, no. 1 (1995): 40–41.

38.   Byron Good and Mary-Jo DelVecchio Good, " 'Learning Medicine': The Constructing of Medical Knowledge at Harvard Medical School," in *Knowledge, Power, and Practice: The Anthropology of Medicine and Everyday Life*, ed. Shirley Lindenbaum and Margaret Lock (Berkeley: University of California Press, 1993), 81–107. In cautioning against "glib characterizations" of large theoretical formulations such as "biomedicine" or "the biomedical model," Good and Good argue for an analysis of medical knowledge that is always "situated, contextualized, and ethnographically rich" (83).

39.   Robert A. Hahn, *Sickness and Healing: An Anthropological Perspective* (New Haven: Yale University Press, 1995), 96–97. Although Hahn includes psychiatry in this small group of specialties, the recent biological revolution in psychiatry makes many psychiatrists increasingly reliant upon chemotherapy and less receptive to psychosocial analysis.

40.   George L. Engel, "The Need for a New Medical Model: A Challenge for Biomedicine," *Science* 196, no. 4286 (1977): 129–36.

41.   On the power of medical metaphors, see Evelyn Fox Keller, *Refiguring Life: Metaphors of Twentieth-Century Biology* (New York: Columbia University Press, 1995). Keller notes how the body as computer is beginning to replace earlier industrial versions of the body as machine.

42.   On a biopsychosocial approach, see Kenneth F. Schaffner, "Philosophy of Medicine," in *Introduction to the Philosophy of Science,* ed. Merrilee H. Salmon et al. (Englewood Cliffs, N.J.: Prentice Hall, 1992), 313–15. For an early and related discussion, see Elliot G. Mishler, "The Social Construction of Illness," in Elliot G. Mishler et al., *Social Contexts of Health, Illness, and Patient Care* (Cambridge: Cambridge University Press, 1981), 141–68.

43.   Poststructuralism, a concept that gets vaguer daily, refers to approaches dispersed widely across areas from feminism to psychoanalysis (see the cross listings in Michael Groden and Martin Kreiswirth, eds., *Johns Hopkins Guide to Literary Theory and Criticism* [Baltimore: Johns Hopkins University Press, 1994]). For an introduction, see John Sturrock, ed., *Structuralism and Since: From Lévi Strauss to Derrida* (Oxford: Oxford University Press, 1979); John Rajchman and Cornel West, eds., *Post-Analytic Philosophy* (New York: Columbia University Press, 1985); Richard Machin and Christopher Norris, eds., *Post-Structuralist Readings of English Poetry* (Cambridge: Cambridge University Press, 1987); and Madan Sarup, *An Introductory Guide to Post-Structuralism and Postmodernism* (Athens: University of Georgia Press, 1989).

44.   "In effect, for poststructuralism, all 'truths' are relative to the frame of reference which contains them; more radically, 'truths' are a function of these frames; and even more radically, these discourses 'constitute' the truths they claim to discover and transmit" (Paul A. Bové, "Discourse," in *Critical Terms for Literary Study,* ed. Frank Lentricchia and Thomas McLaughlin [Chicago: University of Chicago Press, 1990], 56).

45.   Raymond Williams calls "culture" among "the two or three most complicated words in the English language" (*Keywords: A Vocabulary of Culture and Society* [New York: Oxford University Press, 1983], 87). Cecil G. Helman writes: "To some extent, culture can be seen as an inherited 'lens,' through which the individual perceives and understands the world that he inhabits, and learns how to live within it" (*Culture, Health, and Illness: An Introduction for Health Professionals,* 3d ed. [Oxford: Butterworth-Heineman, 1994], 3). Terry Eagleton asks why everyone is talking about culture these days, and he replies that culture is integral to three movements at the forefront of the recent political agenda in the West: "revolutionary nationalism, sexual politics, and ethnic struggle" ("The Contradictions of Postmodernism," *New Literary History* 28, no. 1 [1997]: 1–6).

46. Joel C. Kuipers, "'Medical Discourse' in Anthropological Context: Views of Language and Power," *Medical Anthropology Quarterly* 3, no. 2 (1989): 99–123.

47. Francis L. K. Hsu, "The Self in Cross-Cultural Perspective," in *Culture and Self: Asian and Western Perspectives*, ed. Anthony J. Marsella, George DeVos, and Francis L. K. Hsu (New York: Tavistock Publications, 1985), 24–55.

48. Judith Butler, *The Psychic Life of Power* (Stanford: Stanford University Press, 1997). My belief that an adequate account of selfhood cannot rest on cultural analysis alone but must include biology as well depends partly on research done with twins and with animal cognition, suggesting that selfhood and consciousness are inseparable from genetic endowments distinctive to human biology.

49. On "cultural psychology," see Jerome Bruner, *The Culture of Education* (Cambridge: Harvard University Press, 1996). A "cultural psychology" is not necessarily antibiological, but rather can (in ways Bruner does not pursue) coincide with the approach of evolutionary psychologists, who study how human psychological processes and preferences reflect the development of the brain, over millennia, in specific natural and social environments.

50. Emily Martin, *Flexible Bodies: Tracking Immunity in American Culture— from the Days of Polio to the Age of AIDS* (Boston: Beacon Press, 1994), 23–44; and Donna J. Haraway, "The Biopolitics of Postmodern Bodies: Constitutions of Self in Immune System Discourse," in *Simians, Cyborgs, and Women: The Reinvention of Nature* (New York: Routledge, 1991), 203–30.

CHAPTER THREE: THE WHITE NOISE
OF HEALTH

1. For details in this paragraph, see Harold M. Ginzburg and Eric Reis, "Consequences of the Nuclear Power Plant Accident at Chernobyl," *Public Health Reports* 106, no. 1 (1991): 32–40; "Health and Environmental Consequences of the Chernobyl Nuclear Power Plant Accident," Report DOE/ER-0332 (Washington, D.C.: U.S. Government Printing Office, 1987); Mary Brennan, "USSR: Medical Effects of Chernobyl Disaster," *Lancet* 335, no. 8697 (1990): 1086; Harold M. Ginsburg, "The Psychological Consequences of the Chernobyl Accident—Finding from the International Atomic Energy Agency Study," *Public Health Reports* 108, no. 2 (1993): 184–92.

2. See Neil Everden, *The Social Creation of Nature* (Baltimore: Johns Hopkins University Press, 1992); and Terry Gifford, "The Social Construction of Nature," *ISLE: Interdisciplinary Studies in Literature and Environment* 3, no. 2 (1996): 27–36.

3. Eric Partridge, ed., *The Macmillan Dictionary of Historical Slang* (New York: Macmillan, 1974), s.v. "mad as a hatter."

4.   Gerald Markowitz and David Posner, "Occupational Diseases," in *The Cambridge World History of Human Disease*, ed. Kenneth F. Kiple (New York: Cambridge University Press, 1993), 187–92.

5.   See Barbara Ellen Smith, "Black Lung: The Social Production of Disease," *International Journal of Health Services* 11, no. 3 (1981): 343–59.

6.   Here and throughout the discussion of malaria I am indebted to Laurie Garrett, *The Coming Plague: Newly Emerging Diseases in a World out of Balance* (1994; reprint, New York: Penguin Books, 1995). See also Ellen Ruppel Shell, "Resurgence of a Deadly Disease," *Atlantic Monthly* 280, no. 2 (1997): 45 ff.

7.   Other once feared killers—smallpox, typhoid fever, diphtheria, and cholera—have similarly lost ground to programs of inoculation: smallpox was successfully eradicated by 1980 after a ten-year worldwide campaign. Yet the results are also mixed. As smallpox inoculation declines, seven countries in equatorial Africa have reported outbreaks of human monkeypox disease, against which the smallpox vaccine had offered protection.

8.   See Paul R. Ehrlich and Anne H. Ehrlich, *Healing the Planet: Strategies for Resolving the Environmental Crisis* (New York: Addison-Wesley Publishing, 1991), 39–41.

9.   Henry David Thoreau, *The Journal of Henry David Thoreau*, ed. Bradford Torrey and Francis H. Allen (Boston: Houghton Mifflin, 1906), 11:395. See also Michael P. Branch and Jessica Pierce, "'Another Name for Health': Thoreau and Modern Medicine," *Literature and Medicine* 15, no. 1 (1996): 129–45.

10.   See William Cronon, *Changes in the Land: Indians, Colonists, and the Ecology of New England* (New York: Hill and Wang, 1983). As Cronon writes, "The replacement of Indians by predominantly European populations in New England was as much an ecological as a cultural revolution" (6).

11.   Robin Russell Jones, "Air Pollution Related to Transport," *British Medical Journal* 312, no. 7046 (1996): 1605–6. Asthma attacks apparently can be triggered by changes in climate and air quality, even by thunderstorms, but not without the contribution of other (still debated) factors that raise or lower susceptibility.

12.   R. L. Nagel and A. F. Fleming, "Genetic Epidemiology of the beta s Gene," *Bailliere's Clinical Haematology* 5, no. 2 (1992): 331–65.

13.   Marian Segal, "New Hope for Children with Sickle Cell Disease," *FDA Consumer* 23, no. 2 (1989): 14–18.

14.   See, for example, Theron G. Randolph, *Environmental Medicine: Beginnings and Bibliographies of Clinical Ecology* (Fort Collins, Colo.: Clinical Ecology Publications, 1987); François Ramade, *Ecotoxicology* (1977), trans. L. J. M. Hodgson, 2d ed. (New York: Wiley, 1987); Alyce Bezman Tarcher, ed., *Princi-*

ples and Practice of Environmental Medicine (New York: Plenum Medical Book Co., 1992); and Stuart M. Brooks, *Environmental Medicine* (St. Louis: Mosby, 1995).

15.　See Jonathan Marks, *Human Biodiversity: Genes, Race, and History* (New York: Aldine de Gruyter, 1995), 211–13.

16.　Barbara E. Mahon et al., "Reported Cholera in the United States, 1992–1994: A Reflection of Global Changes in Cholera Epidemiology," *JAMA* 276, no. 4 (1996): 307–12. The total number of reported cases is still small: 160 from 1992 through 1994.

17.　Cited in Ehrlich and Ehrlich, *Healing the Planet*, 5.

18.　Don DeLillo, *White Noise* (New York: Viking Penguin, 1985), 127. Subsequent quotations will be documented within the text.

19.　Thomas J. Ferraro, "Whole Families Shopping at Night," in *New Essays on "White Noise,"* ed. Frank Lentricchia (Cambridge: Cambridge University Press, 1991), 16–17. For helpful analysis, see Frank Lentricchia, ed., *Introducing Don DeLillo* (Durham, N.C.: Duke University Press, 1991)—which reproduces essays in an issue of *South Atlantic Quarterly* devoted to DeLillo (89, no. 2 [1990]); and Paul Civello, *American Literary Naturalism and Its Twentieth-Century Transformations: Frank Norris, Ernest Hemingway, Don DeLillo* (Athens: University of Georgia Press, 1994).

20.　For an illuminating discussion of systems theory and its relation to DeLillo's work, see Tom LeClair, *In the Loop: Don DeLillo and the Systems Novel* (Urbana: University of Illinois Press, 1987).

21.　See Daniel J. Kevles, "Endangered Environmentalists," *New York Review of Books* 44, no. 3 (1997): 31; and John Wargo, *Our Children's Toxic Legacy: How Science and Law Fail to Protect Us from Pesticides* (New Haven: Yale University Press, 1996).

22.　Don DeLillo, quoted in Anthony DeCurtis, "'An Outsider in This Society': An Interview with Don DeLillo," *South Atlantic Quarterly* 89, no. 2 (1990): 295.

23.　Richard Selzer, *Down from Troy: A Doctor Comes of Age* (New York: William Morrow, 1992), 92. Subsequent quotations will be documented within the text.

24.　Stephen Verderber, "Dimensions of Person-Window Transactions in the Hospital Environment," *Environment and Behavior* 18, no. 4 (1986): 450–66.

25.　Roger S. Ulrich, "View through a Window May Influence Recovery from Surgery," *Science* 224, no. 4647 (1984): 420–21.

26.　See Edward O. Wilson, *Biophilia* (Cambridge: Harvard University Press, 1984); Charles J. Lumsden and Edward O. Wilson, "The Relation between Biological and Cultural Evolution," *Journal of Social and Biological Structure* 8, no. 4 (1985): 343–59; and Stephen R. Kellert and Edward O. Wilson, eds., *The Biophilia Hypothesis* (Washington, D.C.: Island Press, 1993).

27.   D. I. Perrett, K. A. May, and S. Yoshikawa, "Facial Shape and Judgements of Female Attractiveness," *Nature* 368, no. 6468 (1994): 239–42. See also Judith Langlois et al., "Facial Diversity and Infant Preferences for Attractive Faces," *Developmental Psychology* 27, no. 1 (1991): 79–84.

28.   See Douglas W. Dockery et al., "An Association between Air Pollution and Mortality in Six U.S. Cities," *New England Journal of Medicine* 329, no. 24 (1993): 1753–59; H. Range Hutson, Deirdre Anglin, and Michael J. Pratts Jr., "Adolescents and Children Injured or Killed in Drive-By Shootings in Los Angeles," *New England Journal of Medicine* 330, no. 5 (1994): 324–27; and Rolv Terje Lie, Allen J. Wilcox, and Rolv Skjærven, "A Population-Based Study of the Risk of Recurrence of Birth Defects," *New England Journal of Medicine* 331, no. 1 (1994): 1–4.

29.   F. J. Malveaux, D. Houlihan, and E. L. Diamond, "Characteristics of Asthma Mortality and Morbidity in African Americans," *Journal of Asthma* 30, no. 6 (1993): 431–37; Sampson B. Sarpong et al., "Socioeconomic Status and Race as Risk Factors for Cockroach Allergen Exposure and Sensitization in Children with Asthma," *Journal of Allergy and Clinical Immunology* 97, no. 6 (1996): 1393–401; and David L. Rosenstreich et al., "The Role of Cockroach Allergy and Exposure to Cockroach Allergen in Causing Morbidity among Inner-City Children with Asthma," *New England Journal of Medicine* 336, no. 19 (1997): 1356–63.

30.   Bunyan I. Bryant and Paul Mohai, *Race and the Incidence of Environmental Hazards: A Time for Discourse* (Boulder: Westview Press, 1992).

31.   Malcom W. Browne, "Land Mines Called a World Menace," *New York Times*, 15 November 1993, A7. Browne cites a 510-page report published by the Arms Project, a branch of the research organization Human Rights Watch.

32.   Peter S. Blair et al., "Smoking and the Sudden Infant Death Syndrome: Results from 1993–5 Case-Control Study for Confidential Inquiry into Stillbirths and Deaths in Infancy," *British Medical Journal* 313, no. 7051 (1996): 195–98. Another indication of cultural influence comes from data showing that low-income groups have higher rates of SIDS (R. P. K. Ford and K. P. Nelson, "Higher Rates of SIDS Persist in Low Income Groups," *Journal of Paediatrics and Child Health* 3, no. 5 [1995]: 408–11).

33.   Garrett, *The Coming Plague*, 11.

34.   Ibid., 644–45, n. 38.

35.   Ibid., 445.

36.   William O. C. M. Cookson and Miriam F. Moffatt, "Asthma: An Epidemic in the Absence of Infection?" *Science* 275, no. 5296 (1997): 41–42.

37.   David V. Bates, "Air Pollution: Time for More Clean Air Legislation?" *British Medical Journal* 312, no. 7032 (1996): 649–50; Joseph F. Albright and Robert A. Goldstein, "Airborne Pollutants and the Immune System," *Otolaryngology—Head and Neck Surgery* 114, no. 2 (1996): 232–38.

38.   Roy Porter, "Diseases of Civilization," in *Companion Encyclopedia of the History of Medicine*, ed. W. F. Bynum and Roy Porter (New York: Routledge, 1993), 1:585–600.

39.   Rae Tyson, "Pollutants Breed Deadly Synthetic: Chemicals May Mimic Hormone," *USA Today*, 21 April 1994, D4.

40.   Data from studies presented at the 1996 International Congress of Endocrinology, quoted in Tim Friend, "Pollutants May Be Raising Rate of Testicular Cancer," *USA Today*, 17 June 1996, D1.

41.   Robert Kunzig, "Twilight of the Cod," *Discover* 16, no. 4 (1995): 44 ff.

42.   Mark Nathan Cohen, *Health and the Rise of Civilization* (New Haven: Yale University Press, 1989), 47. See also Carlo M. Cipolla, *Miasmas and Disease: Public Health and the Environment in the Pre-Industrial Age* (1989), trans. Elizabeth Potter (New Haven: Yale University Press, 1992).

43.   Wallace Stevens, "The Comedian as the Letter C" (1922), in *The Collected Poems of Wallace Stevens*, ed. Holly Stevens (New York: Alfred A. Knopf, 1954), 37.

44.   Eric Chivian et al., *Critical Condition: Human Health and the Environment* (Cambridge: MIT Press, 1993), ix.

CHAPTER FOUR: REINVENTING PAIN

1.   See Elaine Scarry, *The Body in Pain: The Making and Unmaking of the World* (New York: Oxford University Press, 1985). Scarry shows how our awareness of pain is built into even such unlikely areas as product liability law.

2.   John C. Liebeskind, "Pain Can Kill," *Pain* 44, no. 1 (1991): 3–4. Liebeskind reports that pain in rats can depress the immune system and destroy cancer-fighting cells.

3.   In Laura S. Hitchcock, ed., *Living with Chronic Pain: Personal Experiences of Pain Sufferers* (Bethesda, Md.: National Chronic Pain Outreach Association Publishers, 1992), 9.

4.   On the intersubjectivity of pain, see Mark D. Sullivan, "Pain in Language: From Sentience to Sapience," *Pain Forum* 4, no. 1 (1995): 3014; on pain as mystery as opposed to puzzle, see David B. Morris, *The Culture of Pain* (Berkeley: University of California Press, 1991), 23–26. On pain and disability, see Marian Osterweis, Arthur Kleinman, and David Mechanic, eds., *Pain and*

Disability: Clinical, Behavioral, and Public Policy Perspectives (Washington, D.C.: National Academy Press, 1987). On pain and quality of life, see David F. Cella, "Quality of Life: Concepts and Definitions," *Journal of Pain and Symptom Management* 9, no. 3 (1994): 186–92. On chronic pain and depression, see Ann Gamsa and Vaira Vikis-Freibergs, "Psychological Events Are Both Risk Factors in, and Consequences of, Chronic Pain," *Pain* 44, no. 3 (1991): 271–77. Cancer pain, in part because the etiology is clear, appears not to have a strong link with depression (Deborah B. McGuire and Vivian R. Sheidler, "Pain," in *Cancer Nursing: Principles and Practice,* ed. Susan L. Groenwald et al., 3d ed. [Boston: Jones and Bartlett, 1993], 2).

5.   John J. Bonica, "Pain Research and Therapy: History, Current Status, and Future Goals," in *Animal Pain,* ed. Charles E. Short and Alan Van Poznak (New York: Churchill Livingstone, 1992), 2.

6.   Ibid.

7.   Jennifer L. Kelsey and Augustus A. White III, "Epidemiology and Impact of Low Back Pain," *Spine* 5, no. 2 (1980): 133–34.

8.   Norman Cousins, *Anatomy of an Illness as Perceived by the Patient: Reflections on Healing and Regeneration* (New York: W. W. Norton, 1979), 37, 89.

9.   D. Marcer and S. Deighton, "Intractable Pain: A Neglected Area of Medical Education in the UK," *Journal of the Royal Society of Medicine* 81, no. 12 (1988): 698–700.

10.   Bonica, "Pain Research and Therapy," 7.

11.   In Richard S. Weiner, "An Interview with John J. Bonica, M.D.," *Pain Practitioner* 1, no. 1 (1989): 2. Implicitly acknowledging the truth of Bonica's remark, two years later the International Association for the Study of Pain published Howard L. Fields, ed., *Core Curriculum for Professional Education in Pain* (Seattle: IASP Publications, 1991).

12.   C. Stratton Hill Jr., "When Will Adequate Pain Treatment Be the Norm?" *JAMA* 274, no. 23 (1995): 1881.

13.   "Managing Cancer Pain with Opioids: Addiction, Tolerance, and Physical Dependence Defined," *Cancer Pain Release* 7, nos. 2–3 (1994): 2. *Cancer Pain Release* is sponsored by the World Health Organization.

14.   Richard M. Marks and Edward J. Sachar, "Undertreatment of Medical Inpatients with Narcotic Analgesics," *Annals of Internal Medicine* 78, no. 2 (1973): 173–81.

15.   *Management of Cancer Pain* (Washington, D.C.: U.S. Department of Health and Human Services, 1994), iii; Charles S. Cleeland, "The Impact of Pain on the Patient with Cancer," *Cancer* 54, no. 11 (1984): 2635–41, and Charles S. Cleeland et al., "Pain and Its Treatment in Patients with Metastatic Cancer," *New England Journal of Medicine* 330, no. 9 (1994): 592–96; Russell K. Portenoy, "Cancer Pain: Epidemiology and Syndromes," *Cancer* 63, no. 11,

suppl. (1989): 2298–307; The SUPPORT Principal Investigators, "A Controlled Trial to Improve Care for Seriously Ill Hospitalized Patients," *JAMA* 274, no. 20 (1995): 1591–98.

16.   Jane Porter and Hershel Jick, "Addiction Rare in Patients Treated with Narcotics," *New England Journal of Medicine* 302, no. 2 (1988): 123. See also Barry Stimmel, *Pain, Analgesia, and Addiction: The Pharmacologic Treatment of Pain* (New York: Raven Press, 1983).

17.   Hill, "When Will Adequate Pain Treatment Be the Norm?" 1881.

18.   Mayday Fund, "Presentation of Findings," private survey (Washington, D.C.: Mellman-Lazarus-Lake, Inc., 1993).

19.   Ray Tallis, "Terrors of the Body," [London] *Times Literary Supplement*, 1 May 1991, 3.

20.   See Morris, *The Culture of Pain*; two essays by Roy Porter, "Pain and History in the Western World," in *The Puzzle of Pain* (1992), trans. Fideline A. Djité-Bruce (Basel, Switzerland: Gordon and Breach Arts International, 1994), 98–119, and "Pain and Suffering," in *Companion Encyclopedia of the History of Medicine*, ed. W. F. Bynum and Roy Porter (New York: Routledge, 1993), 2:1574–91; and Roselyne Rey, *The History of Pain* (1993), trans. Louis Elliott Wallace, J. A. Cadden, and S. W. Cadden (Cambridge: Harvard University Press, 1995).

21.   Reynolds Price, *A Whole New Life: An Illness and a Healing* (New York: Atheneum, 1994), 108. Subsequent quotations will be documented within the text.

22.   John D. Loeser, "What Is Chronic Pain?" *Theoretical Medicine* 12, no. 3 (1991): 214–15.

23.   Morris, *The Culture of Pain*, passim.

24.   John D. Loeser, "Low Back Pain," in *Pain*, ed. John J. Bonica, Research Publications: Association for Research in Nervous and Mental Disease, vol. 58 (New York: Raven Press, 1980), 363–77.

25.   Michael Von Korff et al., "Effects of Practice Style in Managing Back Pain," *Annals of Internal Medicine* 121, no. 3 (1994): 187–95.

26.   Stanley J. Bigos et al., "A Prospective Study of Work Perceptions and Psychosocial Factors Affecting the Report of a Back Injury," *Spine* 16, no. 1 (1991): 1–6; and T. Dwyer and A. E. Raftery, "Industrial Accidents Are Produced by Social Relations of Work: A Sociological Theory of Industrial Accidents," *Applied Ergonomics* 22, no. 3 (1991): 167–78.

27.   For a review of research, see Ranjan Roy, *The Social Context of the Chronic Pain Sufferer* (Toronto: University of Toronto Press, 1992).

28.   Edward A. Walker et al., "Histories of Sexual Victimization in Patients with Irritable Bowel Syndrome or Inflammatory Bowel Disease," *American Journal of Psychiatry* 150, no. 10 (1993): 1502–6.

29.   Quoted in Gurney Williams III, "Pain! Treating It and Defeating It," *American Health*, November 1991, 46.

30.   IASP Subcommittee on Taxonomy, "Pain Terms: A List with Definitions and Notes on Usage," *Pain* 6, no. 3 (1979): 249–52.

31.   Henry K. Beecher, "Pain in Men Wounded in Battle," *Annals of Surgery* 123, no. 1 (1946): 96–105. For a review based on more recent combat conditions, see Jon W. Blank, "Pain in Men Wounded in Battle: Beecher Revisited," *IASP Newsletter*, January/February 1994, 2–4.

32.   Patrick D. Wall and Mervyn Jones, *Defeating Pain: The War against a Silent Epidemic* (New York: Plenum Press, 1991), 44. See also Patrick D. Wall, "On the Relation of Injury to Pain," *Pain* 6, no. 3 (1979): 253–64. Pain, he says, has only a "weak" relation to injury.

33.   IASP Subcommittee on Taxonomy, "Pain Terms," 250.

34.   Allan I. Basbaum, "Unlocking the Secrets of Pain: The Science," in *1988 Medical and Health Annual*, ed. Ellen Bernstein (Chicago: Encyclopedia Britannica, 1987), 84–103.

35.   Harold Carron, Douglas DeGood, and Raymond Tait, "A Comparison of Low Back Pain Patients in the United States and New Zealand: Psychosocial and Economic Factors Affecting Severity of Disability," *Pain* 21, no. 1 (1985): 77–89; Steven F. Brena, Steven H. Sanders, and Hiroshi Motoyama, "American and Japanese Low Back Pain Patients: Cross-Cultural Similarities and Differences," *Clinical Journal of Pain* 6, no. 2 (1990): 118–24; Steven H. Sanders et al., "Chronic Low Back Pain Patients around the World: Cross-Cultural Similarities and Differences," *Clinical Journal of Pain* 8, no. 4 (1992): 317–23.

36.   Harald Shrader et al., "Natural Evolution of Late Whiplash Syndrome outside the Medicolegal Context," *Lancet* 347, no. 9010 (1996): 1207–11.

37.   Mary-Jo DelVecchio Good et al., eds., *Pain as Human Experience: An Anthropological Perspective* (Berkeley: University of California Press, 1991), 1.

38.   Robert W. Gear et al., "Kappa-Opioids Produce Significantly Greater Analgesia in Women Than in Men," *Nature Medicine* 2, no. 11 (1996): 1248–50.

39.   *The Nuprin Pain Report* (New York: Louis Harris and Associates, 1985), 7; Howard P. Greenwald, "Interethnic Differences in Pain Perception," *Pain* 44, no. 2 (1991): 157–63; Maryann S. Bates, W. Thomas Edwards, and Karen O. Anderson, "Ethnocultural Influences on Variation in Chronic Pain Perception," *Pain* 52, no. 1 (1993): 101–12, and B. Berthold Wolff, "Ethnocultural Factors Influencing Pain and Illness Behavior," *Clinical Journal of Pain* 1, no. 1 (1985): 23–30.

40.   George L. Engel, "'Psychogenic' Pain and the Pain-Prone Patient," *American Journal of Medicine* 26, no. 6 (1959): 899–918. See Pat Califa, "Feminism and Sadomasochism," *CoEvolution Quarterly* 33, no. 2 (1982): 33–40; and

Armando R. Favazza, *Bodies under Siege: Self-Mutilation in Culture and Psychiatry* (Baltimore: Johns Hopkins University Press, 1987).

41.   Timothy Bayer, Paul E. Baer, and Charles Early, "Situational and Psychophysiological Factors in Psychologically Induced Pain," *Pain* 44, no. 1 (1991): 45–50.

42.   Jesse O. Cavenar Jr. and William W. Weddington Jr., "Abdominal Pain in Expectant Fathers," *Psychosomatics* 19, no. 12 (1978): 761–68.

43.   G. Richard Smith Jr., *Somatization Disorder in the Medical Setting* (Washington, D.C.: American Psychiatric Press, 1991), 22; Julia A. Faucett and Jon D. Levine, "The Contributions of Interpersonal Conflict to Chronic Pain in the Presence or Absence of Organic Pathology," *Pain* 44, no. 1 (1991): 35–43; Jay D. Summers et al., "Psychosocial Factors in Chronic Spinal Cord Injury," *Pain* 47, no. 2 (1991): 183–89.

44.   Wilbert E. Fordyce, "Pain Viewed as Learned Behavior," in *Advances in Neurology*, ed. John J. Bonica (New York: Raven Press, 1974), 4:415–22. For a sense of the range of positions on what is learned, see Peter S. Staats, Hamid Hekmat, and Arthur W. Staats, "The Psychological Behaviorism Theory of Pain: A Basis for Unity," *Pain Forum* 5, no. 3 (1996): 194–207.

45.   Donald S. Ciccone and Roy C. Grzesiak, "Cognitive Dimensions of Chronic Pain," *Social Science and Medicine* 19, no. 12 (1984): 1339–45. See also Fordyce, "Pain Viewed as Learned Behavior," 4:415–22; Dennis C. Turk, Donald Meichenbaum, and Myles Genest, *Pain and Behavioral Medicine: A Cognitive-Behavioral Approach* (New York: Guilford Press, 1983); Howard Rachlin, "Pain and Behavior," *The Behavioral and Brain Sciences* 8, no. 1 (1985): 43–53; Gerhard Schüssler, "Coping Strategies and Individual Meanings of Illness," *Social Science and Medicine* 34, no. 4 (1992): 427–32.

46.   See John F. Riley et al., "Chronic Pain and Functional Impairment: Assessing Beliefs about Their Relationship," *Archives of Physical Medicine and Rehabilitation* 69, no. 8 (1988): 573–78; and Lindsey C. Edwards et al., "The Pain Beliefs Questionnaire: An Investigation of Beliefs in the Causes and Consequences of Pain," *Pain* 51, no. 3 (1992): 267–72.

47.   David A. Williams and Beverly Thorn, "An Empirical Assessment of Pain Beliefs," *Pain* 36, no. 3 (1989): 351–58; and David A. Williams and Francis J. Keefe, "Pain Beliefs and the Use of Cognitive-Behavioral Coping Strategies," *Pain* 46, no. 2 (1991): 185–90.

48.   Chris Eccleston, Amanda C. de C. Williams, and Wendy Stainton Rogers, "Patients' and Professionals' Understandings of the Causes of Chronic Pain: Blame, Responsibility, and Identity Protection," *Social Science and Medicine* 45, no. 5 (1997): 699–709.

49.   Mark P. Jensen et al., "Coping with Chronic Pain: A Critical Review of the Literature," *Pain* 47, no. 3 (1991): 249–83; and Mark P. Jensen and Paul

Karoly, "Pain-Specific Beliefs, Perceived Symptom Severity, and Adjustment to Chronic Pain," *Clinical Journal of Pain* 8, no. 2 (1992): 123–30.

50.   Michael S. Shutty Jr., Douglas E. DeGood, and Diane H. Tuttle, "Chronic Pain Patients' Beliefs about Their Pain and Treatment Outcomes," *Archives of Physical Medicine and Rehabilitation* 71, no. 2 (1990): 128–32; and Douglas E. DeGood and Michael S. Shutty Jr., "Assessment of Pain Beliefs, Coping, and Self Efficacy," in *Handbook of Pain Assessment*, ed. Dennis C. Turk and Ronald Melzack (New York: Guilford Press, 1992), 214–34.

51.   E. Nettelbladt, "Subjects on Permanent Disability in Sweden," *Opuscula Medica* [Sweden] 30, no. 2 (1985): 54–56.

52.   Mark D. Sullivan and John D. Loeser, "The Diagnosis of Disability: Treating and Rating Disability in a Pain Clinic," *Archives of Internal Medicine* 152, no. 9 (1992): 1829–35.

53.   George Mendelson, "Compensation and Pain," *Pain* 48, no. 2 (1992): 121–23.

54.   Wilbert E. Fordyce, *Back Pain in the Workplace: Management of Disability in Nonspecific Conditions: A Report of the Task Force on Pain in the Workplace of the International Association for the Study of Pain* (Seattle: IASP Press, 1995).

55.   Nortin M. Hadler, "Backache and Humanism," in *The Adult Spine: Principles and Practice*, ed. John W. Frymoyer (New York: Raven Press, 1991), 2:55–60.

56.   Elizabeth Snead, "Tattooed Scalp Signals a Model of Rebellion," *USA Today*, 23 March 1993, D1.

57.   Mark D. Sullivan, "Pain as Emotion," *Pain Forum* 5, no. 3 (1996): 209.

58.   Janet Boyd, "A Snowball," in *People with Pain Speak Out*, ed. Christine Nyhane and Brian Sardeson (Ballarat East, Australia: Ballarat East Community Health Centre, 1990), 18.

59.   Ronald Melzack, "Central Pain Syndromes and Theories of Pain," in *Pain and Central Nervous System Disease: The Central Pain Syndromes*, ed. Kenneth L. Casey (New York: Raven Press, 1991), 59–64. See also Ronald Melzack, "Gate Control Theory: On the Evolution of Pain Concepts," *Pain Forum* 5, no. 2 (1996): 128–38.

CHAPTER FIVE: UTOPIAN BODIES

1.   Fredric Jameson, "Postmodernism and Utopia," in *Utopia Post Utopia: Configurations of Nature and Culture in Recent Sculpture and Photography* (Cambridge: MIT Press, 1988), 11–32.

2.   See Louis Marin, "Frontiers of Utopia: Past and Present," *Critical Inquiry* 19, no. 3 (1993): 397–420; and Jean Baudrillard, "Utopia Achieved," in

America (1986), trans. Chris Turner (New York: Verso, 1988), 75–105. For a discussion of utopia in the work of the important French postmodern thinker Roland Barthes, see Diana Knight, *Barthes and Utopia: Space, Travel, Writing* (New York: Oxford University Press, 1997).

3. See Krishan Kumar, *Utopia and Anti-Utopia in Modern Times* (Oxford: Basil Blackwell, 1987); Norman Finkelstein, *The Utopian Moment in Contemporary American Poetry* (Lewisburg, Pa.: Bucknell University Press, 1988); Libby Falk Jones and Sarah Webster Goodwin, eds., *Feminism, Utopia, and Narrative* (Knoxville: University of Tennessee Press, 1990); Dragan Klaic, *The Plot of the Future: Utopia and Dystopia in Modern Drama* (Ann Arbor: University of Michigan Press, 1991).

4. Perry Anderson, "Modernism and Revolution," *New Left Review* 144 (March–April 1984): 95–113.

5. Barry Glassner, "Fitness and the Postmodern Self," *Journal of Health and Social Behavior* 30, no. 2 (1989): 189–91.

6. Holly Brubach, "Musclebound," *New Yorker* 68, no. 47 (1993): 32.

7. Gilles Deleuze and Félix Guattari, *Anti-Oedipus: Capitalism and Schizophrenia* (1972), trans. Robert Hurley, Mark Seem, and Helen R. Lane (1977; reprint, Minneapolis: University of Minnesota Press, 1983). See also Arthur W. Frank, "For a Sociology of the Body: An Analytical Review," in *The Body: Social Process and Cultural Theory*, ed. Mike Featherstone, Mike Hepworth, and Bryan S. Turner (Newbury Park, Calif.: Sage Publications, 1991), 36–102.

8. See Frank Dietz, "The Image of Medicine in Utopian and Dystopian Fiction," in *The Body and the Text: Comparative Essays in Literature and Medicine*, ed. Bruce Clarke and Wendell Aycock (Lubbock: Texas Tech University Press, 1990), 115–26; and René J. Dubos, "Medical Utopias," *Daedalus* 88, no. 3 (1959): 410–24.

9. See Sander L. Gilman, *Picturing Health and Illness: Images of Identity and Difference* (Baltimore: Johns Hopkins University Press, 1995).

10. Kathryn Pauly Morgan, "Women and the Knife: Cosmetic Surgery and the Colonization of Women's Bodies," *Hypatia* 6, no. 3 (1991): 25–53. See also Elizabeth Haiken, *Venus Envy: A History of Cosmetic Surgery* (Baltimore: Johns Hopkins University Press, 1997).

11. Geoffrey Cowley, "Attention: Aging Men," *Newsweek*, 16 September 1996, 75. For men, the top procedures are hair replacement and liposuction.

12. See "Bodybuilding: The Good, the Bad, and the Ugly," *Your Health and Fitness*, February/March 1989, 16–17; and, for an anthropological study, Alan M. Klein, *Little Big Men: Bodybuilding Subculture and Gender Construction* (Albany: SUNY Press, 1993).

13. George Hersey, *The Evolution of Allure: Sexual Selection from the Medici Venus to the Incredible Hulk* (Cambridge: MIT Press, 1996). Hersey includes a discussion of Fussell's book.

14. Samuel Wilson Fussell, *Muscle: Confessions of an Unlikely Bodybuilder* (New York: Avon Books, 1991), 23. Subsequent quotations will be documented within the text.

15. Deborah Blum, *Sex on the Brain: The Biological Differences between Men and Women* (New York: Viking, 1997), 100.

16. Sam Fussell, "Bodybuilder Americanus," *Michigan Quarterly Review* 32, no. 4 (1993): 583.

17. See Harold Mersky, "Body-Mind Dilemma in Chronic Pain," in *Chronic Pain: Psychosocial Factors in Rehabilitation*, ed. R. Roy and E. Tunks (Baltimore: Williams and Williams, 1982), 10–19.

18. Edward Shorter, *From Paralysis to Fatigue: A History of Psychosomatic Illness in the Modern Era* (New York: Free Press, 1992).

19. See, for example, Bryan S. Turner, "The Body Question: Recent Developments in Social Theory," in *Regulating Bodies: Essays in Medical Sociology* (New York: Routledge, 1992), 31–66; and Mike Featherstone, Mike Hepworth, and Bryan S. Turner, eds., *The Body: Social Process and Cultural Theory* (Newbury Park, Calif.: Sage Publications, 1991).

20. James H. Jones, *Bad Blood: The Tuskegee Syphilis Experiment* (New York: Free Press, 1981).

21. *Stedman's Medical Dictionary*, 25th ed. (London: Williams and Wilkins, 1990), s.v. "body."

22. See John M. Hoberman, *Mortal Engines: The Science of Performance and the Dehumanization of Sport* (New York: Free Press, 1992)—especially his chapter entitled "Faster, Higher, Stronger: A History of Doping in Sport."

23. "The fifties have seen many changes in the human situation; not least among them are the new attitudes towards those commodities which affect most directly the individual way of life—consumer goods. It is now accepted that saucepans, refrigerators, cars, vacuum cleaners, suitcases, radios, washing machines—all the paraphernalia of mid-century existence—should be designed by a specialist in the look of things" (Richard Hamilton, "Persuading Image" [1959], reprinted in *Collected Works 1953–1982* [London: Thames and Hudson, 1982], 135). See also Sarat Maharaj, "'A Liquid, Elemental Scattering': Marcel Duchamp and Richard Hamilton," in *Richard Hamilton* (London: Tate Gallery Publications, 1992), 40–48.

24. Emily Martin, *The Woman in the Body: A Cultural Analysis of Reproduction* (Boston: Beacon Press, 1987).

25. Nelly Oudshoorn, *Beyond the Natural Body: An Archaeology of Sex Hormones* (New York: Routledge, 1994).

26. Cherry Boone O'Neill, *Starving for Attention* (Minneapolis: CompCare Publishers, 1992), 26. Subsequent quotations will be documented within the text.

27.   Peter N. Stearns, *Fat History: Bodies and Beauty in the Modern West* (New York: New York University Press, 1997), 3.

28.   Leslie Heywood argues that anorexia replicates the binary "male-identified logic" (mind over body, masculine over feminine, white over black, thin over fat) that she identifies as dominant in the modernist aesthetic of Pound, Kafka, and Conrad, but I doubt that many scholars will adopt anorexia as a retrospective metaphor for modernism: misogyny and a rejection of aesthetic excess are as old as Catullus (*Dedication to Hunger: The Anorexic Esthetic in Modern Culture* [Berkeley: University of California Press, 1996]).

29.   Joan Jacobs Brumberg, *Fasting Girls: The Emergence of Anorexia Nervosa as a Modern Disease* (Cambridge: Harvard University Press, 1988). As Brumberg notes, anorexia was known to physicians as early as the 1870s.

30.   T. Gillato, "Mission Impossible," *People Magazine*, 3 June 1996, 71.

31.   Noelle Caskey, "Interpreting Anorexia Nervosa," in *The Female Body in Western Culture: Contemporary Perspectives*, ed. Susan Rubin Suleiman (Cambridge: Harvard University Press, 1986), 175–89.

32.   Noliwe M. Rooks, *Hair Raising: Beauty, Culture, and African American Women* (New Brunswick, N.J.: Rutgers University Press, 1996).

33.   For examples of both approaches, see Naomi Wolf, *The Beauty Myth: How Images of Beauty Are Used against Women* (New York: William Morrow, 1991); and Susan Bordo, *Unbearable Weight: Feminism, Western Culture, and the Body* (Berkeley: University of California Press, 1993).

34.   Kathy Davis, *Reshaping the Female Body: The Dilemma of Cosmetic Surgery* (New York: Routledge, 1995), 51. This paragraph is indebted to Davis's insightful analysis.

35.   Donald W. Lowe, *The Body in Late Capitalist USA* (Durham, N.C.: Duke University Press, 1995), 126.

36.   Rosalind Coward, "'Sexual Liberation' and the Family," *m/f* 1, no. 1 (1978): 16.

37.   Lowe, *The Body in Late Capitalist USA*, 166.

38.   See, among others, Morag MacSween, *Anorexic Bodies: A Feminist and Sociological Perspective on Anorexia Nervosa* (New York: Routledge, 1993).

39.   Jane E. Brody, "Personal Health," *New York Times*, 31 January 1996, B7. For a critique of biological psychiatry in its approach to eating disorders, see Denise Russell, "Female Bodies and Food: A Case of Ethics and Psychiatry," in *Troubled Bodies: Critical Perspectives on Postmodernism, Medical Ethics, and the Body*, ed. Paul A. Komesaroff (Durham, N.C.: Duke University Press, 1995), 222–34.

40.   For a discussion of anorexia as an auto-addiction, see Mary Ann Marrazzi and Elliott D. Luby, "Anorexia Nervosa as an Auto-Addiction: Clinical

and Basic Studies," in *The Psychobiology of Human Eating Disorders: Preclinical and Clinical Perspectives,* ed. Linda H. Schneider, Steven J. Cooper, and Katherine A. Halmi, Annals of the New York Academy of Sciences, vol. 575 (New York: New York Academy of Sciences, 1989), 545–47. For a discussion of the link between eating disorders and neurochemical function, see Bartley G. Hoebel, Sarah F. Leibowitz, and Luis Hernandez, "Neurochemistry of Anorexia and Bulimia," in *The Biology of Feast and Famine: Relevance to Eating Disorders,* ed. G. Harvey Anderson and Sidney H. Kennedy (New York: Academic Press, 1992), 38; and Katherine A. Halmi, ed., *Psychobiology and Treatment of Anorexia Nervosa and Bulimia Nervosa* (Washington, D.C.: American Psychiatric Press, 1992). For a discussion of anorexia and neuropeptide abnormalities, see Walter H. Kaye, "Neurotransmitter Abnormalities in Anorexia and Bulimia Nervosa," in *Biology of Feast and Famine,* 108–10. For a discussion of hyperactivity in anorexics, see Ancel Keys et al., *The Biology of Human Starvation,* 2 vols. (Minneapolis: University of Minnesota Press, 1950). For a discussion of seratonin activity in anorexics, see Kaye, "Neurotransmitter Abnormalities," in *Biology of Feast and Famine,* 111; and Hoebel, Leibowitz, and Hernandez, "Neurochemistry of Anorexia and Bulimia," 35–37. For a discussion of obsessive-compulsive symptoms in anorexics, see James I. Hudson et al., "Phenomenologic Relationship of Eating Disorders to Major Affective Disorder," *Psychiatric Research* 9, no. 4 (1983): 345–54; and Albert Rothenberg, "Differential Diagnosis of Anorexia Nervosa and Depressive Illness: A Review of 11 Studies," *Comparative Psychiatry* 29, no. 4 (1988): 427–32.

41.   Elaine Scarry, *The Body in Pain: The Making and Unmaking of the World* (New York: Oxford University Press, 1985).

42.   Don DeLillo, *White Noise* (New York: Viking Penguin, 1985), 227.

43.   See Michel Foucault, *The Birth of the Clinic: An Archaeology of Medical Perception* (1963), trans. A. M. Sheridan Smith (New York: Pantheon Books, 1973); and Drew Leder, ed., *The Body in Medical Thought and Practice* (Boston: Kluwer Academic Publishers, 1992).

44.   Paul K. Longmore, "Screening Stereotypes: Images of Disabled People in Television and Motion Pictures," in *Images of the Disabled, Disabling Images,* ed. Alan Gartner and Tom Joe (New York: Praeger, 1987), 74. For a historical perspective, see Harlan Hahn, "Disability and the Reproduction of Bodily Images: The Dynamics of Human Appearances," in *The Power of Geography: How Territory Shapes Social Life,* ed. Jennifer Wolch and Michael Dear (Boston: Unwin Hyman, 1989), 370–88.

45.   Roberta Galler, "The Myth of the Perfect Body," in *Pleasure and Danger: Exploring Female Sexuality,* ed. Carole S. Vance (Boston: Routledge and Kegan Paul, 1984), 165–72; and Carol Munter, "Fat and the Fantasy of Perfection," in *Pleasure and Danger,* 225–31.

46. Orlan, quoted in David Gale, "Flesh for Fantasy," *Icon Thoughtstyle Magazine*, June 1997, 119. On Orlan, see also Larissa MacFarquhar, "The Face Age," *New Yorker* 73, no. 20 (1997): 68–70. For a different but related version of the obsolete postmodern body, see Mark Dery, *Escape Velocity: Cyberculture at the End of the Century* (New York: Grove Press, 1996), especially the final chapter entitled "Cyborging the Body Politic: Obsolete Bodies and Posthuman Beings."

47. Jerome E. Bickenbach, *Physical Disability and Social Policy* (Toronto: University of Toronto Press, 1993), 61. See the chapter entitled "The Biomedical Model of Disablement" (61–92). On issues of public policy, see, for example, Marian Osterweis, Arthur Kleinman, and David Mechanic, eds., *Pain and Disability: Clinical, Behavioral, and Public Policy Perspectives* (Washington, D.C.: National Academy Press, 1987); and Han Emanuel, Eric H. de Gier, and Peter A. B. Kalker Konijn, *Disability Benefits: Factors Determining Application and Awards* (Greenwich, Conn.: JAI Press, 1987).

48. Wallace Stevens, "The Poems of Our Climate" (1938), in *The Collected Poems of Wallace Stevens* (New York: Alfred A. Knopf, 1954), 194.

49. Quoted in Deborah Hobler Kahane, *No Less a Woman: Ten Women Shatter the Myths about Breast Cancer* (New York: Prentice Hall Press, 1990), 100. See also Gelya Frank, "Sex Roles and Culture: Social and Personal Reactions to Breast Cancer," in *Women with Disabilities: Essays in Psychology, Culture, and Politics,* ed. Michelle Fine and Adrienne Asch (Philadelphia: Temple University Press, 1988), 72–89.

50. Reynolds Price, *A Whole New Life: An Illness and a Healing* (New York: Atheneum, 1994), 184.

51. K. R. Popper, "Utopia and Violence," *Hibbert Journal* 46 (1948): 115.

CHAPTER SIX: NEUROBIOLOGY
AND THE OBSCENE

1. Steven Lee Meyers, "Police and Music Clash on Obscenity," *New York Times,* 10 January 1992, A14.

2. The most noted feminist opponents of pornography are Andrea Dworkin and Catharine MacKinnon. Susan Sontag argues that "the pornographic imagination says something worth listening to, albeit in a degraded and often unrecognizable form" ("The Pornographic Imagination," in *Styles of Radical Will* [New York: Farrar, Straus and Giroux, 1969], 70). For a range of other perspectives, see Susan Rubin Suleiman, "Pornography, Transgression,

and the Avant Garde: Batailles's *Story of the Eye*," in *The Poetics of Gender*, ed. Nancy K. Miller (New York: Columbia University Press, 1986), 117–36; Lynne Segal, "Does Pornography Cause Violence? The Search for Evidence," in *Dirty Looks: Women, Pornography, Power*, ed. Pamela Church Gibson and Roma Gibson (Bloomington: Indiana University Press, 1993), 5–21; Diana E. H. Russell, ed., *Making Violence Sexy: Feminist Views on Pornography* (New York: Teachers College Press, 1993); Mary Caputi, *Voluptuous Yearnings: A Feminist Theory of the Obscene* (Lanham, Md.: Rowman and Littlefield, 1994); and Laura Kipnis, *Bound and Gagged: Pornography and the Politics of Fantasy in America* (New York: Grove Press, 1996).

3.   Quoted in Meyers, "Police and Music Clash," A14.

4.   Jerome A. Barron and C. Thomas Dienes, *First Amendment Law in a Nutshell* (St. Paul, Minn.: West Publishing Company, 1993), 87. See also Ian Hunter, David Saunders, and Dugald Williamson, *On Pornography: Literature, Sexuality and Obscenity Law* (New York: St. Martin's Press, 1993), 198–228.

5.   Steven Lee Myers, "Obscenity Laws Exist, but What Breaks Them?" *New York Times*, 19 January 1992, A4.

6.   For current biomedical thought, see Gerald S. Golden, "Tourette Syndrome: Recent Advances," *Neurologic Clinics* 8, no. 3 (1990): 705–14. Standard texts are F. S. Abuzzahab and F. O. Anderson, eds., *Gilles de la Tourette's Syndrome* (St. Paul, Minn.: Mason Publishing, 1976); Arnold J. Friedhoff and Thomas N. Chase, eds., *Gilles de la Tourette Syndrome* (New York: Raven Press, 1982); Donald J. Cohen, Ruth D. Brunn, and James F. Leckman, eds., *Tourette's Syndrome and Tic Disorders: Clinical Understanding and Treatment* (New York: John Wiley and Sons, 1988); Arthur K. Shapiro et al., eds., *Gilles de la Tourette Syndrome*, 2d ed. (New York: Raven Press, 1988); and Thomas N. Chase, Arnold J. Friedhoff, and Daniel J. Cohen, eds., *Tourette Syndrome: Genetics, Neurobiology and Treatment* (New York: Raven Press, 1992). Also helpful are two chapters in C. David Marsden and Stanley Fahn, eds., *Movement Disorders* 2 (London: Butterworths, 1987): Joseph Jankovic, "The Neurology of Tics" (383–405), and M. R. Trimble and M. M. Robertson, "The Psychopathology of Tics" (406–22).

7.   See Eric D. Caine, "Gilles de la Tourette's Syndrome: A Review of Clinical and Research Studies and Consideration of Future Directions for Investigation," *Archives of Neurology* 42, no. 4 (1985): 393–97; Harvey S. Singer and John T. Walkup, "Tourette Syndrome and Other Tic Disorders: Diagnosis, Pathophysiology, and Treatment," *Medicine* 70, no. 1 (1991): 15–32.

8.   In 1988 Shapiro et al. reported coprolalia in 32 percent of 213 patients (*Gilles de la Tourette Syndrome*, 2d. ed., 151). In the first edition, Shapiro et al. had reported coprolalia in 60 percent of 145 patients (*Gilles de la Tourette Syn-*

drome [1978], 146). A review article reports that coprolalia occurs in one-third of TS patients in the United Kingdom, 36 percent of Dutch TS patients, 26 percent of Danish TS patients, and 4 percent of Japanese TS patients (Mary M. Robertson, "The Gilles de la Tourette Syndrome: The Current Status," *British Journal of Psychiatry* 154 [February 1989]: 147–69). Joseph Jankovic and Haydee Rohaidy found verbal and mental coprolalia present in 44 percent of 112 patients with Tourette syndrome ("Motor, Behavioral, and Pharmacologic Findings in Tourette's Syndrome," *Canadian Journal of Neurological Sciences* 14, no. 3, suppl. [1987]: 541–46). For the occurrence of coprolalia in other neurological disorders, see Jankovic, "The Neurology of Tics," 394.

9.   For a discussion of the distress caused by coprolalia, see Arthur K. Shapiro et al., "Tourette's Syndrome: Summary of Data on 34 Patients," *Psychosomatic Medicine* 35, no. 5 (1973): 419–35; Shapiro et al., eds., *Gilles de la Tourette Syndrome*, 2d ed., 153.

10.   James F. Leckman et al., "Premonitory Urges in Tourette's Syndrome," *American Journal of Psychiatry* 150, no. 1 (1993): 98–102.

11.   Oliver Sacks, "A Surgeon's Life," *New Yorker* 68, no. 4 (1992): 85–94.

12.   Ruth Dowling Brunn and Cathy L. Budman, "The Natural History of Tourette Syndrome," in *Advances in Neurology*, ed. T. N. Chase, A. J. Friedhoff, and D. J. Cohen (New York: Raven Press, 1992), 58:1–7.

13.   On "gene-culture coevolution," see Charles J. Lumsden and Edward O. Wilson, "The Relation between Biological and Cultural Evolution," *Journal of Social and Biological Structure* 8, no. 4 (1985): 343–59. On "biologically prepared learning," see Roger S. Ulrich, "Biophilia, Biophobia, and Natural Landscapes," in *The Biophilia Hypothesis*, ed. Stephen R. Kellert and Edward O. Wilson (Washington, D.C.: Island Press, 1993), 73–137.

14.   Jankovic and Rohaidy, "Motor, Behavioral, and Pharmacologic Findings in Tourette's Syndrome," 541–46. Brunn and Budman report that patients in Japan show a far lower incidence of coprolalia than do patients in other countries, which, as I indicate later, strongly suggests a cultural influence ("The Natural History of Tourette Syndrome," 2).

15.   For an overview of how the brain processes language, see Sidney J. Segalowitz, ed., *Language Functions and Brain Organization* (New York: Academic Press, 1983); and Alfredo Ardila and Feggy Ostrosky-Solis, eds., *Brain Organization of Language and Cognitive Processes* (New York: Plenum Press, 1989). For evidence that speech perception and production are broadly distributed in the perisylvian area, see Sheila E. Blumstein, "The Neurobiology of the Sound Structure of Language," in *The Cognitive Neurosciences*, ed. Michael S. Gazzaniga (Cambridge: MIT Press, 1995), 927. For discussions of the role of the right hemisphere in language processing, see Monica S.

Hough, "Narrative Comprehension in Adults with Right and Left Hemisphere Brain-Damage: Theme Organization," *Brain and Language* 38, no. 2 (1990): 253–77; Hiram H. Brownell, "The Neuropsychology of Narrative Comprehension," *Aphasiology* 2, nos. 3–4 (1988): 247–50; and Wendy Wapner, Suzanne Hanby, and Howard Gardner, "The Role of the Right Hemisphere in the Apprehension of Complex Linguistic Materials," *Brain and Language* 14, no. 1 (1981): 15–33. For discussions of the importance of subcortical structures to speech, see George A. Ojemann, "Cortical Organization of Language," *Journal of Neuroscience* 11, no. 8 (1991): 2281–87; and Bryan W. Robinson, "Limbic Influences on Human Speech," *Annals of the New York Academy of Sciences* 280 (1976): 761–71. For discussions of category-specific naming deficits, see Harold Goodglass, "Agrammatism," in *Studies in Neurolinguistics*, ed. Haiganoosh Whitaker and Harry A. Whitaker (New York: Academic Press, 1976), 1:237–60; John Hart Jr., Rita Sloan Berndt, and Alfonzo Caramazza, "Category-Specific Naming Deficit Following Cerebral Infarction," *Nature* 316, no. 6027 (1985): 439–40; John Hart Jr. and Barry Gordon, "Neural Subsystems for Object Knowledge," *Nature* 359, no. 6390 (1992): 60–64; and Brenda C. Rapp and Alfonso Caramazza, "Disorders of Lexical Processing and the Lexicon," in *The Cognitive Neurosciences*, ed. Michael S. Gazzaniga (Cambridge: MIT Press, 1995), 905.

16.   J. A. Obeso, J. C. Rothwell, and C. D. Marsden, "Simple Tics in Gilles de la Tourette's Syndrome Are Not Prefaced by a Normal Premovement EEG Potential," *Journal of Neurology, Neurosurgery, and Psychiatry* 44, no. 8 (1981): 735–38.

17.   See John M. Berecz, *Understanding Tourette Syndrome, Obsessive Compulsive Disorder, and Related Problems* (New York: Springer Publishing, 1992), 102–4.

18.   Marc R. Nuwer, "Coprolalia as an Organic Symptom," in *Gilles de la Tourette Syndrome*, ed. Arnold J. Friedhoff and Thomas N. Chase (New York: Raven Press, 1982), 364.

19.   See Colin Martindale, "The Grammar of the Tic in Gilles de la Tourette's Syndrome," *Language and Speech* 19, no. 3 (1976): 266–75.

20.   See Lewis R. Baxter Jr. and Barry H. Guze, "Neuroimaging," in *Handbook of Tourette's Syndrome and Related Tic and Behavioral Disorders*, ed. Roger Kurlan (New York: Marcel Dekker, 1993), 289–304. Chief findings concern cerebral glucose metabolic rates.

21.   Peter Farb, *Word Play: What Happens When People Talk* (New York: Alfred A. Knopf, 1974), 85.

22.   See Timothy B. Jay, "A Maledicta Bibliography," *Maledicta* 9 (1986–1987): 207–24. One exception to the scholarly avoidance or marginalization of the obscene is Peter Michelson's study *Speaking the Unspeakable: A*

Poetics of Obscenity (Albany: SUNY Press, 1993)—a revision of his 1971 text *The Aesthetics of Pornography*.

23. Bruce Feirstein, "I'm No Prude, But . . . ," *TV Guide*, 1 January 1994, 22.

24. Paul Cameron, "Frequency and Kinds of Words in Various Social Settings, or What the Hell's Going On?" *Pacific Sociological Review* 12, no. 2 (1969): 101–4.

25. Murray S. Davis, *Smut: Erotic Reality/Obscene Ideology* (Chicago: University of Chicago Press, 1983), xxiii–xxv.

26. Elliott McGinnies, "Emotionality and Perceptual Defense," *Psychological Review* 56, no. 4 (1949): 244–51; Fred H. Nothman, "The Influence of Response Conditions on Recognition Thresholds for Tabu Words," *Journal of Abnormal and Social Psychology* 65, no. 3 (1962): 154–61; George S. Grosser and Anthony A. Walsh, "Sex Differences in the Differential Recall of Taboo and Neutral Words," *Journal of Psychology* 63 (May 1966): 219–27; Russell Foote and Jack Woodward, "A Preliminary Investigation of Obscene Language," *Journal of Psychology* 83 (March 1973): 263–75.

27. See Edmund Bergler, "Obscene Words," *Psychoanalytic Quarterly* 5 (1936): 226–48; Lawrence Hartmann, "Children's Use of Dirty Words," *Medical Aspects of Human Sexuality* 9 (September 1975): 111–12; Gail B. Butterfield and Earl C. Butterfield, "Lexical Codability and Age," *Journal of Verbal Learning and Verbal Behavior* 16, no. 1 (1977): 113–18.

28. Georges Schaltenbrand, "The Effects on Speech and Language of Stereotactical Stimulation in Thalamus and Corpus Callosum," *Brain and Language* 2, no. 1 (1975): 70–77. See also Bryan W. Robinson, "Limbic Influences on Human Speech," in *Origins and Evolution of Language and Speech*, ed. Stevan R. Harnad et al. (New York: New York Academy of Sciences, 1976), 761–71; and D. Carleton Gajdusek, Guy M. McKhann, and Liana C. Bolis, eds., *Evolution and Neurology of Language*, Discussions in Neuroscience, vol. 10, nos. 1–2 (Amsterdam: Elsevier Science, 1994).

29. See Ronald E. Meyers, "Comparative Neurology of Vocalization and Speech: Proof of a Dichotomy," *Annals of the New York Academy of Sciences* 280 (1976): 745–57. For evidence of prefrontal involvement in the ultrasonic vocalization of rats, see Edward J. Neafsey, "Prefrontal Cortical Control of the Autonomic Nervous System: Anatomical and Physiological Observations," in *The Prefrontal Cortex: Its Structure, Function and Pathology*, ed. H. B. M. Uylings et al., Progress in Brain Research, vol. 85 (New York: Elsevier Science, 1990), 156.

30. Timothy Jay, "The Role of Obscene Speech in Psychology," *Interfaces: Linguistics, Psychology, and Health Therapeutics* 12, no. 3 (1985): 75–91.

31. David E. Comings and Brenda G. Comings, "Tourette Syndrome: Clinical and Psychological Aspects of 250 Cases," *American Journal of Human Ge-*

netics 37, no. 3 (1985): 435–50: "TS can be viewed as a 'disinhibition syndrome' due to release of the inhibiting neuronal pathways" (440).

32.   See, for example, Walle J. H. Nauta, "Limbic Innervation of the Striatum," in *Gilles de la Tourette Syndrome*, ed. Arnold J. Friedhoff and Thomas N. Chase (New York: Raven Press, 1982), 41–47; and Reuven Sandyk, "A Case of Tourette's Syndrome with Midbrain Involvement," *International Journal of Neuroscience* 43, nos. 3–4 (1988): 171–75.

33.   Colin Martindale, "Syntactic and Semantic Correlates of Verbal Tics in Gilles de la Tourette's Syndrome: A Quantitative Case Study," *Brain and Language* 4, no. 2 (1977): 245; Trimble and Robertson, "The Psychopathology of Tics," 420.

34.   Peter Stallybrass and Allon White, *The Politics and Poetics of Transgression* (Ithaca, N.Y.: Cornell University Press, 1986). The pattern persists well outside bourgeois life; obscene narratives are a stronghold of cultural expression from Chaucer to Native American tales. See Panel on Folk Literature and the Obscene, *Journal of American Folklore* 75, no. 297 (1962): 189–226.

35.   Chief Justice Desmond, quoted in Charles Rembar, *The End of Obscenity: The Trials of "Lady Chatterley," "Tropic of Cancer," and "Fanny Hill"* (New York: Random House, 1968), 201. Rembar was the chief defense attorney for Grove Press during these landmark prosecutions.

36.   Henry Miller, *Obscenity and the Law of Reflection* (1945), in *Henry Miller on Writing*, ed. Thomas H. Moore (New York: New Directions, 1964), 186. The best study of Miller and obscenity is still Ihab Hassan's *The Literature of Silence: Henry Miller and Samuel Beckett* (New York: Alfred A. Knopf, 1967).

37.   Nuwer, "Coprolalia as an Organic Symptom," 363–68. In contrast to Nuwer, John M. Berecz has argued recently that Tourette syndrome is a functional rather than biological disorder, properly approached through the paradigm of developmental psychology (*Understanding Tourette Syndrome, Obsessive Compulsive Disorder, and Related Problems: A Developmental and Catastrophic Theory Perspective* [New York: Springer, 1992]).

38.   For a rare biopsychosocial case study of Tourette syndrome, see Bernard C. Meyer and Diane Rose, "Remarks on the Etiology of Gilles de la Tourette's Syndrome," *Journal of Nervous and Mental Disease* 174, no. 7 (1986): 387–96. Oliver Sacks agrees: "Neither a biological nor a psychological nor a moral-social viewpoint is adequate; we must see Tourette's simultaneously from all three perspectives—as a biopsychosocial disorder" ("A Surgeon's Life," 85). See also Sacks's essay "Tourette's Syndrome: A Human Condition," in *Handbook of Tourette Syndrome*, ed. Roger Kurlan (New York: Marcel Dekker, 1993), 509–14.

39.   Henry Miller, *Tropic of Cancer* (1934; reprint, New York: Grove Press, 1961), 249.

40.   Robert A. Hahn and Arthur Kleinman, "Belief as Pathogen, Belief as Medicine: 'Voodoo Death' and the 'Placebo Phenomenon' in Anthropological Perspective," *Medical Anthropology Quarterly* 4, no. 4 (1983): 17.

41.   Henry Miller, "Obscenity in Literature" (1957), in *Henry Miller on Writing,* ed. Thomas H. Moore (New York: New Directions, 1964), 195.

42.   Weston La Barre, "Obscenity: An Anthropological Appraisal," *Law and Contemporary Problems* 20, no. 4 (1955): 541–43.

43.   "Iran Lawmakers Pass Death Penalty for Dealers in Obscene Videos," *New York Times,* 21 December 1993, A4.

44.   Stephen Kaplan and Rachel Kaplan, *Cognition and Environment: Functioning in an Uncertain World* (Ann Arbor, Mich.: Ulrich's Bookstore, 1981), 139. For an extended development of their thinking, see *The Experience of Nature: A Psychological Perspective* (New York: Cambridge University Press, 1989).

45.   Among cognate studies, see Terry Winograd and Fernando Flores, *Understanding Computers and Cognition: A New Foundation for Design* (Norwood, N.J.: Ablex Corporation, 1986); and Humberto R. Maturana and Francisco J. Varela, *The Tree of Knowledge: The Biological Roots of Human Understanding,* rev. ed. (Boston: Shambhala, 1992). For an evolutionary perspective on the development of human language, see Steven Pinker, *The Language Instinct* (New York: William Morrow, 1994).

46.   Ellen Dissanayake, *Homo Aestheticus: Where Art Comes From and Why* (New York: Free Press, 1992), xvi. For a nonbiological view of play and aesthetic behavior, see J. Huizinga, *Homo Ludens: A Study of the Play-Element in Culture* (1944), trans. anon. (1950; reprint, Boston: Beacon Press, 1955); and Jacques Ehrmann, "*Homo Ludens* Revisited," in *Game, Play, Literature,* ed. Jacques Ehrmann (Boston: Beacon Press, 1968), 31–57.

47.   Walter Burkert, *Creation of the Sacred: Tracks of Biology in Early Religions* (Cambridge: Harvard University Press, 1996).

48.   For a comprehensive study of the evidence that underlies evolutionary psychology, see Steven Pinker, *How the Mind Works* (New York: W. W. Norton, 1997).

49.   For an extended study, see Jørgen Rudd, *Taboo: A Study of Malagasy Customs and Beliefs* (New York: Humanities Press, 1960).

50.   Jeffrey A. Gray, *The Neuropsychology of Anxiety: An Enquiry into the Functions of the Septo-Hippocampal System* (Oxford: Clarendon Press, 1982), 443. Gray discusses rituals of anxiety and obsessive-compulsive behavior such as hand washing, rituals that also appear in the various touching and counting manias of Tourette syndrome.

51.   Mary Douglas, *Purity and Danger: An Analysis of the Concepts of Pollution and Taboo* (1966; reprint, New York: Ark Paperbacks, 1984), 35.

52.   Wolf Leslau, "Taboo Expressions in Ethiopia," *American Anthropologist* 61, no. 1 (1959): 105–7.

53.   Mary R. Haas, "Interlingual Word Taboos," *American Anthropologist* 53, no. 3 (1951): 338–44.

54.   "Fear and Loathing in Bochum," *Discover*, 8 April 1997, 22.

55.   "[I]t is important to bear in mind that the feature to be explained need not itself be adaptive. It is sometimes sufficient to be able to demonstrate that the feature, while itself not obviously adaptive, would arise as a by-product of the emergence of other features which are adaptive. This avoids the fallacy sometimes called 'strict adaptationism'" (James R. Hurford, "Evolutionary Modelling of Language," in *Evolution and Neurology of Language*, ed. D. Carleton Gajdusek, Guy M. McKhann, and Liana C. Bolis, Discussions in Neuroscience, vol. 10, nos. 1–2 [Amsterdam: Elsevier Science, 1994], 159). I do not propose to have "demonstrated" the adaptive qualities of obscenity, but I hope my argument will spur the search for additional neurolinguistic and neuropsychological evidence.

56.   For a start, see Geoffrey Hughes, *Swearing: A Social History of Foul Language, Oaths, and Profanity in English* (Oxford: Basil Blackwell, 1991); and David Lawton, *Blasphemy* (Philadelphia: University of Pennsylvania Press, 1993).

57.   Ashley Montagu, *The Anatomy of Swearing* (New York: Macmillan, 1967), 124.

58.   H. L. Mencken, "American Profanity," *American Speech* 19 (1944): 23–24; and Timothy Jay, *Cursing in America* (Philadelphia: John Benjamins Publishing Company, 1992).

59.   *The Compact Edition of the Oxford English Dictionary* (New York: Oxford University Press, 1971), s.v. "bowdlerize" and "prostitute"; Walter M. Kendrick, *The Secret Museum: Pornography in Modern Culture* (New York: Viking, 1987); and, for earlier trends, see Lynn Hunt, ed., *The Invention of Pornography: Obscenity and the Origins of Modernity, 1500–1800* (New York: Zone Books, 1993).

60.   E. Scott Baudhuin, "Obscene Language and Evaluative Response: An Empirical Study," *Psychological Reports* 32, no. 2 (1973): 399–402.

61.   Herbert Basedow, *The Australian Aboriginal* (Adelaide: F. W. Preece and Sons, 1925), 165.

62.   Mervyn S. Sanders et al., "What Is the Significance of Crude Language during Sex Relations?" *Medical Aspects of Human Sexuality* 3, no. 8 (1969): 8–14.

63.   Jane Gross, "School Is Newest Arena for Sex-Harassment Concerns," *New York Times*, 11 March 1992, A16.

64.   Douglas, *Purity and Danger*, 135.

65.   Miller, *Obscenity and the Law of Reflection*, 189.

CHAPTER SEVEN: THE PLOT OF SUFFERING

1.   Larry Kramer, "1,112 and Counting" (1983), reprinted in *Reports from the Holocaust: The Making of an AIDS Activist* (New York: St. Martin's Press, 1989), 33. For a critique of Kramer's manner as inadvertently reinforcing oppressive views of gays, see David Bergman, "Larry Kramer and the Rhetoric of AIDS," in *Gaiety Transfigured: Gay Self-Representation in American Literature* (Madison: University of Wisconsin Press, 1991), 122–38.

2.   World Health Organization, *In Point of Fact*, no. 4 (Geneva: WHO, 1991); U.N. figures were reported on the CBS Evening News, 26 November 1997. See Mirko D. Grmek, *History of AIDS: Emergence and Origin of a Modern Pandemic* (1989), trans. Russell C. Maulitz and Jacalyn Duffin (Princeton: Princeton University Press, 1990). For a critique of analogies that interpret AIDS through past plagues, as if AIDS were radically discontinuous with current patterns of disease, see Elizabeth Fee and Daniel M. Fox, "The Contemporary Historiography of AIDS," *Journal of Social History* 23, no. 2 (1989): 303–14. The quotation in the text comes from Kramer, *Reports from the Holocaust*, 145.

3.   Jacques Derrida, "The Rhetoric of Drugs" (1989), trans. Michael Israel, *differences: A Journal of Feminist Cultural Studies* 5, no. 1 (1993): 20.

4.   See John Preston, ed., *Personal Dispatches: Writers Confront AIDS* (New York: St. Martin's Press, 1989); Franklin Brooks and Timothy F. Murphy, "Annotated Bibliography of AIDS Literature, 1982–91," in *Writing AIDS: Gay Literature, Language, and Analysis*, ed. Timothy F. Murphy and Suzanne Poirier (New York: Columbia University Press, 1993), 321–39; and Anne Hunsaker Hawkins, *Reconstructing Illness: Studies in Pathography* (West Lafayette, Ind.: Purdue University Press, 1993).

5.   Alexandra Juhasz, "Knowing AIDS through the Televised Science Documentary," in *Women and AIDS: Psychological Perspectives*, ed. Corinne Squire (Newbury Park, Calif.: Sage Publications, 1993), 150–64; and Alexandra Juhasz and Catherine Saalfield, *AIDS TV: Identity, Community, and Alternative Video* (Durham, N.C.: Duke University Press, 1995). For early coverage of AIDS on British television, see Simon Watney, "AIDS on Television," in *Policing Desire: Pornography, AIDS, and the Media* (Minneapolis: University of Minnesota Press, 1987), 97–122; for American television, see Paula A. Treichler, "AIDS Narratives on Television: Whose Story?" in *Writing AIDS: Gay Literature, Language, and Analysis*, ed. Timothy F. Murphy and Suzanne Poirier (New York: Columbia University Press, 1993), 161–99; Paula A. Treichler, "Seduced and Terrorized: AIDS and Network Television," in *A Leap in the Dark: AIDS, Art, and Contemporary Cultures*, ed. Allan Klusacek and Ken Morrison (Montreal: Véhicule Press, 1992), 136–51; and James Kinsella, *Covering the Plague: AIDS and the American Media* (New Brunswick, N.J.: Rutgers University Press, 1989).

6.   On cultural aspects, see, among many others, Ronald Frankenberg, "One Epidemic or Three? Cultural, Social, and Historical Aspects of the AIDS Pandemic," in *AIDS: Social Representations, Social Practices*, ed. Peter Aggleton, Graham Hart, and Peter Davies (Philadelphia: Falmer Press, 1989), 21–38.

7.   For the conflict of voices, see Judith Williamson, "Every Virus Tells a Story: The Meanings of HIV and AIDS," in *Taking Liberties: AIDS and Cultural Politics*, ed. Erica Carter and Simon Watney (London: Serpent's Tail, 1989), 69–80; Lee Edelman, "The Plague of Discourse: Politics, Literary Theory, and AIDS," in *Displacing Homophobia: Gay Male Perspectives in Literature and Culture*, ed. Ronald R. Butters, John M. Clum, and Michael Moon (Durham, N.C.: Duke University Press, 1989), 289–305; Thomas Yingling, "AIDS in America: Postmodern Governance, Identity, and Experience," in *Inside/Out: Lesbian Theories, Gay Theories*, ed. Diana Fuss (New York: Routledge, 1991), 291–310; and, on the threats to subjectivity, Alexander García Düttmann, *At Odds with AIDS: Thinking and Talking about a Virus*, trans. Peter Gilgen and Conrad Scott-Curtis (Stanford: Stanford University Press, 1996). For the visual rhetoric of public health posters, see Sander L. Gilman, "The Beautiful Body and AIDS: The Image of the Body at Risk at the Close of the Twentieth Century," in *Picturing Health and Illness: Images of Identity and Difference* (Baltimore: Johns Hopkins University Press, 1995), 115–72.

8.   Paula A. Treichler, "AIDS, Homophobia, and Biomedical Discourse: An Epidemic of Signification," *Cultural Studies* 1, no. 3 (1987): 263–305; "AIDS, Gender, and Biomedical Discourse: Current Contests for Meaning," in *AIDS: The Burdens of History*, ed. Elizabeth Fee and Daniel M. Fox (Berkeley: University of California Press, 1988), 190–266; "AIDS, HIV, and the Cultural Construction of Reality," in *The Time of AIDS: Social Analysis, Theory, and Method* (Newbury Park, Calif.: Sage Publications, 1992), 65–98; and "How to Use a Condom: Bedtime Stories for the Transcendental Signifier," in *Disciplinarity and Dissent in Cultural Studies*, ed. Cary Nelson and Dilip Parameshwar Gaonkar (New York: Routledge, 1996), 347–96. A collection of Treichler's work is forthcoming in *How to Have Theory in an Epidemic: Cultural Chronicles of AIDS* (Durham, N.C.: Duke University Press).

9.   For important work within the medical community, see Arthur Kleinman, *The Illness Narratives: Suffering, Healing, and the Human Condition* (New York: Basic Books, 1988); Eric J. Cassell, *The Nature of Suffering and the Goals of Medicine* (New York: Oxford University Press, 1991); and Nathan I. Cherney, Nessa Coyle, and Kathleen M. Foley, "Suffering in the Advanced Cancer Patient: A Definition and Taxonomy," *Journal of Palliative Care* 10, no. 2 (1994): 57–70. The best discussion of religious views is still John Bowker, *Problems of Suffering in Religions of the World* (Cambridge: Cambridge University Press, 1970).

10.   Jay M. Weiss, "Psychological Factors in Stress and Disease," *Scientific American* 226, no. 6 (1972): 104–13. See especially Christopher Peterson, Steven F. Maier, and Martin E. P. Seligman, "The Biology of Learned Helplessness," in *Learned Helplessness: A Theory for the Age of Personal Control* (New York: Oxford University Press, 1993), 60–97. Also, Martin E. P. Seligman, *Helplessness: On Depression, Development, and Death* (1975; reprint, New York: W. H. Freeman, 1992); and Mario Mikulincer, *Human Learned Helplessness: A Coping Perspective* (New York: Plenum Press, 1994).

11.   C. Richard Chapman and Jonathan Gavrin, "Suffering and Its Relationship to Pain," *Journal of Palliative Care* 9, no. 2 (1993): 5–13.

12.   Laurel Archer Copp, "The Spectrum of Suffering" (1974), reprinted in *American Journal of Nursing* 90, no. 8 (1990): 35–39; Patrick L. Starck and John P. McGovern, eds., *The Hidden Dimension of Illness: Human Suffering* (New York: National League for Nursing Press, 1992); and Judith M. Saunders, "HIV/AIDS and Suffering," in *Suffering*, ed. Betty Rolling Ferrell (Boston: Jones and Bartlett, 1996), 95–119.

13.   Walter J. Slatoff, *The Look of Distance: Reflections on Suffering and Sympathy in Modern Literature—Auden to Agee, Whitman to Woolf* (Columbus: Ohio State University Press, 1985), 233.

14.   See David H. Richter, *Falling into Theory: Conflicting Views on Reading Literature* (New York: St. Martin's Press, 1994).

15.   For explorations into narrative and suffering, see Kleinman, *The Illness Narratives*; Harold Schweitzer, *Suffering and the Remedy of Art* (Albany: SUNY Press, 1997); and, most important, Arthur Kleinman, Veena Das, and Margaret Lock, eds., *Social Suffering* (Berkeley: University of California Press, 1997).

16.   T. S. Eliot, "The Three Voices of Poetry" (1953), in *On Poetry and Poets* (New York: Farrar, Straus and Cudahy, 1957).

17.   Donald Wesling and Tadeusz Slawek discuss "postmodern indeterminate voice" in *Literary Voice: The Calling of Jonah* (Albany: SUNY Press, 1995), 184–202. For a more philosophical discussion, attractively rooted in the physiology of human vocalization, see David Applebaum, *Voice* (Albany: SUNY Press, 1990).

18.   On silence, see Elaine Scarry, *The Body in Pain: The Making and Unmaking of the World* (New York: Oxford University Press, 1985), 42–45. Voice and representation are discussed by several contributors in Mary-Jo DelVecchio Good et al., eds., *Pain as Human Experience: An Anthropological Perspective* (Berkeley: University of California Press, 1992).

19.   On suffering, see Thomas Dilworth, "Auden's 'Musée des Beaux Arts,'" *Explicator* 49, no. 3 (1991): 181–83.

20.   Elisabeth Hansot, "A Letter from a Patient's Daughter," *Annals of Internal Medicine* 125, no. 2 (1996): 149–51.

21.   On suffering, see Cho-hee Joh, "Beckett's Capacity for Differentiation: Some Observations on Reading His Works," *Journal of English Language and Literature* 35, no. 4 (1989): 759–73.

22.   See Paul Fussell, *The Great War and Modern Memory* (New York: Oxford University Press, 1975).

23.   See Susan Sipple, "'Witness [to] the Suffering of Women': Poverty and Sexual Transgression in Meridel le Sueur's *Women on the Breadlines*," in *Feminism, Bakhtin, and the Dialogic*, ed. Dale M. Bauer and Susan Jarret McKinstry (Albany: SUNY Press, 1991), 135–53; John Knott, *Discourses of Martyrdom in English Literature, 1563–1694* (Cambridge: Cambridge University Press, 1994); and Katherine Heinrichs, "Love and Hell: The Denizens of Hades in the Love Poems of the Middle Ages," *Neophilologus* 73, no. 4 (1989): 593–604.

24.   Joyce Carol Oates, "Remarks . . . Accepting the National Book Award in Fiction" (1970), in Mary Kathryn Grant, *The Tragic Vision of Joyce Carol Oates* (Durham, N.C.: Duke University Press, 1978), 164.

25.   See Larry Dossey, *Healing Words: The Power of Prayer and the Practice of Medicine* (San Francisco: Harper San Francisco, 1993) and *Prayer Is Good Medicine* (San Francisco: Harper San Francisco, 1996).

26.   M. M. Bakhtin, *Speech Genres and Other Late Essays*, ed. Caryl Emerson and Michael Holquist, trans. Vern W. McGee (Austin: University of Texas Press, 1986).

27.   Jacques Derrida, "The Law of Genre," *Critical Inquiry* 7, no. 1 (1980): 65. Derrida offers this view as a "hypothesis."

28.   On genre and narrative change, see Ralph Cohen, "History and Genre," *New Literary History* 17, no. 2 (1986): 203–18.

29.   Lawrence L. Langer, *Holocaust Testimonies: The Ruins of Memory* (New Haven: Yale University Press, 1991), 35. Langer emphasizes the difference between written (literary) accounts by Holocaust survivors and oral accounts (129), but he also observes how interviewers can "control and shape" (9) the memories of Holocaust survivors, how survivors lean forward to address both the camera and posterity (19), how interviewer and survivor duel about where a testimony should end (28), how interviews almost always begin and end in the same way (67). "Survivor testimony" is now a distinct postmodern subgenre, born of our specific historical experience with the disasters of World War II, adhering to informal conventions governing questions, content, setting, gesture, emotion, and even camera angle (since historians and archivists now often work with film).

30.   E. D. Hirsch Jr., *Validity in Interpretation* (New Haven: Yale University Press, 1967), 4.

31.   See Thomas O. Beebee, *The Ideology of Genre: A Comparative Study of Generic Instability* (University Park: Penn State University Press, 1994).

32.   See two books by Hayden White, *Metahistory: The Historical Imagination in Nineteenth-Century Europe* (Baltimore: Johns Hopkins University Press, 1974) and *The Content of the Form: Narrative Discourse and Historical Representation* (Baltimore: Johns Hopkins University Press, 1987).

33.   Thomas Gould, *The Ancient Quarrel between Poetry and Philosophy* (Princeton: Princeton University Press, 1990), ix.

34.   For a non-Western view, see Gananath Obeyesekere, "Depression, Buddhism, and the Work of Culture in Sri Lanka," in *Culture and Depression: Studies in the Anthropology and Cross-Cultural Psychiatry of Affect and Disorder,* ed. Arthur Kleinman and Byron Good (Berkeley: University of California Press, 1985), 134–52.

35.   M. M. Bakhtin, *The Dialogic Imagination: Four Essays by M. M. Bakhtin,* ed. Michael Holquist, trans. Caryl Emerson and Michael Holquist (Austin: University of Texas Press, 1981); and Tzvetan Todorov, *Mikhail Bakhtin: The Dialogical Principle* (1981), trans. Wlad Godzich (Minneapolis: University of Minnesota Press, 1984).

36.   "Clarification" is one definition of the notorious and much debated Aristotelian term *catharsis* (see *Aristotle's Poetics: A Translation and a Commentary for Students of Literature,* trans. Leon Golden, commentary by O. B. Hardison Jr. [Englewood Cliffs, N.J.: Prentice-Hall, 1968]).

37.   Gustavo Gutiérrez, *A Theology of Liberation: History, Politics, and Salvation* (1971), trans. Caridad Inda and John Eagleson (Maryknoll, N.Y.: Orbis Books, 1973).

38.   See Elizabeth Fee and Daniel M. Fox, eds., *AIDS: The Burdens of History* (Berkeley: University of California Press, 1988); Douglas Crimp, ed., *AIDS: Cultural Analysis/Cultural Activism* (Cambridge: MIT Press, 1988); Richard A. Berk, *The Social Impact of AIDS in the U.S.* (Cambridge, Mass.: Abt Books, 1988); Ronald Byer, *Private Acts, Social Consequences: AIDS and the Politics of Public Health* (New York: Free Press, 1989); Douglas A. Feldman, ed., *Culture and AIDS* (New York: Praeger, 1990); Richard Ulack and William F. Skinner, eds., *AIDS and the Social Sciences* (Lexington: University Press of Kentucky, 1991); Marie A. Muir, *The Environmental Context of AIDS* (New York: Praeger, 1991); Joan Huber and Beth E. Schneider, eds., *The Social Context of AIDS* (Newbury Park, Calif.: Sage Publications, 1992); Michaël Pollak, with Geneviève Paicheler and Janine Pierret, *AIDS: A Problem for Sociological Research* (Newbury Park, Calif.: Sage Publications, 1992); and Hung Fan, Ross F. Conner, and Luis P. Villarreal, *AIDS: Science and Society* (Boston: Jones and Bartlett, 1996).

39.   Charles E. Rosenberg, *Explaining Epidemics and Other Studies in the History of Medicine* (Cambridge: Cambridge University Press, 1992), 292.

40.   Susan Sontag, *AIDS and Its Metaphors* (New York: Farrar, Straus and Giroux, 1989), 17.

41.   Michael D. Quam, "The Sick Role, Stigma, and Pollution: The Case of AIDS," in *Culture and AIDS*, ed. Douglas A. Feldman (New York: Praeger, 1990), 45–54. See also Gregory M. Herek, ed., *Stigma and Sexual Orientation: Understanding Prejudice against Lesbians, Gay Men, and Bisexuals* (Thousand Oaks, Calif.: Sage Publications, 1998).

42.   S. C. McCombie, "AIDS in Cultural, Historic, and Epidemiologic Context," in *Culture and AIDS*, ed. Douglas A. Feldman (New York: Praeger, 1990), 15–16.

43.   Paul E. Farmer, *AIDS and Accusation: Haiti and the Geography of Blame* (Berkeley: University of California Press, 1992). See also Paula A. Treichler, "AIDS and HIV Infection in the Third World: A First World Chronicle," in *Remaking History*, ed. Barbara Kruger and Phil Mariani, Dia Art Foundation Discussions in Contemporary Culture, no. 4 (Seattle: Bay Press, 1989), 31–86.

44.   Christopher C. Taylor, "AIDS and the Pathogenesis of Metaphor," in *Culture and AIDS*, ed. Douglas A. Feldman (New York: Praeger, 1990), 58.

45.   Quoted in Mary Fisher, *I'll Not Go Quietly: Mary Fisher Speaks Out* (New York: Scribner, 1995), 92.

46.   Cindy Patton, " 'With Champagne and Roses': Women at Risk from/in AIDS Discourse," in *Women and AIDS: Psychological Perspectives*, ed. Corinne Squire (Newbury Park, Calif.: Sage Publications, 1993), 165–87; and Jenny Kitzinger, "Visible and Invisible Women in AIDS Discourses," in *AIDS: Setting a Feminist Agenda*, ed. Lesley Doyal, Jennie Naidoo, and Tamsin Wilton (London: Taylor and Francis, 1994), 95–109.

47.   "The Denver Principles: Founding Statement of People with AIDS/ARC" (1983), in The ACT UP/New York Women and AIDS Book Group, *Women, AIDS, and Activism* (Boston: South End Press, 1990), 239–40.

48.   Randy Shilts, "AIDSpeak Spoken Here," in *And the Band Played On: Politics, People, and the AIDS Epidemic* (New York: St. Martin's Press, 1987), 314–23. Shilts notes: "the new syntax allowed gay political leaders to address and largely determine public health policy in the coming years, because public health officials quickly mastered AIDSpeak, and it was fundamentally a political tongue" (315).

49.   Max Navarre, "Fighting the Victim Label," in *AIDS: Cultural Analysis/Cultural Activism*, ed. Douglas Crimp (Cambridge: MIT Press, 1988), 145. Douglas Crimp argues for the combination of mourning *and* activism ("Mourning and Militancy," *October* 51 [1989]: 3–18).

50.   Arthur W. Frank, *The Wounded Storyteller: Body, Illness, and Ethics* (Chicago: University of Chicago Press, 1995), 97–114.

51.   Judy Elsley, "The Rhetoric of the NAMES Project AIDS Quilt: Reading the Text(ile)," in *AIDS: The Literary Response*, ed. Emmanuel S. Nelson (New York: Twayne Publishers, 1992), 187–96.

52.   Gregory Woods, "AIDS to Remembrance: The Uses of Elegy," in *AIDS:*

The Literary Response, ed. Emmanuel S. Nelson (New York: Twayne Publishers, 1992), 155–66.

53. George M. Carter, *ACT UP: The AIDS War and Activism,* Open Magazine Pamphlet Series, no. 15 (Westfield, N.J.: Open Media, 1992), 18.

54. Fan, Conner, and Villarreal, *AIDS: Science and Society,* 204–5. See also, Gilbert Elbaz, *New York ACT UP* (Ph.D. diss., City University of New York, 1993). ACT UP also lobbied in a fairly traditional and effective manner for changes in government health care policies.

55. John M. Clum, "'And Once I Had It All': AIDS Narratives and Memories of an American Dream," in *Writing AIDS: Gay Literature, Language, and Analysis,* ed. Timothy F. Murphy and Suzanne Poirier (New York: Columbia University Press, 1993), 220. This paragraph is indebted to Clum's account.

56. Stanley Aronowitz, "Against the Liberal State: ACT-UP and the Emergence of Postmodern Politics," in *Social Postmodernism: Beyond Identity Politics,* ed. Linda Nicholson and Steven Seidman (Cambridge: Cambridge University Press, 1995), 361.

57. See Arthur Kleinman and Joan Kleinman, "The Appeal of Experience; The Dismay of Images: Cultural Appropriations of Suffering in Our Times," in *Social Suffering,* ed. Arthur Kleinman, Veena Das, and Margaret Lock (Berkeley: University of California Press, 1997), 1–23.

58. On moral community, see Tom Regan, *The Thee Generation: Reflections on the Coming Revolution* (Philadelphia: Temple University Press, 1991), 20.

CHAPTER EIGHT: ILLNESS IN THE TIME
OF DISNEY

1. Jean Baudrillard, *America* (1986), trans. Chris Word (New York: Verso, 1988), 55; Umberto Eco, "Travels in Hyperreality," in *Travels in Hyperreality: Essays* (1983), trans. William Weaver (New York: Harcourt Brace Jovanovich, 1986), 43–48; and Louis Marin, *Utopics: Spatial Play* (1973), trans. Robert A. Vollrath (Atlantic Highlands, N.J.: Humanities Press, 1984), 239–57.

2. Douglas Gomery, "Disney's Business History: A Reinterpretation," in *Disney Discourse: Producing the Magic Kingdom,* ed. Eric Smoodin (New York: Routledge, 1994), 71–86.

3. Mitsuhiro Yoshimoto, "Images of Empire: Tokyo Disneyland and Japanese Cultural Imperialism," in *Disney Discourse: Producing the Magic Kingdom,* ed. Eric Smoodin (New York: Routledge, 1994), 186.

4. Marin, *Utopics,* 240; Eco, "Travels in Hyperreality," 44; Baudrillard, *America,* 55.

5. Michael Wood, *America in the Movies* (New York: Basic Books, 1975), 18.

6. Joseph Turow and Lisa Coe, "Curing Television's Ills: The Portrayal of

Health Care," *Journal of Communication* 35, no. 4 (1985): 36–51. See also Nancy Signorelli, "Television and Health: Images and Impact," in *Mass Communication and Public Health: Complexities and Conflicts,* ed. Charles Atkin and Lawrence Wallack (Newbury Park, Calif.: Sage Publications, 1990), 96–113.

7.   Among the few exceptions, see Dena Andre, Philip Brookman, and Jane Livingston, eds., *Hospice: A Photographic Inquiry* (Boston: Little Brown and Company, 1996).

8.   Sherwin B. Nuland, *How We Die: Reflections on Life's Final Chapter* (New York: Alfred A. Knopf, 1994), 67.

9.   Douglas J. Lanska, "Geographic Distribution of Stroke Mortality among Immigrants to the United States," *Stroke* 28, no. 1 (1997): 53–57.

10.   George Howard et al., "Role of Social Class in Excess Black Stroke Mortality," *Stroke* 26, no. 10 (1995): 1759–63.

11.   Angela Colantonio et al., "Psychosocial Predictors of Stroke Outcomes in an Elderly Population," *Journal of Gerontology* 48, no. 5 (1993): S261–S268; Sheldon Cohen et al., "Social Ties and Susceptibility to the Common Cold," *JAMA* 277, no. 24 (1997): 1940–44; Thomas A. Glass and George L. Maddox, "The Quality and Quantity of Social Support: Stroke Recovery as Psycho-Social Transition," *Social Science and Medicine* 34, no. 11 (1992): 1249–61; Philip L. P. Morris et al., "The Relationship between the Perception of Social Support and Post-Stroke Depression in Hospitalized Patients," *Psychiatry* 54, no. 3 (1991): 306–16.

12.   Gary M. Williams and Ernst L. Wynder, "Diet and Cancer: A Synopsis of Causes and Prevention Strategies," in *Nutrition and Cancer Prevention,* ed. Ronald R. Watson and Siraj I. Mufti (New York: CRC Press, 1996), 2.

13.   "Cancer Prevention Awareness," NIH Publication no. 90–2039 (March 1990): 10.

14.   Sam Shapiro, "Evidence on Screening for Breast Cancer from a Randomized Trial," *Cancer* 39, no. 6 (1977): 2772–82. According to the American Medical Association, 90 percent of women whose breast cancer is detected at an early stage are cancer-free after five years of treatment and considered cured (Ramona I. Slupik, ed., *Complete Guide to Women's Health* [New York: Random House, 1996], 272).

15.   Ronald Ross et al., "Serum Testosterone Levels in Healthy Young Black and White Men," *Journal of the National Cancer Institute* 76, no. 1 (1986): 45–48. Testosterone has been hypothesized to play a role in the etiology of prostate cancer.

16.   Meinir Krishnasamy, "Social Support and the Patient with Cancer: A Consideration of the Literature," *Journal of Advanced Nursing* 23, no. 4 (1996): 757–62.

17.   D. C. Greenwood et al., "Coronary Heart Disease: A Review of the Role

of Psychosocial Stress and Social Support," *Journal of Public Health Medicine* 18, no. 2 (1996): 221–31.

18. On controversy concerning the relation between diet and heart disease, see Elizabeth Rieger, "The Diet-Heart Disease Hypothesis: A Response to Atrens," *Social Science and Medicine* 42, no. 9 (1996): 1227–33. For evidence that eating thirty-five grams of fish daily reduces the risk of heart attack by 44 percent, see Martha L. Daviglus et al., "Fish Consumption and the Thirty-Year Risk of Fatal Myocardial Infarction," *New England Journal of Medicine* 336, no. 15 (1997): 1046–53.

19. Veronika Brezinka and France Kittel, "Psychosocial Factors of Coronary Heart Disease in Women: A Review," *Social Science and Medicine* 42, no. 10 (1996): 1351–65; John B. McKinlay, "Some Contributions from the Social System to Gender Inequalities in Heart Disease," *Journal of Health and Social Behavior* 37, no. 1 (1996): 1–26; and Andrea Z. LaCroix, "Psychosocial Factors and Risk of Coronary Heart Disease in Women: An Epidemiologic Perspective," *Fertility and Sterility* 62 (suppl. 2), no. 6 (1994): S133–S139.

20. Sarah H. Wild et al., "Mortality from Coronary Heart Disease and Stroke for Six Ethnic Groups in California, 1985 to 1990," *Annals of Epidemiology* 5, no. 6 (1995): 432–39.

21. Youlian Liao and Richard S. Cooper, "Continued Adverse Trends in Coronary Heart Disease Mortality among Blacks, 1980–91," *Public Health Reports* 110, no. 5 (1995): 572–79.

22. Charlie Davison, Stephen Frankel, and George Davey Smith, " 'To Hell with Tomorrow': Coronary Heart Disease Risk and the Ethnography of Fatalism," in *Private Risks and Public Dangers*, ed. Sue Scott et al., Explorations in Sociology, no. 43 (Aldershot, U.K.: Avebury, 1992), 96; Nuland, *How We Die*, 19.

23. Project on Disney, *Inside the Mouse: Work and Play at Disney World* (Durham, N.C.: Duke University Press, 1995), 115.

24. Wayne Katon and Herbert Schulberg, "Epidemiology of Depression in Primary Care," *General Hospital Psychiatry* 14, no. 4 (1992): 237–47. See also J. Angst, "Epidemiology of Depression," *Psychopharmacology* 106, suppl. (1992): S71–S74.

25. William R. Beardslee et al., "The Impact of Parental Affective Disorder on Depression in Offspring: A Longitudinal Follow-Up in a Nonreferred Sample," *Journal of the American Academy of Child and Adolescent Psychiatry* 32, no. 4 (1993): 723–30; and Myrna M. Weissman, Philip J. Leaf, and Martha Livingston Bruce, "Single Parent Women," *Social Psychiatry* 22, no. 1 (1987): 29–36.

26. Earl Ubell, "You CAN Fight Depression," *Parade*, 8 May 1988, unpaginated reprint.

27. For an overview, see John A. Talbott, Robert E. Hales, and Stuart C.

Yudofsky, eds., *Textbook of Psychiatry* (Washington, D.C.: American Psychiatric Press, 1988), 403–41. For competing accounts, see Aaron T. Beck et al., eds., *Cognitive Therapy of Depression* (New York: Guilford Press, 1979); Joseph J. Schildkraut and Seymour S. Kety, "Biogenic Amines and Emotion," *Science* 156, no. 3771 (1967): 21–30; Edward Bibring, "The Mechanism of Depression," in *Affective Disorders: Psychoanalytic Contribution to Their Study*, ed. Phyllis Greenacre (New York: International Universities Press, 1953), 13–48; and Marc Ansseau, Remy von Frenckell, and Georges Franck, eds., *Biological Markers of Depression: State of the Art* (London: Excerpta Medica, 1991).

28.   Arthur Kleinman and Byron Good, "Introduction: Culture and Depression," in *Culture and Depression: Studies in the Anthropology and Cross-Cultural Psychiatry of Affect and Disorder*, ed. Arthur Kleinman and Byron Good (Berkeley: University of California Press, 1985), 5.

29.   H. Marmanidis, G. Holme, and R. J. Hafner, "Depression and Somatic Symptoms: A Cross-Cultural Study," *Australian and New Zealand Journal of Psychiatry* 28, no. 2 (1994): 274–78; Dykes M. Young, "Depression," in *Culture and Psychopathology: A Guide to Clinical Assessment*, ed. Wen-Shing Tseng and Jon Streltzer (New York: Brunner/Mazel, 1997), 28–45.

30.   Kleinman and Good, "Introduction," 3.

31.   A. Furnham and R. Malik, "Cross-Cultural Beliefs about 'Depression,'" *International Journal of Social Psychiatry* 40, no. 2 (1994): 106–23.

32.   E. S. Paykel et al., "Life Events, Social Support, and Marital Relationships in the Outcome of Severe Depression," *Psychological Medicine* 26, no. 1 (1996): 121–33; and Cathy Donald Sherborne, Ron D. Hays, and Kenneth B. Wells, "Personal and Psychosocial Risk Factors for Physical and Mental Health Outcomes and Course of Depression among Depressed Patients," *Journal of Consulting and Clinical Psychology* 63, no. 3 (1995): 345–55.

33.   "Plain Talk about Depression," NIH Publication no. 93–3561 (April 1993), 2.

34.   William Styron, *Darkness Visible: A Memoir of Madness* (New York: Random House, 1990), 7. Subsequent references will be documented within the text.

35.   I. Pilowsky and D. L. Bassett, "Pain and Depression," *British Journal of Psychiatry* 141 (July 1982): 30–36; Ranjan Roy, M. Thomas, and M. Matas, "Chronic Pain and Depression: A Review," *Comprehensive Psychiatry* 25, no. 1 (1984): 96–105; Joan M. Romano and Judith A. Turner, "Chronic Pain and Depression: Does the Evidence Support a Relationship?" *Psychological Bulletin* 97, no. 1 (1985): 18–34; I. Pilowsky, "Affective Disorders and Pain," in *Pain Research and Clinical Management*, ed. R. Dubner, G. Gebhart, and M. Bond (Amsterdam: Elsevier, 1988), 3:263–74; Jennifer A. Haythornthwaite, William J. Sieber, and Robert D. Kerns, "Depression and the Chronic Pain Experi-

ence," *Pain* 46, no. 2 (1991): 177–84; and Ann Gamsa and Vaira Vikis-Freibergs, "Psychological Events Are Both Risk Factors in, and Consequences of, Chronic Pain," *Pain* 44, no. 3 (1991): 271–77. Cancer pain, unlike many types of chronic pain, is a special case because diagnosis and etiology are generally clear; cancer appears not to have a *strong* link with depression (Deborah B. McGuire and Vivian R. Sheidler, "Pain," in *Cancer Nursing: Principles and Practice,* ed. Susan L. Groenwald et al., 3d ed. [Boston: Jones and Bartlett, 1993], 505).

36.   "Depression Fact Sheet," Eli Lilly and Company, Indianapolis, Ind., 18 September 1991; and the issue on "Depression," *CQ Researcher* 2, no. 37 (1992): 857–80.

37.   Manfred Bergener, "Introduction," in *Treating Alzheimer's and Other Dementias: Clinical Application of Recent Research Advances,* ed. Manfred Bergener and Sanford I. Finkel (New York: Springer Publishing, 1995), xxi.

38.   Quoted in Stephen G. Post, *The Moral Challenge of Alzheimer Disease* (Baltimore: Johns Hopkins University Press, 1995), 8. I have transformed the text to dialogue, but the words are identical.

39.   Ming-Xin Tang et al., "Effect of Age, Ethnicity, and Head Injury on the Association between APOE Genotypes and Alzheimer's Disease," *Annals of the New York Academy of Sciences* 802 (16 December 1996): 6–15; and Nuland, *How We Die,* 89–117.

40.   Mike Featherstone and Andrew Wernick, "Introduction," in *Images of Aging: Cultural Representations of Later Life,* ed. Mike Featherstone and Andrew Wernick (New York: Routledge, 1995), 2–3. On current stereotypes of aging, see Richard H. Davis and James A. Davis, *TV's Image of the Elderly: A Practical Guide for Change* (Lexington, Mass.: Lexington Books, 1985).

41.   Maurice Jackson, Bohdan Kolody, and James L. Wood, "To Be Old and Black: The Case for Double Jeopardy on Income and Health," in *Minority Aging: Sociological and Social Psychological Issues,* ed. Ron C. Manuel, Contributions in Ethnic Studies, no. 8 (Westport, Conn.: Greenwood Press, 1982), 77–82.

42.   Thomas R. Cole, *The Journey of Life: A Cultural History of Aging in America* (Cambridge: Cambridge University Press, 1992), 229.

43.   Stephen Katz, "Imagining the Life-Span: From Premodern Miracles to Postmodern Fantasies," in *Images of Aging: Cultural Representations of Later Life,* ed. Mike Featherstone and Andrew Wernick (New York: Routledge, 1995), 70. For a critique of current biomedical thought and practices related to old age, see Katz's *Disciplining Old Age: The Formation of Gerontological Knowledge* (Charlottesville: University Press of Virginia, 1996), with its extensive bibliography of current research.

44.   Ann Robertson, "The Politics of Alzheimer's Disease: A Case Study in

Apocalyptic Demography," *International Journal of Health Services* 20, no. 3 (1990): 429–42. See also, Haim Hazan, *Old Age: Constructions and Deconstructions* (Cambridge: Cambridge University Press, 1994); Thomas R. Cole et al., eds., *Voices and Visions of Aging: Toward a Critical Gerontology* (New York: Springer Publishing, 1993); Thomas R. Cole, David D. van Tassel, and Robert Kastenbaum, eds., *Handbook of Humanities and Aging* (New York: Springer Publishing, 1992); Kathleen M. Woodward, *Aging and Its Discontents: Freud and Other Fictions* (Bloomington: Indiana University Press, 1991); and Stuart F. Spicker, Kathleen M. Woodward, and David D. van Tassel, eds., *Aging and the Elderly: Humanistic Perspectives in Gerontology* (Atlantic Highlands, N.J.: Humanities Press, 1978).

45.   Julia Neuberger, "Cultural Issues in Palliative Care," in *Oxford Textbook of Palliative Medicine*, ed. Derek Doyle, Geoffrey W. C. Hanks, and Neil MacDonald (Oxford: Oxford University Press, 1993), 505–14; Marguerite M. Coke and James A. Twaite, *The Black Elderly: Satisfaction and Quality of Later Life* (New York: Hayworth Press, 1995), 99.

46.   Zygmunt Bauman, *Mortality, Immortality, and Other Life Strategies* (Stanford: Stanford University Press, 1992), especially chapter four.

47.   The SUPPORT Principal Investigators, "A Controlled Trial to Improve Care for Seriously Ill Hospitalized Patients," *JAMA* 274, no. 20 (1995): 1591–98.

48.   Ira Byock, *Dying Well: The Prospects for Growth at the End of Life* (New York: Riverhead Books, 1997), 35.

49.   Ibid., 33.

50.   Dame Cicely Saunders, "The Evolution of the Hospices," in *The History of the Management of Pain: From Early Principles to Present Practice*, ed. Ronald D. Mann (Park Ridge, N.J.: Parthenon Publishing Group, 1988), 167–78; and David A. Bennahum, "The Historical Development of Hospice and Palliative Care," in *Hospice and Palliative Care: Concepts and Practice*, ed. Denice C. Sheehan and Walter B. Forman (Sudbury, Mass.: Jones and Bartlett, 1996), 1–10.

51.   John Naisbitt, *Megatrends: Ten New Directions Transforming Our Lives* (New York: Warner Books, 1982), 139–40.

52.   Hans-Georg Gadamer, *The Enigma of Health: The Art of Healing in a Scientific Age* (1993), trans. Jason Gaiger and Nicholas Walker (Stanford: Stanford University Press, 1996), 96.

53.   Arthur L. Caplan, "The Concepts of Health, Illness, and Disease," in *Companion Encyclopedia of the History of Medicine*, ed. W. F. Bynum and Roy Porter (New York: Routledge, 1993), 1:238.

54.   *The Columbia Dictionary of Quotations* (New York: Columbia University Press, 1993), s.v. "health."

55.   See, for example, *The Wellness Encyclopedia* (Boston: Houghton Mifflin, 1991).

56.   Christopher Boorse, "Health as a Theoretical Concept," *Philosophy of Science* 44, no. 4 (1977): 542–73. Boorse's view is endorsed by H. Tristram Engelhardt Jr. in *The Foundations of Bioethics* (New York: Oxford University Press, 1986), 378. See also Arthur W. Frank, "From Sick Role to Health Role: Deconstructing Parsons," in *Talcott Parsons: Theorist of Modernity*, ed. Roland Robertson and Bryan S. Turner (Newbury Park, Calif.: Sage Publications, 1991), 205–16.

57.   Figures come mostly from "Current Estimates from the National Health Interview Survey, 1994," *Vital and Health Statistics*, series 10, no. 193 (1995): 83–84; and *Statistical Abstract of the United States 1996* (Washington, D.C.: U.S. Department of Commerce, 1996), 141–42.

58.   This hypothetical figure adjusts the population estimate for 1990 made by the U.S. Bureau of the Census (248,718,301)—including "count resolution corrections" through December 1995—with the 1996 population estimate of 265,890,998 in the *Information Please Almanac*, ed. Otto Johnson (Boston: Houghton Mifflin, 1997).

59.   For a rejection of the conventional dichotomy between health and disease, see Aaron Antonovsky, "Toward a New View of Health and Illness," in *Unraveling the Mystery of Health: How People Manage Stress and Stay Well* (San Francisco: Jossey-Bass, 1987), 1–14.

60.   Lisa Cartwright and Brian Goldfarb, "Cultural Contagion: On Disney's Health Education Films for Latin America," in *Disney Discourse: Producing the Magic Kingdom*, ed. Eric Smoodin (New York: Routledge, 1994), 169–80.

61.   Sergei Eisenstein, *Eisenstein on Disney*, ed. Jay Leyda, trans. Alan Upchurch (London: Methuen 1988), 63.

CONCLUSION: NARRATIVE BIOETHICS

1.   Leslie Marmon Silko, *Ceremony* (New York: Viking Penguin, 1977), 2. For the wider context of Silko's link between health and narrative, see Roma Heilig Morris, "The Whole Story: Nature, Healing, and Narrative in the Native American Wisdom Tradition," *Literature and Medicine* 15, no. 1 (1996): 94–111.

2.   Don DeLillo, quoted in Anthony DeCurtis, "'An Outsider in This Society': An Interview with Don DeLillo," *South Atlantic Quarterly* 89, no. 2 (1990): 293.

3.   Ibid., 286.

4. Anthony DePalma, "In Mexico, Pain Relief Is a Medical and Political Issue," *New York Times*, 9 June 1996, A6. The figures, cited for 1994, come from the University of Wisconsin Pain Research Center.

5. E. M. Forster, *Aspects of the Novel* (New York: Harcourt, Brace and Company, 1927), 44.

6. Martin Kreisworth, "Trusting the Tale: The Narrativist Turn in the Human Sciences," *New Literary History* 23, no. 3 (1992): 629-57. For a sample of interest in narrative from various disciplines, see Paul Ricoeur, *Time and Narrative* (1983), trans. Kathleen McLaughlin/Blamey and David Pellauer, 3 vols. (Chicago: University of Chicago Press, 1984-88); Donald P. Spence, *Narrative Truth and Historical Truth: Meaning and Interpretation in Psychoanalysis* (New York: W. W. Norton, 1982); Wallace Martin, *Recent Theories of Narrative* (Ithaca, N.Y.: Cornell University Press, 1986); Hayden White, *The Content of the Form: Narrative Discourse and Historical Representation* (Baltimore: Johns Hopkins University Press, 1987); Donald E. Polkinghorne, *Narrative Knowing and the Human Sciences* (Albany: SUNY Press, 1988); Personal Narratives Group, ed., *Interpreting Women's Lives: Feminist Theory and Personal Narratives* (Bloomington: Indiana University Press, 1989); Jerome Bruner, *Acts of Meaning* (Cambridge: Harvard University Press, 1990); Ivan Brady, ed., *Anthropological Poetics* (Savage, Md.: Rowman and Littlefield, 1991); and George C. Rosenwald and Richard L. Ochberg, eds., *Storied Lives: The Cultural Politics of Self Understanding* (New Haven: Yale University Press, 1992).

7. Warren Thomas Reich, "Introduction," in *Encyclopedia of Bioethics*, ed. William Thomas Reich, rev. ed. (New York: Simon and Schuster Macmillan, 1995), 1:xx. For the history of ethical concerns in medicine stretching back to the Hippocratic oath, see Robert Baker, "The History of Medical Ethics," in *Companion Encyclopedia of the History of Medicine*, ed. W. F. Bynum and Roy Porter (New York: Routledge, 1993), 2:852-87.

8. Barry Saunders, M.D., personal correspondence with author, 9 April 1997.

9. Richard Stone, quoted by Will Hermes in "Too Many Stories," *Utne Reader*, September-October 1997, 40. Stone is author of *The Healing Art of Storytelling* (Los Angeles: Hyperion, 1997). Although its impact on daily courtroom activity is still minimal, one sign of change is the academic movement known as "narrative law," or "law and literature," where legal scholars argue for narrative as an alternative to the traditional presentation of facts (see Paul Gewirtz, *Law's Stories: Narrative and Rhetoric in the Law* [New Haven: Yale University Press, 1996]). On medicine and narrative, see, among many others, Kathryn Montgomery Hunter, *Doctors' Stories: The Narrative Structure of Medical Knowledge* (Princeton: Princeton University Press, 1991); Robert

Coles, *The Call of Stories* (Boston: Houghton Mifflin, 1989); Arthur Kleinman, *The Illness Narratives: Suffering, Healing, and the Human Condition* (New York: Basic Books, 1988); Howard Brody, *Stories of Sickness* (New Haven: Yale University Press, 1987); and Oliver Sacks, "Preface," in *The Man Who Mistook His Wife for a Hat and Other Clinical Tales* (New York: Simon and Schuster, 1985). On narrative bioethics, see Hilde Lindemann Nelson, ed., *Stories and Their Limits: Narrative Approaches to Bioethics* (New York: Routledge, 1997); Anne Hudson Jones, "Literature and Medicine: Narrative Ethics," *Lancet* 349, no. 9060 (1997): 1243–46; and Kathryn Montgomery Hunter, "Overview: 'The Whole Story,'" *Second Opinion* 19, no. 2 (1993): 97–103.

10.   See Michael S. Gazzaniga and Joseph E. LeDoux, *The Integrated Mind* (New York: Plenum Press, 1978), 149. The relation of this experiment to narrative was described by historian of science Anne Harrington in "The Brain as Story-Teller: Historical Questions on the Place of Narrative in Neurobiology," a paper delivered at a March 1992 conference entitled "Neurobiology and Narrative: Goals and Levels of Explanation in Neuroscience, Psychology, and Psychiatry" at the University of Notre Dame.

11.   Leslie Marmon Silko, *Ceremony* (New York: Viking Penguin, 1977), 2.

12.   See Arthur Kleinman and Byron Good, eds., *Culture and Depression: Studies in the Anthropology and Cross-Cultural Psychiatry of Affect and Disorder* (Berkeley: University of California Press, 1985); David B. Morris, *The Culture of Pain* (Berkeley: University of California Press, 1991); Ranjan Roy, *The Social Context of the Chronic Pain Sufferer* (Toronto: University of Toronto Press, 1992); and Mary-Jo DelVecchio Good et al., eds., *Pain as Human Experience: An Anthropological Perspective* (Berkeley: University of California Press, 1992).

13.   Tod Chambers, "From the Ethicist's Point of View: The Literary Nature of Ethical Inquiry," *Hastings Center Report* 26, no. 1 (1996): 25.

14.   See, for example, Drew Leder, "Toward a Hermeneutical Bioethics," in *A Matter of Principles? Ferment in U.S. Bioethics,* ed. Edwin R. DuBose, Ronald P. Hamel, and Laurence J. O'Connell (Valley Forge, Pa.: Trinity Press International, 1994), 240–59; and the entire issue on literature and medical ethics in *Journal of Medicine and Philosophy* 21, no. 3 (1996), including a dissenting view from K. Danner Clouser ("Philosophy, Literature, and Ethics: Let the Engagement Begin," 321–40).

15.   See Brody, *Stories of Sickness* and "'My Story Is Broken; Can You Help Me Fix It?' Medical Ethics and the Joint Construction of Narrative," *Literature and Medicine* 13, no. 1 (1994): 79–92; Arthur Kleinman, *The Illness Narratives*; and Rita Charon, "Narrative Contributions to Medical Ethics: Recognition, Formulation, Interpretation, and Validation in the Practice of the Ethicist," in *A Matter of Principles? Ferment in U.S. Bioethics,* ed. Edwin R. DuBose, Ronald

P. Hamel, and Laurence J. O'Connell (Valley Forge, Pa.: Trinity Press International, 1994), 260–83.

16.   Kathryn Montgomery Hunter, "Narrative," in *Encyclopedia of Bioethics,* ed. William Thomas Reich, rev. ed. (New York: Simon and Schuster Macmillan, 1995), 4:1789–94.

17.   Arthur W. Frank, *The Wounded Storyteller: Body, Illness, and Ethics* (Chicago: University of Chicago Press, 1995). Quotations will be documented within the text.

18.   Leslie J. Blackhall et al. show that Korean Americans and Mexican Americans over age sixty-five were more likely to hold a "family-centered" model of medical decision making than a (Western) patient-autonomy model ("Ethnicity and Attitudes toward Patient Autonomy," *JAMA* 274, no. 10 [1995]: 820–25).

19.   See Howard M. Spiro et al., eds., *Empathy and the Practice of Medicine: Beyond Pills and the Scalpel* (New Haven: Yale University Press, 1993).

20.   Martha Craven Nussbaum, "Flawed Crystals: James's *The Golden Bowl* and Literature as Moral Philosophy," *New Literary History* 15, no. 1 (1983): 25–50. The essay is reprinted in her book *Love's Knowledge: Essays on Philosophy and Literature* (New York: Oxford University Press, 1990). See also Donald G. Marshall, ed., *Literature as Philosophy, Philosophy as Literature* (Iowa City: University of Iowa Press, 1987).

21.   Martha C. Nussbaum, *The Fragility of Goodness: Luck and Ethics in Greek Tragedy and Philosophy* (Cambridge: Cambridge University Press, 1986).

22.   Richard Rorty, ed., *The Linguistic Turn: Recent Essays in Philosophical Method* (Chicago: University of Chicago Press, 1967). For a recent exploration, see Arthur Danto, "Philosophy as/and/of Literature," in *Post-Analytic Philosophy,* ed. John Rajchman and Cornel West (New York: Columbia University Press, 1985), 63–83.

23.   Nussbaum, *The Fragility of Goodness,* 15–16.

24.   For a skeptical reading of Nussbaum, see Richard A. Posner, "Against Ethical Criticism," *Philosophy and Literature* 21, no. 1 (1997): 1–27.

25.   See Rom Harré, ed., *The Social Construction of Emotions* (Oxford: Basil Blackwell, 1986); and James A. Russell, "Culture and the Categorization of Emotions," *Psychological Bulletin* 110, no. 3 (1991): 426–50.

26.   Antonio R. Damasio, *Descartes' Error: Emotion, Reason, and the Human Brain* (New York: Putnam, 1994), 45.

27.   The major texts by Bakhtin on which I base my comments here are *Problems of Dostoevsky's Poetics* (1929), trans. Caryl Emerson (Minneapolis: University of Minnesota Press, 1984); *Rabelais and His World* (1940), trans. Helen Iswolsky (Cambridge: Harvard University Press, 1969); and *The Dialogic*

Imagination: Four Essays by M. M. Bakhtin, ed. Michael Holquist, trans. Caryl Emerson and Michael Holquist (Austin: University of Texas Press, 1981). On the application and extension of Bakhtin's thought, see Ken Hirschkop and David Shepherd, eds., *Bakhtin and Cultural Theory* (Manchester, U.K.: Manchester University Press, 1989); Gary Saul Morson and Caryl Emerson, eds., *Rethinking Bakhtin: Extensions and Challenges* (Evanston, Ill.: Northwestern University Press, 1989); and Michael Holquist, *Dialogism: Bakhtin and His World* (New York: Routledge, 1990).

28.   Bakhtin, "Discourse in the Novel" (1934–35), in *The Dialogic Imagination: Four Essays by M. M. Bakhtin*, ed. Michael Holquist, trans. Caryl Emerson and Michael Holquist (Austin: University of Texas Press, 1981), 262. I quote the translation of this passage in Tzvetan Todorov, *Mikhail Bakhtin: The Dialogical Principle* (1981), trans. Wlad Godzich (Minneapolis: University of Minnesota Press, 1984), 56.

29.   Frank, *The Wounded Storyteller*, 25.

30.   David Armstrong, "The Patient's View," *Social Science and Medicine* 18, no. 9 (1984): 737–44. I am indebted to Armstrong's discussion of the change from a visual to an auditory concept of illness.

31.   "The ability to communicate effectively with patients and families or legal surrogates is one of the most vital professional skills in appropriate decision making" (John Edward Ruark, Thomas Alfred Raffin, and the Stanford University Medical Center Committee on Ethics, "Initiating and Withdrawing Life Support," *New England Journal of Medicine* 318, no. 1 [1988]: 26).

32.   Howard B. Beckman and Richard M. Frankel, "The Effect of Physician Behavior on the Collection of Data," *Annals of Internal Medicine* 101, no. 5 (1984): 692–96. For another influential account of medical failures to listen, see Candace West, *Routine Complications: Troubles with Talk between Doctors and Patients* (Bloomington: Indiana University Press, 1984). The topic has been revived recently in Bernard Lown, *The Lost Art of Healing* (Boston: Houghton-Mifflin, 1996).

33.   Tony Realini, Adina Kalet, and Joyce Sparling, "Interruption in the Medical Interaction," *Archives of Family Medicine* 4, no. 12 (1995): 1028–33. Another 1995 study found that patients engaged in significantly more interruptive and overlapping speech than physicians did; the few gender differences emerging did not indicate a clear pattern of male dominance (J. T. Irish and J. A. Hall, "Interruptive Patterns in Medical Visits: The Effects of Role, Status, and Gender," *Social Science and Medicine* 41, no. 6 [1995]: 873–81).

34.   Kathryn Montgomery Hunter, Rita Charon, and John L. Coulehan, "The Study of Literature in Medical Education," *Academic Medicine* 70, no. 9 (1995): 788.

35. Stanley Cavell, "The Uncanniness of the Ordinary" (1986), in *In Quest of the Ordinary: Lines of Skepticism and Romanticism* (Chicago: University of Chicago Press, 1988), 176. On the complications of Cavell's thinking and its engagement with philosophers such as Kant, Hume, Wittgenstein, and Heidegger, to which I cannot possibly do justice here, see Stephen Mulhall, *Stanley Cavell: Philosophy's Recounting of the Ordinary* (Oxford: Clarendon Press, 1994).

36. In *The Claim of Reason: Wittgenstein, Skepticism, Morality, and Tragedy* (Oxford: Oxford University Press, 1979), Cavell devotes the entire third section to knowledge and the concept of morality, but he calls it the "most thesis-bound" (xii) portion of the book, for it consists mainly in refuting the positions of "emotivism" and "prescriptivism" characteristic of analytic moral philosophy until, say, 1960. I would argue that his subsequent ongoing discussion of "the everyday" constitutes a subtle, implicit, and far more important contribution to ethical thinking.

37. Mary Devereaux, "Neighboring the World: Movies as a Subject for Philosophy," in *The Senses of Stanley Cavell*, ed. Richard Fleming and Michael Payne (Lewisburg, Pa.: Bucknell University Press, 1989), 186–99.

38. Cavell, "The Uncanniness of the Ordinary," 175. For his ongoing engagement with Thoreau, see Cavell, *The Senses of Walden: An Expanded Edition* (San Francisco: North Point Press, 1981).

39. Stanley Cavell, "The Ordinary as the Uneventful" (1980), in *The Cavell Reader*, ed. Stephen Mulhall (Oxford: Blackwell Publishers, 1996), 253–59. For a psychology to complement a philosophy of the everyday, see Mihaly Csikszentmihalyi, *Flow: The Psychology of Optimal Experience* (New York: Harper and Row, 1990): *flow* is "the state in which people are so involved in an activity that nothing else seems to matter" (4).

40. Paul A. Komesaroff, "From Bioethics to Microethics: Ethical Debate and Clinical Medicine," in *Troubled Bodies: Critical Perspectives on Postmodernism, Medical Ethics, and the Body*, ed. Paul A. Komesaroff (Durham. N.C.: Duke University Press, 1995), 62–86.

41. Susan Sontag, *AIDS and Its Metaphors* (New York: Farrar, Straus and Giroux, 1989), 14–15.

42. See M. E. Opler, "The Concept of Supernatural Power among the Chiricahua and Mescalero Apaches," *American Anthropologist* 37, no. 1 (1935): 65–70; Eric Stone, *Medicine among the American Indians* (New York: Hafner, 1962); Henrietta H. Stockel, *Survival of the Spirit: Chiricahua Apaches in Captivity* (Reno: University of Nevada Press, 1993); and David B. Morris, "Placebo, Pain, and Belief," in *The Placebo Effect: An Interdisciplinary Exploration*, ed. Anne Harrington (Cambridge: Harvard University Press, 1997), 187–207.

43.   Cavell, "The Uncanniness of the Ordinary," 171. Cavell cites Hume's *Treatise of Human Nature* (1739–40), I.iv.2.

44.   Cavell, "The Uncanniness of the Ordinary," 165. Cavell cites Ludwig Wittgenstein's *Philosophical Investigations* (#195), which was written between 1945 and 1949. For an ongoing engagement with skepticism and loss through Wittgenstein, Emerson, and the everyday, see Stanley Cavell, *This New Yet Unapproachable America: Lectures after Emerson and Wittgenstein* (Albuquerque: Living Batch Press, 1989).

45.   Don DeLillo, quoted in Anthony DeCurtis, "An Outsider in This Society," 301.

46.   Audre Lorde, *The Cancer Journals* (Argyle, N.Y.: Spinsters, Ink, 1980), 52.

47.   Andy Warhol, *The Philosophy of Andy Warhol (From A to B and Back Again)* (New York: Harcourt Brace Jovanovich, 1975), 110.

48.   Philippe Ariès, *The Hour of Our Death* (1977), trans. Helen Weaver (New York: Alfred A. Knopf, 1981), 607.

49.   "Pragmatism . . . asks its usual question. 'Grant an idea or belief to be true,' it says, 'what concrete difference will its being true make in anyone's actual life? How will the truth be realized? What experiences will be different from those which would obtain if the belief were false? What, in short, is the truth's cash-value in experiential terms?'" (William James, "Pragmatism's Conception of Truth," in *Pragmatism* [1907], ed. Fredson Bowers and Ignas K. Skrupskelis [Cambridge: Harvard University Press, 1975], 97).

50.   Ezekiel J. Emanuel and Linda L. Emanuel argue that cost savings from hospice-style care at the end of life may reach only 40 percent over conventional care, but 40 percent is still a huge savings ("The Economics of Dying: The Illusion of Cost Savings at the End of Life," *New England Journal of Medicine* 330, no. 8 [1994]: 540–44). For comments and discussion, see *New England Journal of Medicine* 331, no. 7 (1994): 477–79.

Index

access to medical care, 13, 102, 222–25
acquired immunodeficiency syndrome, 12,
    40, 59–60, 65, 100–102, 190–92, 208–17,
    315n2, 320n48; AIDSpeak, 212–13,
    320n48; vs. classical disease, 290n22;
    metaphors of, 209–10; socially con-
    structed, 209; victimization and, 211–17;
    women and, 212
activism: ACT UP lobbying, 321n54; mourn-
    ing and, 320n49; silence = death, 201
ACT UP (AIDS Coalition to Unleash
    Power), 214–17, 321n54
acupuncture, 15, 70
AD. See Alzheimer's disease
addiction: anorexia and, 157, 305–6n40;
    heroin, TB, and, 101; hospital patients,
    113; sex addicts, 64
advance directive, 16
aging, 2–3, 28, 63, 77, 128–29, 150, 159;
    Alzheimer's disease, 234–37; critique of
    biomedical approach toward, 325n43;

pneumonia and, 103; sexuality and, 236;
    stereotypes of, 325n40; stroke and social
    support, 223
AIDS. See acquired immunodeficiency syn-
    drome
AIDS Memorial Quilt, 59, 213–14
alcoholism, 14, 39, 63, 77, 88, 285n30
allergies, 64; bronchial asthma, 99; diesel
    fuel and, 86
alternative medicine, 15, 69–70
Alzheimer's disease, 234–37; Reagan and,
    63; selfhood and, 57
ambiguities: AIDS and, 192; confusion of
    postmodern period, 17; medicine and,
    18, 39; narrative and, 265; the unknown,
    274
amenorrhea, 157
American Board of Internal Medicine, 265
analgesia, 97; costs of, 111; opioids and,
    109, 112, 115, 124; pervasiveness of, 134;
    uneven distribution, 249. See also pain

335

Compositor:	Impressions Book and Journal Services, Inc.
Text:	10/14 Palatino
Display:	Snell Roundhand Script and Bauer Bodoni